Rapid Review
Pharmacology

Rapid Review Series

Series Editor
Edward F. Goljan, MD

Behavioral Science, Second Edition
Vivian M. Stevens, PhD; Susan K. Redwood, PhD; Jackie L. Neel, DO;
Richard H. Bost, PhD; Nancy W. Van Winkle, PhD; Michael H. Pollak, PhD

Biochemistry, Second Edition
John W. Pelley, PhD; Edward F. Goljan, MD

Gross and Developmental Anatomy, Second Edition
N. Anthony Moore, PhD; William A. Roy, PhD, PT

Histology and Cell Biology, Second Edition
E. Robert Burns, PhD; M. Donald Cave, PhD

Microbiology and Immunology, Second Edition
Ken S. Rosenthal, PhD; James S. Tan, MD

Neuroscience
James A. Weyhenmeyer, PhD; Eve A. Gallman, PhD

Pathology, Second Edition
Edward F. Goljan, MD

Pharmacology, Second Edition
Thomas L. Pazdernik, PhD; Laszlo Kerecsen, MD

Physiology
Thomas A. Brown, MD

USMLE Step 2
Michael W. Lawlor, MD, PhD

USMLE Step 3
David Rolston, MD; Craig Nielsen, MD

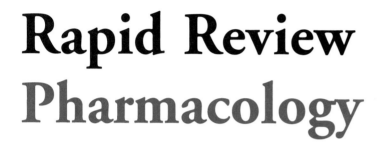

Rapid Review
Pharmacology

SECOND EDITION

Thomas L. Pazdernik, PhD
Professor
Pharmacology, Toxicology, and Therapeutics
University of Kansas Medical Center
Kansas City, Kansas

Laszlo Kerecsen, MD
Professor
Department of Pharmacology
Arizona College of Osteopathic Medicine
Midwestern University
Glendale, Arizona

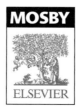

MOSBY

ELSEVIER

MOSBY
ELSEVIER

1600 John F. Kennedy Blvd.
Suite 1800
Philadelphia, PA 19103-2899

RAPID REVIEW PHARMACOLOGY, Second Edition   ISBN-10: 0-323-04550-2
Copyright © 2007, 2003 by Mosby, Inc., an affiliate of Elsevier Inc.   ISBN-13: 978-0-323-04550-6

NOTICE

Knowledge and best practice in this field are constantly changing. As new research and experience broaden our knowledge, changes in practice, treatment and drug therapy may become necessary or appropriate. Readers are advised to check the most current information provided (i) on procedures featured or (ii) by the manufacturer of each product to be administered, to verify the recommended dose or formula, the method and duration of administration, and contraindications. It is the responsibility of the practitioner, relying on their own experience and knowledge of the patient, to make diagnoses, to determine dosages and the best treatment for each individual patient, and to take all appropriate safety precautions. To the fullest extent of the law, neither the Publisher nor the Authors assume any liability for any injury and/or damage to persons or property arising out or related to any use of the material contained in this book.

Library of Congress Cataloging-in-Publication Data

Pazdernik, Thomas.
    Pharmacology / Thomas L. Pazdernik, Laszlo Kerecsen.—2nd ed.
      p. ; cm.—(Rapid review series)
    Includes index.
    ISBN 0-323-04550-2
      1. Pharmacology—Examinations, questions, etc. I. Kerecsen, Laszlo. II. Title.
    III. Series.
      [DNLM: 1. Pharmaceutical Preparations—Examination Questions. 2. Pharmaceutical Preparations—Outlines. 3. Drug Therapy—Examination Questions. 4. Drug Therapy—Outlines. QV 18.2 P348p 2007]
    RM105.P39 2007
    615′.1076—dc22
                                                        2006041871

Publishing Director: Linda Belfus
Acquisitions Editor: James Merritt
Developmental Editor: Katie DeFrancesco
Design Direction: Steven Stave

Printed in the United States of America.

Last digit is the print number: 9 8 7 6 5 4 3 2 1

*To my wife, Betty; my daughter Nancy, her husband, Billy,
and my granddaughter Rebecca Irene; my daughter Lisa and
her husband, Chris; and my triplet grandchildren, Cassidy Rae,
Thomas Pazdernik, and Isabel Mari*

TLP

To Gabor and Tamas, my sons

LK

Series Preface

The First Editions of the *Rapid Review Series* have received high critical acclaim from students studying for the United States Medical Licensing Examination (USMLE) Step 1 and high ratings in *First Aid for the USMLE Step 1*. The Second Editions continue to be invaluable resources for time-pressed students. As a result of reader feedback, we have improved upon an already successful formula. We have created a learning system, including a print and electronic package, that is easier to use and more concise than other review products on the market.

SPECIAL FEATURES

Book

- **Outline format:** Concise, high-yield subject matter is presented in a study-friendly format.
- **High-yield margin notes:** Key content that is most likely to appear on the exam is reinforced in the margin notes.
- **Visual elements:** Abundant two-color schematics, black and white images, and summary tables enhance your study experience.
- **Two-color design:** Colored text and headings make studying more efficient and pleasing.
- **Two practice examinations:** Two sets of 50 USMLE Step 1–type clinically oriented, multiple-choice questions (including images where necessary) and complete discussions (rationales) for all options are included.

New! Online Study and Testing Tool

- **350 USMLE Step 1–type MCQs:** Clinically oriented, multiple-choice questions that mimic the current board format are presented. These include images where necessary, and complete rationales for all answer options. All the questions from the book

are included so you can study them in the most effective mode for you!
- **Test mode:** Select from randomized 50-question sets or by subject topics for an exam-like review session. This mode features a 60-minute timer to simulate the actual exam, a detailed assessment report that can be printed or saved to your hard drive, and direct links to all or only incorrect questions. The links include your answer, the correct answer, and full rationales for all answer options, so you can fully analyze your test session and learn from your mistakes.
- **Study mode:** Like the test mode, in the study mode you can select from randomized 50-question sets or by subject topics to create a dynamic study session. This mode features unlimited attempts at each question, instant feedback (either on selection of the correct answer or when using the "Show Answer" feature), complete rationales for all answer options, and a detailed progress report that can be printed or saved to your hard drive.
- **Online access:** Online access allows you to study from an internet-enabled computer wherever and whenever it is convenient. This access is activated through registration on www.studentconsult.com with the pincode printed inside the front cover.

Student Consult

- **Full online access:** You can access the complete text and illustrations of this book on www.studentconsult.com.
- **Save content to your PDA:** Through our unique Pocket Consult platform, you can clip selected text and illustrations and save them to your PDA for study on the fly!
- **Free content:** An interactive community center with a wealth of additional valuable resources is available.

Acknowledgment of Reviewers

The publisher expresses sincere thanks to the medical students and faculty who provided many useful comments and suggestions for improving both the text and the questions. Our publishing program will continue to benefit from the combined insight and experience provided by your reviews. For always encouraging us to focus on our target, the USMLE Step 1, we thank the following:

Patricia C. Daniel, PhD, Kansas University Medical Center

Steven J. Engman, Loyola University Chicago Stritch School of Medicine

Omar A. Khan, University of Vermont College of Medicine

Michael W. Lawlor, Loyola University Chicago Stritch School of Medicine

Lillian Liang, Jefferson Medical College

Erica L. Magers, Michigan State University College of Human Medicine

Acknowledgments

The authors wish to acknowledge Jim Merritt, acquisitions editor, Katie DeFrancesco, developmental editor, and Joan Sinclair, project manager, at Elsevier. We also thank Mary Durkin and Martha Cushman for editing the text; Donna Frassetto and Sharon Maddox for editing the questions; and Matt Chansky for his excellent illustrations. We give a special thanks to Tibor Rozman, MD, for his contributions to the development of clinically relevant questions and to Tamas Kerecsen for processing the questions. We also thank the faculty of the Department of Pharmacology, Toxicology, and Therapeutics at the University of Kansas Medical Center and the faculty of the Department of Pharmacology at Arizona College of Osteopathic Medicine, Midwestern University, for their superb contributions to the development of materials for our teaching programs. Finally, we thank the numerous medical students who, over the years, have been our inspiration for developing teaching materials.

Thomas L. Pazdernik, PhD
Laszlo Kerecsen, MD

Contents

CHAPTER

1

Pharmacokinetics

I. Definition
- Pharmacokinetics is the fate of drugs within the body.
- Pharmacokinetics involves absorption, distribution, metabolism, and excretion (ADME) of drugs (Fig. 1-1).

Pharmacokinetics: absorption, distribution, metabolism, excretion (ADME)

II. Drug Permeation
- Passage of drug molecules across biological membranes
- Important for pharmacokinetic and pharmacodynamic features of drugs
  A. Processes of permeation
    1. Passive diffusion
       a. Characteristics
          (1) Does *not* make use of a carrier
          (2) Not saturable
          (3) Low structural specificity
          (4) Driven by concentration gradient
       b. Aqueous diffusion: passage through central pores in cell membranes
          - Possible for low-molecular-weight substances
       c. Lipid diffusion: direct passage through lipid bilayer
          - Facilitated by increased degree of lipid solubility
          - Driven by a concentration gradient (nonionized forms move most easily)
          (1) Lipid solubility is the most important limiting factor for drug permeation; a large number of lipid barriers separate body compartments.
          (2) Lipid to aqueous partition coefficient determines how readily a drug molecule moves between lipid and aqueous media.

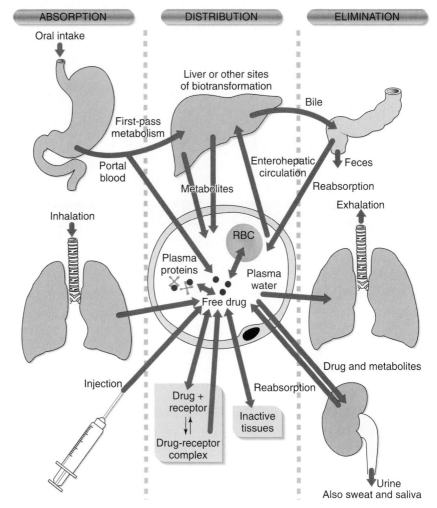

1-1: *Schematic representation of the fate of a drug in the body (pharmacokinetics). Orange arrows indicate passage of drug through the body (intake to output). Orange circles represent drug molecules. RBC, red blood cell.*

2. Active transport
   a. Characteristics
      (1) Carrier-mediated
      (2) Structural selectivity
      (3) Competition by similar molecules
      (4) Energy-dependent
      (5) Saturable
      (6) Movement occurs against a concentration or electrochemical gradient
      (7) Rapid
   b. Sites of active transport: neuronal membranes, choroid plexus, renal tubular cells, hepatocytes

Active transport requires energy to move molecules against concentration gradient.

3. Facilitated diffusion
   - Carrier-mediated process that does *not* require energy
   - Involves movement along a concentration or electrochemical gradient
4. Pinocytosis
   - Process in which a cell engulfs extracellular material within membrane vesicles
   - Used by exceptionally large molecules (molecular weight > 1000), such as iron-transferrin complex and vitamin B_{12}–intrinsic factor complex

III. Absorption
   - Absorption involves the process by which drugs enter into the body.
   A. Factors that affect absorption
   1. Solubility
      a. Drugs in aqueous solutions mix more readily with the aqueous phase at absorptive sites, so they are absorbed more rapidly than those in oily solutions.
      b. Drugs in suspension or solid form are dependent on the rate of dissolution before they can mix with the aqueous phase at absorptive sites.
   2. Concentration
      - Drugs in highly concentrated solutions are absorbed more readily than those in dilute concentrations.
   3. Blood flow
      - Greater blood flow means higher rates of drug absorption (e.g., absorption is greater in muscle tissue than in subcutaneous sites).
   4. Absorbing surface
      - Organs with large surface areas, such as the lungs and intestines, have more rapid drug absorption (e.g., absorption is greater in the intestine than in the stomach).
   5. Contact time
      - The greater the time, the greater the amount of drug absorbed.
   6. pH
      - For weak acids and weak bases, the pH determines the relative amount of drug in ionized or nonionized form, which in turn affects solubility.
      a. Weak organic acids donate a proton to form anions (Fig. 1-2), as shown in the following equation:

$$HA \leftrightarrow H^+ + A^-$$

where

$$HA = \text{weak acid}$$
$$H^+ = \text{proton}$$
$$A^- = \text{anion}$$

   b. Weak organic bases accept a proton to form cations (see Fig. 1-2), as shown in the following equation:

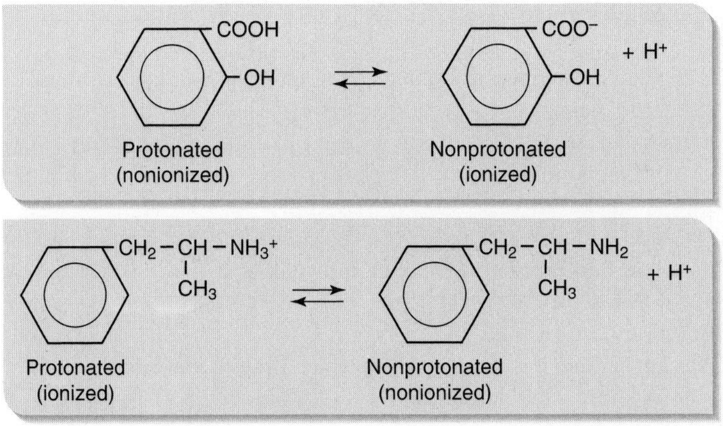

1-2: *Examples of the ionization of a weak organic acid (salicylate, top) and a weak organic base (amphetamine, bottom).*

$$HB^+ \leftrightarrow B + H^+$$

where

$$B = \text{weak base}$$
$$H^+ = \text{proton}$$
$$HB^+ = \text{cation}$$

    c. Only the nonionized form of a drug can readily cross cell membranes.

    d. The ratio of ionized versus nonionized forms is a function of pK_a (measure of drug acidity) and the pH of the environment. When $pH = pK_a$, a compound is 50% ionized and 50% nonionized; protonated form dominates at pH less than pK_a; unprotonated form dominates at pH greater than pK_a.

- The Henderson-Hasselbalch equation can be used to determine the ratio of the nonionized form to the ionized form.

$$\log \frac{[\text{protonated form}]}{[\text{unprotonated form}]} = pK_a - pH$$

IV. Bioavailability
- Bioavailability is the relative amount of the administered drug that reaches the general circulation.
- Several factors influence bioavailability.
  A. First-pass metabolism
  - Enzymes in the intestinal flora, intestinal mucosa, and liver metabolize drugs before they reach the general circulation, significantly decreasing systemic bioavailability.
  B. Drug formulation
  - Bioavailability after oral administration is affected by the extent of disintegration of a particular drug formulation.
  C. Route of administration (Table 1-1)

Weak organic acids pass through membranes best in acidic environments.

Weak organic bases pass through membranes best in basic environments.

Bioavailability depends on the extent of absorption.

Sublingual nitroglycerin avoids first-pass metabolism, promoting rapid absorption.

D. Bioequivalence
- Two drug formulations with the same bioavailability (extent of absorption) and rate of absorption are bioequivalent.

V. Distribution
- Distribution is the delivery of a drug from systemic circulation to tissues.
- Drugs may distribute into certain body compartments (Table 1-2).
  A. Apparent volume of distribution (V_d): space in the body into which the drug appears to disseminate
    1. The V_d is calculated according to the following equation:

$$V_d = \frac{\text{Amount of drug given by IV injection}}{C_0}$$

where

C_0 = concentration of drug in plasma at time 0 after equilibration.

2. A large V_d means that a drug is concentrated in tissues.
3. A small V_d means that a drug is in the extracellular fluid or plasma; that is, the V_d is inversely related to plasma drug concentration.
  B. Factors that affect distribution: plasma protein and tissue binding, gender, age, amount of body fat, relative blood flow, size, and lipid solubility
    1. Plasma protein binding
      a. Drugs with high plasma protein binding remain in plasma; thus, they have a low V_d and a prolonged half-life.
      b. Binding acts as a drug reservoir, slowing onset and prolonging duration of action.
      c. Many drugs bind reversibly with one or more plasma proteins (e.g., albumin) in the vascular compartment.
      d. Disease states (e.g., liver disease, which affects albumin concentration) and drugs that alter protein binding influence the concentration of other drugs.
    2. Sites of drug concentration (Table 1-3)
      a. Redistribution
        (1) Intravenous thiopental is initially distributed to areas of highest blood flow, such as the brain, liver, and kidneys.
        (2) The drug is then redistributed to and stored first in muscle, and then in adipose tissue.
      b. Ion trapping
        (1) Weak organic acids are trapped in basic environments.
        (2) Weak organic bases are trapped in acidic environments.
      c. Sites of drug exclusion (places where it is difficult for drugs to enter)
        - Cerebrospinal, ocular, lymph, pleural, and fetal fluids

VI. Biotransformation: Metabolism
- The primary site of biotransformation, or metabolism, is the liver, and the primary goal is drug inactivation.

**TABLE 1-1:
Routes of
Administration**

Route	Advantages	Disadvantages
Enteral		
Oral	Most convenient Produces slow, uniform absorption Relatively safe Economical	Poor absorption of large and charged particles Destruction of drug by enzymes or low pH (e.g., peptides, proteins, penicillins) Drugs bind or complex with gastrointestinal contents (e.g., calcium binds to tetracycline) Cannot be used for drugs that irritate the intestine
Rectal	Limited first-pass metabolism Useful when oral route precluded	Absorption often irregular and incomplete May cause irritation to rectal mucosa
Sublingual/buccal	Rapid absorption Avoids first-pass metabolism	Absorption of only small amounts (e.g., nitroglycerin)
Parenteral		
Intravenous	Most direct route Bypasses barriers to absorption (immediate effect) Suitable for large volumes Dosage easily adjusted	Increased risk of adverse effects from high concentration immediately after injection Not suitable for oily substances or suspensions
Intramuscular	Quickly and easily administered Possible rapid absorption May use as depot Suitable for oily substances and suspensions	Painful Bleeding May lead to nerve injury
Subcutaneous	Quickly and easily administered Fairly rapid absorption Suitable for suspensions and pellets	Painful Large amounts cannot be given
Inhalation	Used for volatile compounds (e.g., halothane and amyl nitrite) and drugs that can be administered by aerosol (e.g., albuterol) Rapid absorption due to large surface area of alveolar membranes and high blood flow through lungs Aerosol delivers drug directly to site of action and may minimize systemic side effects	Variable systemic distribution
Topical	Application to specific surface (skin, eye, nose, vagina) allows local effects	May irritate surface
Transdermal	Allows controlled permeation through skin (e.g., nicotine, estrogen, testosterone, fentanyl, scopolamine, clonidine)	May irritate surface

Compartment	Volume (L/kg)	Liters in 70-kg Human	Drug Type
Plasma water	0.045	3	Strongly plasma–protein bound drugs and very large drugs (e.g., heparin)
Extracellular body water	0.20	14	Large water-soluble drugs (e.g., mannitol)
Total body water	0.60	42	Small water-soluble drugs (e.g., ethanol)
Tissue	>0.70	>49	Drugs that avidly bind to tissue (e.g., chloroquine; 115 L/kg)

TABLE 1-2:
Body Compartments in Which Drugs May Distribute

Site	Characteristics
Fat	Stores lipid-soluble drugs
Tissue	May represent sizable reservoir, depending on mass, as with muscle
	Several drugs accumulate in liver
Bone	Tetracyclines are deposited in calcium-rich regions (bones, teeth)
Transcellular reservoirs	Gastrointestinal tract serves as transcellular reservoir for drugs that are slowly absorbed or that are undergoing enterohepatic circulation

TABLE 1-3:
Sites of Drug Concentration

A. Products of drug metabolism
  • Products are usually less active pharmacologically.
  • However, products also are sometimes active drugs, in which the prodrug form is inactive and the metabolite is active.

L-DOPA → dopamine

B. Phase I biotransformation (oxidation, reduction, hydrolysis)
  1. The products are usually more polar metabolites, resulting from introducing or unmasking a function group ($-OH$, $-NH_2$, $-SH$, $-COO^-$).
  2. The process involves enzymes located in the smooth endoplasmic reticulum.
  3. Oxidation usually occurs via a cytochrome P-450 system.
  4. The estimated percentage of drugs metabolized by the major P-450 enzymes (Fig. 1-3)
C. Phase II biotransformation
  • Involves conjugation, in which an endogenous substance, such as glucuronic acid, combines with a drug or phase I metabolite to form a conjugate with high polarity
  1. Glucuronidation
    • A major route of metabolism for drugs and endogenous compounds (steroids, bilirubin)
    • Occurs in the endoplasmic reticulum
  2. Sulfation
    • A major route of drug metabolism
    • Occurs in the cytoplasm

Conjugation reactions (e.g., glucuronidation, sulfation) usually make drugs more water soluble and more excretable.

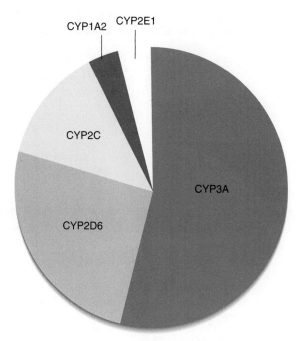

1-3: *Diagram showing the estimated percentage of drugs metabolized by the major cytochrome P-450 enzymes.*

Methylation and acetylation reactions often make drugs less water soluble.

3. Methylation and acetylation reactions
   - Involve the conjugation of drugs (by transferases) with other substances (e.g., methyl, acetyl) to metabolites, thereby decreasing drug activity
D. Phase III processes
   - Transporters responsible for influx and efflux of molecules involved in absorption, distribution, and elimination
E. Drug interactions
   - May occur as a result of changes to the cytochrome P-450 enzyme system
   1. Inducers of cytochrome P-450
      - Hasten metabolism of drugs
      - Examples: phenobarbital, phenytoin, rifampin, carbamazepine, St. John's wort
   2. Inhibitors of cytochrome P-450
      - Decreases metabolism of drugs
      - Examples: cimetidine, ketoconazole, erythromycin
   3. Inhibitors of intestinal P-glycoprotein
      - Drugs that inhibit this transporter increase bioavailability, thus resulting in potential toxicity.
      - Examples of inhibitors: verapamil, grapefruit juice
      - Examples of drugs made more toxic: digoxin, cyclosporine, saquinavir
F. Genetic polymorphisms
   - Influence the metabolism of a drug, thereby altering its effects (Table 1-4)

TABLE 1-4: Genetic Polymorphisms and Drug Metabolism

Predisposing Factor	Drug	Clinical Effect
G6PD deficiency	Primaquine, sulfonamides	Acute hemolytic anemia
Slow N-acetylation	Isoniazid	Peripheral neuropathy
Slow N-acetylation	Hydralazine	Lupus syndrome
Slow ester hydrolysis	Succinylcholine	Prolonged apnea
Slow oxidation	Tolbutamide	Cardiotoxicity
Slow acetaldehyde oxidation	Ethanol	Facial flushing

G6PD, glucose-6-phosphate dehydrogenase.

G. Reactive metabolite intermediates
  - Are responsible for mutagenic, carcinogenic, and teratogenic effects, as well as specific organ-directed toxicity
  - Examples of resulting conditions: acetaminophen-induced hepatotoxicity, aflatoxin-induced tumors, cyclophosphamide-induced cystitis

VII. Excretion
  - Excretion is the amount of drug and drug metabolites excreted by any process per unit time.
  A. Excretion processes in kidney
    1. Glomerular filtration rate
      - Depends on the size, charge, and protein binding of a particular drug
      - Is lower for highly protein-bound drugs
      - Drugs that are *not* protein bound or *not* reabsorbed are eliminated at a rate equal to the creatinine clearance rate (125 mL/min).
    2. Tubular secretion
      - Occurs in the middle segment of the proximal convoluted tubule
      - Provides transporters for anions (e.g., penicillins, cephalosporins, salicylates) and cations (e.g., pyridostigmine)
      - Can be used to increase drug concentration by use of another drug that competes for the transporter (e.g., probenecid inhibits penicillin secretion)
      - Has a rate that approaches renal plasma flow (660 mL/min)
      a. Characteristics of tubular secretion
        (1) Competition for the transporter
        (2) Saturation of the transporter
        (3) High plasma protein binding favors increased tubular secretion because the affinity of the solute is greater for the transporter than for the plasma protein
      b. Examples of drugs that undergo tubular secretion: penicillin, cephalosporins, salicylates, thiazide diuretics, uric acid
    3. Passive tubular reabsorption
      a. Uncharged drugs can be reabsorbed into the systemic circulation in the distal tubule.
      b. Ion trapping
        - Trapping of the ionized form of drugs in the urine

A drug with a larger V_d is eliminated more slowly than one with a smaller V_d.

Excretion by tubular secretion is rapid, but capacity limited.

(1) With weak acids (phenobarbital, methotrexate, aspirin), alkalinization of urine (sodium bicarbonate) increases renal excretion.

(2) With weak bases (amphetamine, phencyclidine), acidification of urine (ammonium chloride) increases renal excretion.

B. Excretion processes in the liver

1. Large polar compounds (molecular weight > 325) may be actively secreted into bile.

- Separate transporters for anions (e.g., glucuronide conjugates), neutral molecules (e.g., ouabain), and cations (e.g., tubocurarine)

2. These large drugs often undergo enterohepatic recycling, in which drugs secreted in the bile are again reabsorbed in the small intestine.

Enterohepatic recycling prolongs the duration of action.

- The enterohepatic cycle can be interrupted by agents that bind drugs in the intestine (e.g., charcoal, cholestyramine).

C. Other sites of excretion

- Example: excretion of gaseous anesthetics by the lungs

VIII. Kinetic Processes

- The therapeutic utility of a drug depends on the rate and extent of input, distribution, and loss.

A. Clearance kinetics

1. Clearance

- The volume of plasma from which a substance is removed per unit time
- To calculate clearance, divide the rate of drug elimination by the plasma concentration of the drug.

2. Total body clearance

- Is calculated using the following equation:

$$Cl = V_d \times K_{el}$$

where

V_d = volume of distribution

K_{el} = elimination rate

3. Renal clearance

- Is calculated using the following equation:

$$Cl_r = \frac{U \times C_{ur}}{C_p}$$

where

U = urine flow (mL/min)

C_{ur} = urine concentration of a drug

C_p = plasma concentration of a drug

B. Elimination kinetics

1. Zero-order kinetics

- The elimination of a constant amount of drug per unit time
- Examples: ethanol, heparin, phenytoin (at high doses), salicylates (at high doses)

a. Important characteristics of zero-order kinetics
 (1) Rate is independent of drug concentration.
 (2) Elimination pseudo–half-life is proportional to drug concentration.
 (3) Small increase in dose can produce larger increase in concentration.
 (4) Process only occurs when enzymes or transporters are saturated.
b. Graphically, plasma drug concentration versus time yields a straight line (Fig. 1-4A).

Zero-order: dose-dependent pharmacokinetics

2. First-order kinetics
 • The elimination of a constant percentage of drug per unit time
 • Examples: most drugs (unless given at very high concentrations)
a. Important characteristics of first-order kinetics
 (1) Rate of elimination is proportional to drug concentration.
 (2) Drug concentration changes by some constant fraction per unit time (i.e., 0.1/hr).
 (3) Half-life ($t_{1/2}$) is constant (i.e., independent of dose).

First-order: dose-independent pharmacokinetics

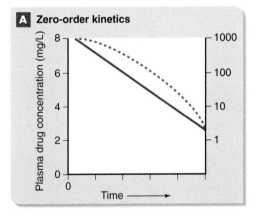

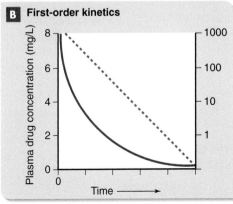

1-4: *Kinetic order of drug disappearance from the plasma. Note that the scale on the left x-axis (**A**) is arithmetic, yielding a relationship shown by the* solid *line, and the scale on the right x-axis (**B**) is logarithmic, yielding a relationship shown by the* dashed *line.*

   b. Graphically, a semilogarithmic plot of plasma drug concentration versus time yields a straight line (Fig. 1-4B).
   c. Elimination rate constant (K_{el})
   • Sum of all rate constants due to metabolism and excretion

$$K_{el} = K_m + K_{ex}$$

where

$$K_m = \text{metabolic rate constant}$$
$$K_{ex} = \text{excretion rate constant}$$
$$K_{el} = \text{elimination rate constant}$$

   d. Biologic or elimination half-life
   • Time required for drug concentration to drop by one half; independent of dose.
   • Is calculated using the following equation:

$$t_{1/2} = \frac{0.693}{K_{el}}$$

where

$$K_{el} = \text{elimination rate constant}$$

3. Repetitive dosing kinetics
   • The attainment of a steady state of plasma concentration of a drug following first-order kinetics when a fixed drug dose is given at constant time interval
   a. Concentration at steady state (C_{ss}) occurs when input equals output, as indicated by the following equation:

$$C_{ss} = \frac{\text{Input}}{\text{Output}} = \frac{F \times D/\tau}{Cl}$$

where

$$F = \text{bioavailability}$$
$$D = \text{dose}$$
$$\tau = \text{dosing interval}$$
$$Cl = \text{clearance}$$

   b. The time required to reach the steady-state condition is $4\frac{1}{2} - 5 \times t_{1/2}$ (Table 1-5).

TABLE 1-5:
Number of Half-Lives ($t_{1/2}$) Required to Reach Steady-State Concentration (C_{ss})

% C_{ss}	Number of $t_{1/2}$
50.0	1
75.0	2
87.5	3
93.8	4
98.0	5

c. The loading dose necessary to reach the steady-state condition immediately can be calculated using the following equation:

$$LD = 1.44 C_{ss} \times \frac{V_d}{F}$$

where

LD = loading dose
C_{ss} = concentration at steady
V_d = volume of distribution
F = bioavailability

4. Amount of drug in body at any time:

$$X_b = V_d \times C_p$$

where

X_b = amount of drug in the body
V_d = volume of distribution
C_p = concentration in plasma

2

Pharmacodynamics

I. Definition
   - Pharmacodynamics involves the biochemical and physiologic effects of drugs on the body.

II. Dose-Response Relationships
   A. These relationships are usually expressed as a log dose-response (LDR) curve.
   B. Properties of LDR curves
      - LDR curves are typically S-shaped.
      - A steep slope in the midportion of the "S" indicates that a small increase in dosage will produce a large increase in response.
      1. Graded response (Fig. 2-1): response in one subject or test system
         - Median effective concentration (EC_{50}): concentration that corresponds to 50% of the maximal response
      2. All-or-none (quantal) response: number of individuals within a group responding to a given dose
         - The end point is set, and an individual is either a responder or a nonresponder.
         a. This response is expressed as a normal histogram or cumulative distribution profile (Fig. 2-2).
            - The normal histogram is usually bell-shaped.
         b. Median effective dose (ED_{50}): dose to which 50% of subjects respond
         c. The therapeutic index (TI) and the margin of safety (MS) are based on quantal responses.
            - TI: ratio of the lethal dose in 50% of the population (LD_{50}) divided by the effective dose for 50% of the population

Graded response measures degree of change; quantal measures frequency of response.

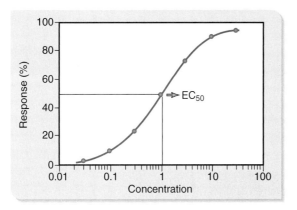

2-1: *Log dose-response curve for an agonist-induced response. The median effective concentration (EC$_{50}$) is the concentration that results in a 50% maximal response.*

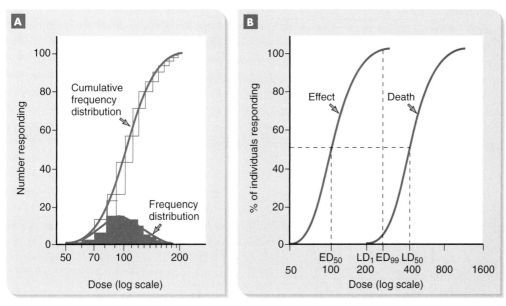

2-2: A, *Cumulative frequency distribution and frequency distribution curves for a drug using a logarithmic dose scale.* **B,** *Cumulative frequency distribution curves for the therapeutic and lethal effects of a drug using a logarithmic dose scale.*

(ED$_{50}$), or

$$TI = \frac{LD_{50}}{ED_{50}}$$

- MS: ratio of the lethal dose for 1% of the population (LD$_1$) divided by the effective dose for 99% of the population (LD$_{99}$), or

$$MS = \frac{LD_1}{ED_{99}}$$

TABLE 2-1:
Drug Receptors and Mechanisms of Signal Transduction

Receptor	Ligand	Mechanism	Time
G Protein–Coupled Receptors			
α₁-Adrenergic receptors	Phenylephrine (agonist) Prazosin (antagonist)	Activation of phospholipase C	Sec
α₂-Adrenergic receptors	Clonidine (agonist) Yohimbine (antagonist)	Inhibition of adenylyl cyclase	Sec
β-Adrenergic receptors	Isoproterenol (agonist) Propranolol (antagonist)	Stimulation of adenylyl cyclase	Sec
Muscarinic receptors	Pilocarpine (agonist) Atropine (antagonist)	Activation of phospholipase C	Sec
Ligand-Gated Ion Channels			
GABA_A receptors	Benzodiazepines (agonists) Flumazenil (antagonist)	Chloride flux	Msec
Nicotinic ACh receptors	Nicotine (agonist) Tubocurarine (antagonist)	Sodium flux	Msec
Membrane-Bound Enzymes			
Insulin receptors	Insulin	Activation of tyrosine kinase	Min
Cytokine receptors	Interleukin-2	Activation of tyrosine kinase	Min
Cytoplasmic Receptors			
Cytoplasmic guanylyl cyclase	Nitroglycerin	Activation of guanylyl cyclase	Min
Nuclear Receptors			
Steroid receptors	Adrenal and gonadal steroids	Activation of gene transcription	Hr
Thyroid hormone receptors	Thyroxine	Activation of gene transcription	Hr

ACh, acetylcholine; GABA, γ-aminobutyric acid.

III. Drug Receptors
- Drug receptors are biologic components on the surface of or within cells that bind with drugs, resulting in molecular changes that produce a certain response.
  A. Types of receptors and their signaling mechanisms (Table 2-1)
    1. Membrane receptors are coupled with a G protein, an ion channel, or an enzyme.
      a. G protein–coupled receptors (see Table 2-1)
        - These receptors are a superfamily of diverse guanosine triphosphate (GTP)–binding proteins that couple to "serpentine" transmembrane receptors (Fig. 2-3).
      b. Ligand-gated channels (see Table 2-1)

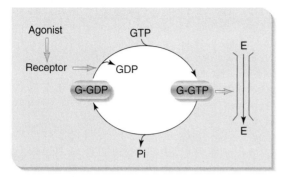

2-3: *The guanine nucleotide–dependent activation-inactivation cycle of G proteins. The agonist activates the receptor, releasing GDP from the G protein and allowing GTP to bind to the G protein. The G protein, in its G-GTP state, regulates activity of an effector enzyme or ion channel (E). The signal is terminated by the hydrolysis of GTP, yielding GDP bound to the G protein. GDP, guanosine diphosphate; GTP, guanosine triphosphate; Pi, inorganic phosphate.*

        (1) Signals cross membranes due to changes in ion conductance and alter the electrical potential of cells.

        (2) The speed of the response is rapid.

     c. Receptor-linked enzymes (see Table 2-1)

  2. Intracellular receptors (inside cells)

     • Cytoplasmic guanylyl cyclase is activated by nitric oxide.

     a. Ligand-responsive transcription factors alter gene expression and protein synthesis.

     b. Other intracellular sites can serve as targets for drug molecules crossing cell membranes (e.g., structural proteins, DNA, RNA).

     c. Drugs using these mechanisms include steroids, lipid-soluble drugs, nitric oxide.

B. Degree of receptor binding

  1. Drug molecules bind to receptors at a rate that is dependent on drug concentration.

  2. The dissociation constant ($K_D = k_{-1}/k_1$) of the drug-receptor complex is inversely related to the affinity of the drug for the receptor.

     • A drug with a K_D of 10^{-7} M has a higher affinity than a drug with a K_D of 10^{-6} M.

     • k_1 is the rate of onset, and k_{-1} is the rate of offset for receptor occupancy.

  3. The intensity of response is proportional to the number of receptors occupied.

C. Terms used to describe drug-receptor interactions

  1. Affinity

     • Propensity of a drug to bind with a given receptor

  2. Potency

     • Comparative expression that relates the dose required to produce a particular effect of a given intensity relative to a standard reference (Fig. 2-4)

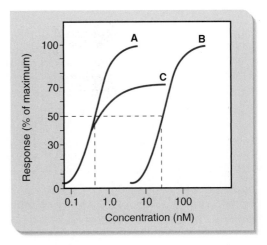

2-4: *Dose-response curves of three agonists with differing potency and efficacy. Agonists A and B have the same efficacy but different potency; A is more potent than B. Agonists A and C have the same potency but different efficacy; A is more efficacious than C.*

3. Efficacy (intrinsic activity)
   - Maximal response resulting from binding of drug to its receptor (see Fig. 2-4)
4. Full agonist
   - Drug that stimulates a receptor, provoking a maximal biologic response
5. Partial agonist
   - Drug that provokes a submaximal response
   - In Figure 2-4, drug C is a partial agonist.
6. Inverse agonist
   - Drug that stimulates a receptor, provoking a negative biologic response (e.g., a decrease in basal activity)
7. Antagonist
   - Drug that interacts with a receptor but does not result in a biologic response (no intrinsic activity)
   a. Competitive antagonist (Fig. 2-5)
      - Binds reversibly to the same receptor site as an agonist
      (1) Effect can be overcome by increasing the dose of the agonist (reversible effect).
      (2) A fixed dose of a competitive antagonist causes the log dose-response curve of an agonist to make a parallel shift to the right.
      (3) A partial agonist may act as a competitive inhibitor to a full agonist.
   b. Noncompetitive antagonist (Fig. 2-6)
      - Binds irreversibly to the receptor site for the agonist
      (1) Its effects cannot be overcome completely by increasing the concentration of the agonist.

Be able to compare affinities, potencies, and intrinsic activities of drugs from LDR curves.

Propranolol is a competitive antagonist of epinephrine at β-adrenergic receptors.

Phenoxybenzamine is a noncompetitive antagonist of epinephrine at α-adrenergic receptors.

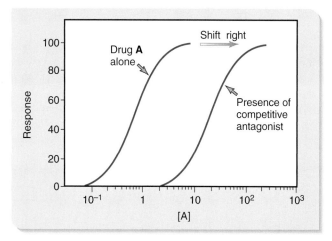

2-5: *Competitive antagonism. The log dose-response curve for drug A shifts to the right in the presence of a fixed dose of a competitive antagonist.*

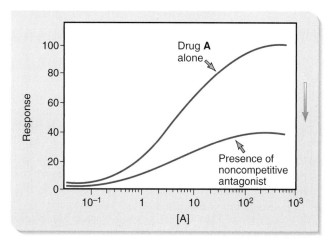

2-6: *Noncompetitive antagonism. The log dose-response curve for drug A shifts to the right and downward in the presence of a fixed dose of a noncompetitive antagonist.*

        (2) A fixed dose of a noncompetitive antagonist causes a nonparallel, downward shift of the log dose-response curve of the agonist to the right.

IV. Pharmacodynamically Altered Responses
    A. Decreased drug activity
        1. Antagonism resulting from drug interactions
            a. Physiologic (functional) antagonism
              • This response occurs when two agonists with opposing physiologic effects are administered together.

Be able to depict drug potentiation, competitive antagonism, and noncompetitive antagonism from LDR curves.

- Examples: histamine (vasodilation), norepinephrine (vasoconstriction)
  - b. Competitive antagonism
    - This response occurs when a receptor antagonist is administered with an agonist.
    - Examples:
    - (1) Naloxone, when blocking the effects of morphine
    - (2) Atropine, when blocking the effects of acetylcholine (ACh) at a muscarinic receptor
    - (3) Flumazenil, when blocking the effects of diazepam at a benzodiazepine receptor
  2. Tolerance definition: diminished response to the same dose of a drug over time
    - a. Mechanisms of tolerance
      - (1) Desensitization
        - Rapid process involving continuous exposure to a drug, altering the receptor so that it cannot produce a response
        - Continuous exposure to β-adrenergic agonist (e.g., use of albuterol in asthma) results in decreased responsiveness.
      - (2) Down-regulation: decrease in number of receptors caused by high doses of agonists over prolonged periods
      - (3) Tachyphylaxis: rapid development of tolerance
        - (a) Indirect-acting amines (e.g., tyramine, amphetamine) exert effects by releasing monoamines.
        - (b) Several doses given over a short time deplete the monoamine pool, reducing the response to successive doses.

B. Increased drug activity
  1. Supersensitivity or hyperactivity
    - Enhanced response to a drug may be due to an increase in the number of receptors (up-regulation).
    - Antagonists cause up-regulation of receptors.
  2. Potentiation
    - Enhancement of the effect of one drug, which has no effect by itself, when combined with a second drug (e.g., 0 + 5 = 20, not 5)
    - Produces a shift of the log dose-response curve to the left
    - Examples:
    - a. Physostigmine, an acetylcholinesterase inhibtor (AChEI), potentiates the response to acetylcholine (ACh).
    - b. Cocaine (an uptake I blocker) potentiates the response to norepinephrine (NE).
  3. Synergism
    - Production of a greater response than of two drugs that act individually (e.g., 2 + 5 = 15, not 7)

C. Dependence
  1. Physical dependence
    - Repeated use produces an altered or adaptive physiologic state if the drug is not present.

Continuous use of β-adrenergic agonists involves both desensitization and down-regulation.

Drugs that may lead to dependence: alcohol, barbiturates, benzodiazepines, narcotic analgesics

2. Psychological dependence: compulsive drug-seeking behavior
   - Individuals use a drug repeatedly for personal satisfaction.
3. Substance dependence (addiction)
   - Individuals continue substance use despite significant substance-related problems.

3 **CHAPTER**

Introduction to Autonomic and Neuromuscular Pharmacology

TARGET TOPICS

- Parasympathetic nervous system
- Sympathetic nervous system
- Neurochemistry of the autonomic nervous system
- Drugs that affect the cholinergic system
- Drugs that affect the adrenergic system
- Physiologic aspects of autonomic nerve activity

I. Divisions of the Efferent Autonomic Nervous System (ANS) (Fig. 3-1)
   A. Parasympathetic nervous system (PSNS): craniosacral division of the ANS
      1. Origin: midbrain, medulla oblongata, sacral cord
      2. Nerve fibers: long preganglionic nerve fibers, short postganglionic nerve fibers
      3. Neurotransmitter
         - Acetylcholine (ACh) is the neurotransmitter both at the ganglia (stimulates nicotinic receptors) and at the neuroeffector junction (stimulates muscarinic receptors).
      4. Associated processes: digestion, conservation of energy, maintenance of organ function
   B. Sympathetic nervous system (SNS): thoracolumbar division of the ANS
      1. Origin: thoracic and upper lumbar regions of spinal cord
      2. Nerve fibers
         a. Short preganglionic nerve fibers, which synapse in the paravertebral ganglionic chain
         b. Long postganglionic nerve fibers

PSNS = craniosacral origin

ACh stimulates both nicotinic and muscarinic receptors.

SNS = thoracolumbar origin

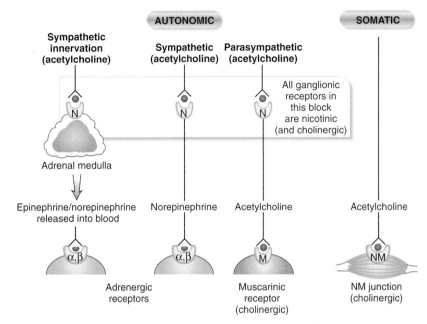

3-1: Schematic representation of sympathetic, parasympathetic, and somatic efferent neurons. α, α-adrenoreceptor; β, β-adrenoreceptor; M, muscarinic receptor; N, nicotinic receptor; NM, neuromuscular.

3. Neurotransmitters
   a. ACh is the neurotransmitter at the ganglia (stimulates nicotinic receptors).
   b. Norepinephrine is usually the neurotransmitter at the neuroeffector junction (stimulates α- or β-adrenergic receptors).
      • Exception: ACh is a neurotransmitter found in sympathetic nerve endings at thermoregulatory sweat glands.
4. Associated processes: mobilizing the body's resources to respond to fear and anxiety ("fight-or-flight" response)

II. Neurochemistry of the Autonomic Nervous System
   A. Cholinergic pathways
      1. Cholinergic fibers
         a. Synthesis, storage, and release (Fig. 3-2A)
         b. Receptor activation and signal transduction
            • ACh activates nicotinic or muscarinic receptors (Table 3-1).
         c. Inactivation
            • ACh is metabolized to acetate and choline
            (1) Occurs by acetylcholinesterase (AChE) in the synapse
            (2) Occurs by pseudocholinesterase in the blood and liver
      2. Drugs that affect cholinergic pathways (Table 3-2)
         a. Botulinum toxin
            (1) Mechanism of action: blocks release of ACh, inhibiting neurotransmitter transmission

> Epinephrine and norepinephrine both stimulate α- and β-adrenergic receptors.

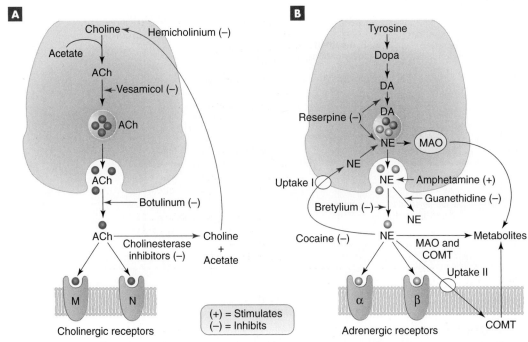

3-2: *Cholinergic and adrenergic neurotransmission and sites of drug action.* **A,** *Illustration of the synthesis, storage, release, inactivation, and postsynaptic receptor activation of cholinergic neurotransmission.* **B,** *Illustration of the synthesis, storage, release, termination of action, and postsynaptic action of adrenergic neurotransmission. Uptake I is a transporter that transports NE into the presynaptic neuron. Uptake II is a transporter that transports NE into the postsynaptic neuron. α, α-adrenoreceptor; β, β-adrenoreceptor; ACh, acetylcholine; COMT, catechol-O-methyltransferase; DA, dopamine; M, muscarinic receptor; MAO, monoamine oxidase; N, nicotinic receptor; NE, norepinephrine.*

      (2) Uses
         (a) Localized spasms of ocular and facial muscles
         (b) Lower esophageal sphincter spasm in achalasia
         (c) Spasticity resulting from central nervous system (CNS) disorders
    b. Cholinesterase inhibitors
      (1) Mechanism of action: prevent breakdown of ACh
      (2) Examples: indirect-acting cholinergic receptor agonists (e.g., neostigmine, physostigmine, pyridostigmine, donepezil)
    c. Cholinergic receptor antagonists
      (1) Muscarinic receptor antagonists such as atropine
      (2) Nicotinic receptor antagonists such as the ganglionic blocker trimethaphan and the neuromuscular blocker tubocurarine
  B. Adrenergic pathways
    1. Adrenergic fibers
      a. Synthesis, storage, and release (Fig. 3-2B)
      b. Receptor activation and signal transduction
        • Norepinephrine or epinephrine binds to α or β receptors on postsynaptic effector cells (Table 3-3).

Physostigmine reverses the CNS effects of atropine poisoning.

TABLE 3-1:
**Properties of
Cholinergic
Receptors**

Type of Receptor	Principal Locations	Mechanism of Signal Transduction	Effects
Muscarinic			
M_1	Autonomic ganglia Presynaptic nerve terminals CNS neurons	Increased IP_3 and DAG Increased intracellular calcium	Modulation of neurotransmission
M_2	Cardiac tissue (sinoatrial and atrioventricular nodes) Nerves	Increased potassium efflux Inhibition of cAMP	Slowing of heart rate and conduction
M_3	Smooth muscles and glands	Increased IP_3 and DAG Increased intracellular calcium	Contraction of smooth muscles Stimulation of glandular secretions
	Endothelium	Increased nitric oxide formation	Nitric oxide vasodilation
	Vascular smooth muscle	Increased cGMP (from nitric oxide)	
Nicotinic			
N_M (muscle type)	Skeletal neuromuscular junctions	Increased sodium influx	Muscle contraction
N_N (neuron type)	Postganglionic cell body Dendrites	Increased sodium influx	Excitation of postganglionic neurons

cAMP, cyclic adenosine monophosphate; cGMP, cyclic guanosine monophosphate; CNS, central nervous system; DAG, diacylglycerol; IP_3, inositol triphosphate.

TABLE 3-2:
**Drugs that Affect
Autonomic
Neurotransmission**

Mechanism	Drugs that Affect Cholinergic Neurotransmission	Drugs that Affect Adrenergic Neurotransmission
Inhibit synthesis of neurotransmitter	Hemicholinium*	Metyrosine
Prevent vesicular storage of neurotransmitter	Vesamicol*	Reserpine
Inhibit release of neurotransmitter	Botulinum toxin	Bretylium Guanethidine
Stimulate release of neurotransmitter	Black widow spider venom*	Amphetamine Tyramine
Inhibit reuptake of neurotransmitter	—	Tricyclic antidepressants Cocaine
Inhibit metabolism of neurotransmitter	Cholinesterase inhibitors (physostigmine, neostigmine)	Monoamine oxidase inhibitors (tranylcypromine)
Activate postsynaptic receptors	Acetylcholine (M, N) Bethanechol (M) Pilocarpine (M)	Albuterol (β_2) Dobutamine (β_1) Epinephrine (α, β)
Block postsynaptic receptors	Atropine (muscarinic receptors) and tubocurarine (nicotinic receptors)	Phentolamine (α-adrenergic receptors) and propranolol (β-adrenergic receptors)

*Used experimentally but not therapeutically.
M, muscarinic receptor; N, nicotinic receptor.

**TABLE 3-3:
Properties of
Adrenergic
Receptors**

Type of Receptor	Mechanism of Signal Transduction	Effects
α_1	Increased IP$_3$ and DAG	Contraction of smooth muscles
α_2	Decreased cAMP	Inhibited norepinephrine release Decrease in aqueous humor secretion Decrease in insulin secretion Mediation of platelet aggregation and mediation of CNS effects
β_1	Increased cAMP	Increase in secretion of renin Increase in heart rate, contractility, and conduction
β_2	Increased cAMP	Glycogenolysis Relaxation of smooth muscles Uptake of potassium in smooth muscles
β_3	Increased cAMP	Lipolysis

cAMP, cyclic adenosine monophosphate; CNS, central nervous system; DAG, diacylglycerol; IP$_3$, inositol triphosphate.

   c. Termination of action: reuptake
- Reuptake by active transport (uptake I) is the primary mechanism for removal of norepinephrine from the synaptic cleft.
   (1) Monoamine oxidase (MAO) is an enzyme located in the mitochondria of presynaptic adrenergic neuron and liver.
   (2) Catechol-*O*-methyltransferase (COMT) is an enzyme located in the cytoplasm of autonomic effector cells and liver.
2. Drugs that affect adrenergic pathways (see Fig. 3-2 and Table 3-2)
   a. Guanethidine
- Uptake involves active transport into the peripheral adrenergic neuron by the norepinephrine reuptake system (uptake I).
   (1) Mechanism of action
     (a) Guanethidine eventually depletes the nerve endings of norepinephrine by replacing norepinephrine in the storage granules.
     (b) Its uptake is blocked by reuptake inhibitors (e.g., cocaine, tricyclic antidepressants such as imipramine).
   (2) Use: hypertension (discontinued in United States)
   b. Reserpine
   (1) Mechanism of action
     (a) Depletes storage granules of catecholamines by binding to granules and preventing uptake and storage of norepinephrine
     (b) Acts centrally also to produce sedation, depression, and parkinsonian symptoms (due to depletion of norepinephrine, serotonin, and dopamine)
   (2) Use: mild hypertension (rarely used today)
   (3) Adverse effects: pseudoparkinsonism
   c. Adrenergic receptor antagonists
   (1) May be nonselective or selective for either α or β receptors

(2) May be selective for a particular subtype of α or β receptor (see Chapter 5)

III. Physiologic Considerations
  A. Dual innervation
   • Most visceral organs are innervated only by both the sympathetic and parasympathetic nervous systems.
   • Most blood vessels are innervated by the sympathetic system
  B. Physiologic effects of autonomic nerve activity (Table 3-4)
   • α responses: usually excitatory (contraction of smooth muscle)
   • β_1 responses: located in the heart and are excitatory; cause renin secretion in the kidney
   • β_2 responses: usually inhibitory (relaxation of smooth muscle)

   1. Adrenal medulla
    a. This modified sympathetic ganglion releases epinephrine and norepinephrine.
    b. These circulating hormones can affect α and β responses throughout the body.
   2. Heart
    a. Sympathetic effects increase cardiac output.
     (1) Positive chronotropic effect (increased heart rate)
     (2) Positive inotropic effect (increased force of contraction)
     (3) Positive dromotropic effect (increased speed of conduction of excitation)
    b. Parasympathetic effects (M_2) decrease heart rate and cardiac output.
     (1) Negative chronotropic effect (decreased heart rate)
     (2) Negative inotropic effect (decreased force of contraction)
      • Exogenous ACh only (no vagal innervation of the ventricular muscle)
     (3) Negative dromotropic effect (decreased velocity of conduction of excitation)
   3. Blood pressure
    • The overall effects of autonomic drugs on blood pressure are complex and are determined by at least four parameters.
    a. Direct effects on the heart
     (1) β_1 stimulation leads to an increased heart rate, and increased force means increased blood pressure.
     (2) Muscarinic stimulation leads to a decreased heart rate, and decreased force means decreased blood pressure.
    b. Vascular effects
     (1) Muscarinic stimulation results in dilation, which decreases blood pressure.
     (2) Alpha (α) stimulation results in constriction, which increases blood pressure.
     (3) Beta (β_2) stimulation results in dilation, which decreases blood pressure.

The only tone to the vasculature is sympathetic.

At rest, the predominant tone to the heart is parasympathetic.

TABLE 3-4:
Direct Effects of Autonomic Nerve Activity on Body Systems

| Organ/Tissue | SYMPATHETIC RESPONSE | | PARASYMPATHETIC RESPONSE | |
	Action	Receptor	Action	Receptor
Eye: Iris				
Radial muscle	Contracts (mydriasis)	α_1	—	—
Circular muscle	—	—	Contracts	M_3
Ciliary muscle	Relaxes for far vision	β_2	Contracts	M_3
Heart				
Sinoatrial node	Accelerates	$\beta_1 > \beta_2$	Decelerates	M_2
Ectopic pacemakers	Accelerates	$\beta_1 > \beta_2$	—	—
Contractility	Increases	$\beta_1 > \beta_2$	Decreases (atria)	M_2
Arterioles				
Coronary	Dilation	β_2	Dilation	M
	Constriction	$\alpha_1 > \alpha_2$	—	—
Skin and mucosa	Constriction	$\alpha_1 > \alpha_2$	Dilation	M
Skeletal muscle	Constriction	$\alpha_1 > \alpha_2$	Dilation	M*
	Dilation	β_2, M†	—	—
Splanchnic	Constriction	$\alpha_1 > \alpha_2$	Dilation	M*
Renal and mesenteric	Dilation	Dopamine, β_2	—	—
	Constriction	$\alpha_1 > \alpha_2$	—	—
Veins				
Systemic	Dilation	β_2	—	—
	Constriction	$\alpha_1 > \alpha_2$	—	—
Bronchiolar Muscle	Relaxes	β_2	Contracts	M
GI Tract				
Smooth muscle				
Walls	Relaxes	α_2, β_2	Contracts	M
Sphincters	Contracts	α_1	Relaxes	M
Secretion	Inhibits	α_2	Increases	M
Genitourinary Smooth Muscle				
Bladder wall	Relaxes	β_2	Contracts	M
Sphincter	Contracts	α_1	Relaxes	M
Uterus, pregnant	Relaxes	β_2	—	—
	Contracts	α_1	—	—
Penis, seminal vesicles	Ejaculation	α_2	Erection	M
Skin				
Pilomotor smooth muscle	Contracts	α_1	—	—
Sweat glands				
Thermoregulatory	Increases	M	—	—
Apocrine (stress)	Increases	α_1	—	—
Other Functions				
Muscle	Promotes K^+ uptake	β_2	—	—
Liver	Gluconeogenesis	α, β_2	—	—
	Glycogenolysis	α_1, β_2	—	—
Fat cells	Lipolysis	β_3	—	—
Kidney	Renin release	β_1, α_1†	—	—
	Sodium reabsorption	α_1	—	—

*The endothelium of most blood vessels releases endothelium-derived releasing factor (EDRF), which causes vasodilation in response to muscarinic stimuli. However, these muscarinic receptors are not innervated and respond only to *circulating muscarinic agonists.*
†Vascular smooth muscle has sympathetic cholinergic dilator fibers.
‡α_1 inhibits; β_1 stimulates.
GI, gastrointestinal; M, muscarinic.

  c. Redistribution of blood
  (1) With increased sympathetic activity, the blood is shunted away from organs and tissues such as the skin, gastrointestinal tract, and glands and toward the heart and voluntary (e.g., skeletal) muscles.
  (2) This process occurs as a result of a predominance of β_2 vasodilation rather than α_1 constriction at these sites.
  d. Reflex phenomena
  (1) A decrease in blood pressure, sensed by baroreceptors in the carotid sinus and aortic arch, causes reflex tachycardia.
  (2) An increase in blood pressure causes reflex bradycardia.

4. Eye
  a. Pupil (iris)
  (1) Sympathetic effects contract (mydriasis) radial muscle (α-adrenergic receptor).
  (2) Parasympathomimetic effects contract (miosis) circular muscle (M_3-muscarinic receptors).
  b. Ciliary muscle
  (1) Sympathetic (β-adrenergic receptors) causes relaxation and facilitates the secretion of aqueous humor.
  (2) Parasympathetic (M_3-muscarinic receptors) causes contraction (accommodation for near vision) and opens pores facilitating outflow of aqueous humor into canal of Schlemm.

Fall in blood pressure produces reflex tachycardia.

Elevation in blood pressure produces reflex bradycardia.

Cholinergic Drugs

TARGET TOPICS

- Muscarinic receptor agonists
- Cholinesterase inhibitors
- Ganglionic stimulants
- Muscarinic receptor antagonists
- Nicotinic receptor antagonists

I. Cholinoreceptor Agonists
  A. Muscarinic receptor agonists (Box 4-1)
    - Physiologic muscarinic effects (Table 4-1)
    1. Pharmacokinetics
      a. Choline esters: quaternary ammonium compounds
        - Do *not* readily cross the blood-brain barrier
        - Inactivated by acetylcholinesterase (AChE) or pseudocholinesterase
      b. Plant alkaloids
        - Muscarine is used experimentally to investigate muscarinic receptors.
        - Pilocarpine, a tertiary amine, can enter the central nervous system (CNS) and is used to treat glaucoma.
    2. Mechanism of action: directly stimulate muscarinic receptors
    3. Uses
      a. Bethanechol (selectively acts on smooth muscle of the gastrointestinal tract and the urinary bladder)
        (1) Urinary retention in the absence of obstruction
        (2) Postoperative ileus
        (3) Gastric atony and retention after bilateral vagotomy
      b. Pilocarpine
        (1) Glaucoma (ophthalmic preparation)
        (2) Xerostomia (dry mouth): given orally to stimulate salivary gland secretion
    4. Adverse effects: nausea, vomiting, diarrhea, salivation
      a. Due to overstimulation of parasympathetic effector organs
      b. Treatment of overdose
        (1) Atropine to counteract muscarinic effects
        (2) Epinephrine to overcome severe cardiovascular reactions or bronchoconstriction

Overstimulation of muscarinic receptors leads to DUMBELS: defecation, urination, miosis, bronchoconstriction, emesis, lacrimation, salivation.

BOX 4-1

MUSCARINIC AND NICOTINIC RECEPTOR AGONISTS

Choline Esters

Acetylcholine (M, N)
Bethanechol (M)
Carbachol (M)

Plant Alkaloids

Muscarine (M)
Nicotine (N)
Pilocarpine (M)

M, muscarinic; N, nicotinic.

TABLE 4-1: Effects of Muscarinic Receptor Agonists

Organ/Organ System	Effects
Cardiovascular	Hypotension from direct vasodilation Bradycardia at high doses Slowed conduction and prolonged refractory period of atrioventricular node
Gastrointestinal	Increased tone and increased contractile activity of gut Increased acid secretion Nausea, vomiting, cramps, and diarrhea
Genitourinary	Involuntary urination from increased bladder motility and relaxation of sphincter Penile erection
Eye	Miosis: contraction of sphincter muscle, resulting in reduced intraocular pressure Contraction of ciliary muscle; accommodated for near vision
Respiratory system	Bronchoconstriction
Glands	Increased secretory activity, resulting in increased salivation, lacrimation, and sweating

   B. Cholinesterase inhibitors (Box 4-2; see also Fig. 3-2A)
      1. Pharmacokinetics
         a. Edrophonium is rapid and short-acting (i.e., effects last only about 10 min after injection).
         b. Physostigmine crosses the blood-brain barrier.
         c. Drugs used in Alzheimer's disease cross the blood-brain barrier.
      2. Mechanism of action
         • Bind to and inhibit AChE, increasing the concentration of acetylcholine (ACh) in the synaptic cleft

---

BOX 4-2

CHOLINESTERASE INHIBITORS

Reversible Inhibitors

Donepezil (A)
Edrophonium (MG)
Galantamine (A)
Neostigmine (C, MG)
Physostigmine (C)
Pyridostigmine (C, MG)
Rivastigmine (A,C)
Tacrine (A)

Irreversible Inhibitors

Echothiophate
Isoflurophate
Malathion
Parathion
Sarin

C, carbamate structure; A, used in Alzheimer's disease; MG, used in myasthenia gravis.

- Stimulate responses at the muscarinic receptors as well as at the neuromuscular junction (NMJ)
- Stimulate responses at nicotinic receptors in the ganglia at higher doses
  a. Reversible inhibitors
     (1) Truly reversible; compete with ACh at the enzyme active site: edrophonium, tacrine, donepezil, galantamine
     (2) Carbamates; carbamoylate the serine hydroxyl at active site of enzyme which is rapidly hydrolyzed (pseudoreversible): physostigmine, pyridostigmine, neostigmine, rivastigmine
  b. Irreversible inhibitors (organophosphates); phosphorylate the serine hydroxyl at active site of enzyme: echothiophate, isoflurophate, malathion, parathion, sarin
     - The phosphoryl group is not readily cleaved from the cholinesterase, but the enzyme can be reactivated by the early use of pralidoxime.
  3. Uses
     a. Alzheimer's disease: donepezil, tacrine, rivastigmine, galantamine
     b. Paralytic ileus and urine retention: neostigmine
     c. Glaucoma: physostigmine, echothiophate
     d. Myasthenia gravis: edrophonium (short-acting; diagnosis only), pyridostigmine (treatment), neostigmine (treatment)

Tacrine may cause hepatotoxicity.

e. Insecticides and chemical warfare: organophosphates used as insecticides (malathion, parathion) and as components in nerve gases (sarin)

4. Adverse effects: nausea, vomiting, diarrhea, salivation, lacrimation, constricted pupils

   a. Due to overstimulation of parasympathetic effector organs

   b. Treatment

     (1) Atropine to counteract muscarinic effects

     (2) Pralidoxime to reactivate enzyme if toxicity due to an organophosphate; contraindicated for reversible inhibitors

     (3) Supportive therapy (check and support vital signs)

C. Ganglionic stimulants

- Effects depend on the predominant autonomic tone at the organ system being assessed.

1. ACh

- Much higher levels of ACh are required to stimulate nicotinic receptors in ganglia than muscarinic receptors at the neuroeffector junction.

2. Nicotine

- Stimulates the ganglia at low doses and blocks the ganglia at higher doses by persistent depolarization of nicotinic receptors and secondary desensitization of receptors.

- Uses

   a. Experimentally to investigate the ANS

   b. Clinically as a drug to help smokers quit smoking

   c. As an adjunct to haloperidol in the treatment of Tourette's syndrome

3. Cholinesterase inhibitors

- Increase the concentration of ACh at the ganglia

II. Cholinoreceptor Antagonists

A. Muscarinic receptor antagonists (Box 4-3)

- Belladonna alkaloids
- Synthetic muscarinic antagonists
- Other classes of drugs with atropine-like effects, such as antihistamines, antipsychotics, tricyclic antidepressants, and antiparkinsonian drugs

1. Mechanism of action: competitive inhibition of ACh at the muscarinic receptor

2. Uses

   a. Chronic obstructive pulmonary disease (COPD) (ipratropium and tiotropium)

   b. Asthma prophylaxis (ipratropium)

   c. Bradycardia (atropine)

   d. Motion sickness (scopolamine)

   e. Parkinson's disease (benztropine, trihexyphenidyl)

   f. Bladder or bowel spasms and incontinence (oxybutynin, tolterodine)

   g. Ophthalmic uses: facilitation of ophthalmoscopic examinations when prolonged dilation is needed; iridocyclitis (tropicamide, homatropine)

   h. "Colds" (over-the-counter remedies)

Drugs used in the management of myasthenia gravis: neostigmine, pyridostigmine, edrophonium (diagnosis)

BOX 4-3

MUSCARINIC RECEPTOR ANTAGONISTS

Belladonna Alkaloids

Atropine
Hyoscyamine
Scopolamine

Synthetic Muscarinic Antagonists

Benztropine
Homatropine
Ipratropium
Oxybutynin
Tiotropium
Trihexyphenidyl
Tolterodine
Tropicamide

---

       (1) Some symptomatic relief as the result of a drying effect
       (2) Useful as sleep aids
    i. Parasympathomimetic toxicity: atropine
       (1) Overdose of AChE inhibitors
       (2) Mushroom *(Amanita muscaria)* poisoning
  3. Adverse effects
    a. Overdose
       (1) Common signs: dry mouth; dilated pupils; blurring of vision; hot, dry, flushed skin; tachycardia; fever; CNS changes
       (2) Death follows coma and respiratory depression.
    b. Treatment of overdose
       (1) Gastric lavage
       (2) Supportive therapy
       (3) Diazepam to control excitement and seizures
       (4) Effects of muscarinic receptor antagonists may be overcome by increasing levels of ACh in the synaptic cleft (usually by administration of AChE inhibitors such as physostigmine); physostigmine used only for pure anticholinergics and not for poisoning with antihistamines, antipsychotics, or tricyclic antidepressant drugs.
  B. Nicotinic receptor antagonists
    1. Ganglionic blockers
      • Block nicotinic receptor at ganglion
      • Primarily used in mechanistic studies

Atropine toxicity: "mad as a hatter, dry as a bone, blind as a bat, red as a beet, hot as hell"

    a. Hexamethonium: prototypic ganglionic blocking agent; used experimentally

    b. Trimethaphan: used to control blood pressure during surgery (discontinued in United States)

2. Neuromuscular blockers

    a. Mechanism of action: block nicotinic receptors at the neuromuscular junction (e.g., atracurium, d-tubocurarine) (see Chapter 6)

    b. Use: relaxation of striated muscle

       • Relaxation may be reversed by cholinesterase inhibitors (neostigmine or pyridostigmine).

Adrenergic Drugs

I. Adrenoreceptor Agonists
- Physiologic effects (Table 5-1)
  A. Selected catecholamines (Box 5-1)
  - Endogenous catecholamines (norepinephrine, epinephrine, and dopamine) are found in peripheral sympathetic nerve endings, the adrenal medulla, and the brain.
  - Catecholamines affect blood pressure and heart rate (Fig. 5-1).
  - Monoamine oxidase (MAO) inhibitors, catechol-O-methyltransferase (COMT) inhibitors, tricyclic antidepressants, and cocaine potentiate the effects of catecholamines.
  1. Norepinephrine (NE)
     - Use: blood pressure elevation, resulting from the ability of the drug to increase total peripheral resistance through arteriolar constriction
  2. Epinephrine (EPI)
     a. Pharmacokinetics
        (1) Usually injected subcutaneously
        (2) Intracardiac or intravenous route used in cardiac arrest
     b. Uses
        (1) Treatment of asthma
        (2) Treatment of anaphylactic shock or angioedema
        (3) Prolongation of action of local anesthetics, due to the vasoconstrictive properties of epinephrine
        (4) Treatment of cardiac arrest, bradycardia, and complete heart block in emergencies

Potency of α_1-adrenoreceptor agonists: EPI > NE >> DA >>>> ISO

Potency of β_1-adrenoreceptor agonists: ISO >> EPI > NE = DA

TABLE 5-1:
**Pharmacologic
Effects and Clinical
Uses of
Adrenoreceptor
Agonists**

Drug	Effect and Receptor Selectivity	Clinical Application
Direct-Acting Adrenoreceptor Agonists		
Catecholamines		
Dobutamine	Cardiac stimulation (β_1) $\beta_1 > \beta_2$	Shock, heart failure
Dopamine	Renal vasodilation (D_1) Cardiac stimulation (β_1) Increased blood pressure (α_1) $D_1 = D_2 > \beta > \alpha$	Shock, heart failure
Epinephrine	Increased blood pressure (α_1) Cardiac stimulation (β_1) Bronchodilation (β_2) General agonist (α_1, α_2, β_1, β_2)	Anaphylaxis, open-angle glaucoma, asthma, hypotension, cardiac arrest, ventricular fibrillation, reduction in bleeding in surgery, prolongation of local anesthetic action
Isoproterenol	Cardiac stimulation (β_1) $\beta_1 = \beta_2$	Atrioventricular block, bradycardia
Norepinephrine	Increased blood pressure (α_1) α_1, α_2, β_1	Hypotension, shock
Noncatecholamines		
Albuterol	Bronchodilation (β_2) $\beta_2 > \beta_1$	Asthma
Clonidine	Decreased sympathetic outflow (α_2)	Chronic hypertension
Oxymetazoline	Vasoconstriction (α_1)	Decongestant
Phenylephrine	Vasoconstriction, increased blood pressure, and mydriasis (α_1) $\alpha_1 > \alpha_2$	Pupil dilation, decongestion, mydriasis, neurogenic shock, blood pressure maintenance during surgery
Ritodrine	Bronchodilation and uterine relaxation (β_2)	Premature labor
Terbutaline	Bronchodilation and uterine relaxation (β_2) $\beta_2 > \beta_1$	Asthma, premature labor
Fenoldopam	Dilates renal and mesenteric vascular beds D_1-agonist	Hypertensive emergency
Indirect-Acting Adrenoreceptor Agonists		
Amphetamine	Increased norepinephrine release General agonist (α_1, α_2, β_1, β_2)	Narcolepsy, obesity, attention deficit disorder
Cocaine	Inhibited norepinephrine reuptake General agonist (α_1, α_2, β_1, β_2)	Local anesthesia
Mixed-Acting Adrenoreceptor Agonists		
Ephedrine	Vasoconstriction (α_1) General agonist (α_1, α_2, β_1, β_2)	Decongestant, urine incontinence, hypotension
Phenylpropanolamine	Vasoconstriction (α_1)	Decongestant, no longer used because it may cause higher incidence of stroke
Pseudoephedrine	Vasoconstriction (α_1)	Decongestant

BOX 5-1

ADRENORECEPTOR AGONISTS

Direct-Acting Agonists and Receptor Selectivity

Catecholamines

Dobutamine	β_1 (α_1)
Dopamine (DA)	D_1 (α_1 and β_1 at high doses)
Epinephrine (EPI)	α_1, α_2, β_1, β_2
Isoproterenol (ISO)	β_1, β_2
Norepinephrine (NE)	α_1, α_2, β_1

Noncatecholamines

Albuterol	β_2
Clonidine	α_2
Methoxamine	α_1
Methyldopa	α_2
Oxymetazoline	α_1, α_2
Phenylephrine	α_1
Ritodrine	β_2
Salmeterol	β_2
Terbutaline	β_2

Indirect-Acting Agonists

Releasers
Amphetamine
Tyramine

Monoamine Oxidase Inhibitors
Phenelzine (MAO-A, -B)
Selegiline (MAO-B)
Tranylcypromine (MAO-A, -B)

Catechol-O-methyltransferase Inhibitors
Entacapone
Tolcapone

Reuptake Inhibitors
Cocaine
Imipramine

Mixed-Acting Agonists
Ephedrine

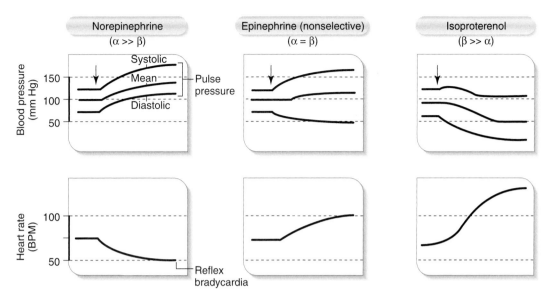

5-1: *Graphic representations of the effects of catecholamines on blood pressure and heart rate. Note that the pulse pressure is greatly increased with epinephrine and isoproterenol. Norepinephrine causes reflex bradycardia.*

3. Dopamine (DA)
   a. Mechanism of action: stimulates D_1 specific dopamine receptors on renal vasculature, and at higher doses it also stimulates β_1- and α_1-adrenergic receptors
      (1) Low doses stimulate primarily renal dopamine receptors (0.5-2 μg/kg/min) causing vasodilation in the kidney.
      (2) Moderate doses also stimulate β_1-adrenergic receptors (2-10 μg/kg/min) increasing cardiac contractility.
      (3) High doses also stimulate α_1-adrenergic receptors (>10 μg/kg/min) causing vasoconstriction.
   b. Use: cardiogenic and noncardiogenic shock (dopamine increases blood flow through the kidneys)
   c. Adverse effects
      (1) Premature ventricular tachycardia, sinus tachycardia
      (2) Angina pectoris
B. α-Adrenergic receptor agonists (see Box 5-1)
   1. α_1-Adrenergic receptor agonists
      • Examples: methoxamine, phenylephrine
      a. Mechanism of action: directly stimulate α_1-receptors
      b. Uses (similar effects to those that occur after an injection of norepinephrine)
         (1) Blood pressure elevation
         (2) Nasal decongestant
         (3) Mydriasis induction
   2. α_2-Adrenergic receptor agonists

Potency of β_2-adrenoreceptor agonists: ISO > EPI >> NE > DA

- Examples: methyldopa, clonidine
- Used to treat hypertension (see Chapter 13)

C. β-Adrenergic receptor agonists (see Box 5-1)

  1. β_1-Adrenergic receptor agonists

    a. Example: dobutamine

    b. Use: selective inotropic agent in the management of advanced cardiovascular failure associated with low cardiac output

  2. β_2-Adrenergic receptor agonists

    a. Examples: terbutaline, albuterol, salmeterol

    b. Uses

      (1) Asthma and chronic obstructive pulmonary disease (COPD) (albuterol, salmeterol)

      (2) Hyperkalemia (terbutaline)

      (3) Delay of premature labor (terbutaline, ritodrine)

    c. Adverse effects

      (1) Fine skeletal muscle tremor (most common)

      (2) Minimal cardiac adverse effects (palpitations)

      (3) Nervousness

D. Dopamine D_1 agonist

  1. Fenoldopam

- An intravenous dopamine D_1 agonist used for the acute treatment of severe hypertension

E. Indirect stimulants (see Box 5-1)

  1. Tyramine

- Releases norepinephrine from storage granules, thus producing both α and β stimulation

    a. Leads to tachyphylaxis, because of depletion of norepinephrine stores after repeated use

    b. Results in hypertensive crisis in patients who are taking MAO inhibitors when tyramine is ingested (foods, wine)

  2. Amphetamine

- Indirect-acting amine that releases norepinephrine and epinephrine

    a. Uses

      (1) Central nervous system (CNS) stimulant: stimulates mood and alertness

      (2) Appetite suppression

      (3) Attention-deficit hyperactivity/attention deficit disorder in children (methylphenidate is preferable)

    b. Adverse effects (due to sympathomimetic effects)

      (1) Nervousness, insomnia, anorexia

      (2) Growth inhibition (children)

  3. Monoamine oxidase (MAO) inhibitors

    a. Examples: phenelzine, tranylcypromine, selegiline

    b. Use: occasional treatment of depression and Parkinson's disease (see Chapters 10 and 11)

  4. Catechol-O-methyltransferase inhibitors

    a. Examples: tolcapone, entacapone

Hypertensive crisis: MAO inhibitors and tyramine-rich foods ("cheese effect")

    b. Use: Parkinson's disease (see Chapter 11)

   5. Norepinephrine reuptake (uptake I) inhibitors

    a. Examples: cocaine, imipramine

    b. Potentiate effects of norepinephrine, epinephrine, and dopamine, but not isoproterenol (not taken up by uptake I) (see Fig. 3-2B)

 F. Direct and indirect stimulants (see Box 5-1)

   1. Example: ephedrine

   2. Mechanism of action

    a. Releases norepinephrine (like tyramine)

    b. Also has a direct effect on α-adrenergic receptors

   3. Uses: mild asthma, nasal decongestion

II. Adrenoreceptor Antagonists

 A. α-Adrenergic receptor antagonists

   • Mechanism of action: block α-mediated effects of sympathomimetic drugs or sympathetic nerve stimulation

   1. Nonselective α-adrenergic receptor antagonists (Box 5-2)

    a. Phentolamine

     (1) Pharmacokinetics: reversible, short-acting

     (2) Uses

      (a) Diagnosis and treatment of pheochromocytoma

      (b) Reversal of effects resulting from accidental subcutaneous injection of epinephrine

    b. Phenoxybenzamine

     (1) Pharmacokinetics: irreversible, long-acting

     (2) Use: preoperative management of pheochromocytoma

   2. Selective α_1-adrenergic receptor antagonists (see Box 5-2)

    • Examples: doxazosin, prazosin, terazosin, tamsulosin

    a. Mechanism of action: block α_1 receptors selectively on arterioles and venules, producing less reflex tachycardia than nonselective α-receptor antagonists

    b. Uses

     (1) Hypertension (doxazosin, prazosin, terazosin)

     (2) Benign prostatic hyperplasia (BPH) (doxazosin, tamsulosin)

    c. Adverse effects

     (1) Orthostatic hypotension

     (2) Impaired ejaculation

   3. Selective α_2-adrenergic receptor antagonist: yohimbine

    • No clinical use (ingredient in herbal preparations; marketed for treatment of impotence)

    • May inhibit the hypotensive effect of clonidine or methyldopa

 B. β-Adrenergic receptor antagonists (beta blockers)

   1. Pharmacologic properties

    a. Mechanism of action

     (1) Block β-receptor sympathomimetic effects

     (2) Exert cardiovascular effects: decreased cardiac output and renin secretion

Note: -sin ending

Tamsulosin, which relaxes the bladder neck and the prostate, is used to treat BPH.

Large "first-dose" effect

Note: -olol ending

> ## BOX 5-2
>
> ### ADRENORECEPTOR ANTAGONISTS
>
> **Nonselective α-Receptor Antagonists**
> Phenoxybenzamine
> Phentolamine
>
> **α_1-Receptor Antagonists**
> Doxazosin
> Prazosin
> Terazosin
> Tamsulosin (prostate specific)
>
> **α_2-Receptor Antagonists**
> Yohimbine
>
> **Nonselective β-Receptor Antagonists**
> Propranolol
> Timolol
>
> **β_1-Receptor Antagonists**
> Atenolol
> Esmolol
> Metoprolol
>
> **Nonselective α- and β-Receptor Antagonists**
> Carvedilol
> Labetalol
>
> **β-Receptor Antagonists with Intrinsic Sympathomimetic Activity (ISA)**
> Acebutolol (β_1-selective)
> Pindolol (nonselective)

      (a) Decreased vasodilation
      (b) Decreased salt and water retention
      (c) Decreased heart and vascular remodeling
   b. Uses
     (1) Cardiac problems: arrhythmias, "classical" angina (angina of effort), hypertension, moderate heart failure
     (2) Thyrotoxicosis
     (3) Performance anxiety
     (4) Essential tremor
     (5) Migraine (prevention; propranolol, timolol)

   c. Adverse effects
- (1) Bradycardia, heart block
- (2) Bronchiolar constriction
- (3) Increased triglycerides, decreased high-density lipoprotein (HDL) levels
- (4) Mask symptoms of hypoglycemia (in diabetics)
- (5) Sedation; "tired or exhausted feeling"
- (6) Depression

   d. Precautions
- (1) Abrupt withdrawal of β-adrenoreceptor antagonists can produce nervousness, increased heart rate, and increased blood pressure.
- (2) These drugs should be used with caution in patients with asthma, heart block, COPD, and diabetes.

2. Nonselective β-adrenergic receptor antagonists (see Box 5-2)

   a. Propranolol: β_1- and β_2-receptor antagonist
- (1) Mechanism of action
  - (a) Decreases heart rate and contractility
  - (b) Decreases cardiac output, thus reducing blood pressure
  - (c) Decreases renin release
- (2) Uses: arrhythmias, hypertension, angina, heart failure, tremor, migraine prophylaxis, and pheochromocytoma

   b. Timolol
- (1) Mechanism of action: lowers intraocular pressure, presumably by reducing production of aqueous humor
- (2) Uses: wide-angle glaucoma (topical preparation), migraine prophylaxis, hypertension

3. Selective β_1-adrenergic receptor antagonists (see Box 5-2)

   a. Metoprolol and atenolol: cardioselective β_1-adrenergic blockers
- (1) Uses
  - (a) Hypertension, angina, acute myocardial infarction (MI), heart failure, tachycardia
  - (b) MI (prevention)
- (2) These β_1-adrenergic blockers may be safer than propranolol for patients who experience bronchoconstriction because they produce less blockade of β_2-receptors.

   b. Esmolol
- (1) Pharmacokinetics
  - (a) Short half-life (9 min)
  - (b) Given by intravenous infusion
- (2) Uses: hypertensive crisis, acute supraventricular tachycardia

4. Nonselective β- and α_1-adrenergic receptor antagonists (see Box 5-2)

   a. Labetalol
- (1) Mechanism of action: α and β blockade (β blockade is predominant)
  - Reduces blood pressure without a substantial decrease in resting heart rate, cardiac output, or stroke volume

---

Use beta blockers with caution in the following conditions: heart block, asthma, COPD, diabetes

Contraindication to use of nonselective β-adrenergic receptor antagonists: asthma

Use selective β_1-adrenergic receptor antagonists with caution in the following conditions: asthma, COPD

           (2) Uses

               (a) Hypertension and hypertensive emergencies

               (b) Pheochromocytoma

       b. Carvedilol

           (1) Mechanism of action: α and β blockade

           (2) Use: heart failure

5. β-Adrenoreceptor antagonists with intrinsic sympathomimetic activity (ISA) (see Box 5-2)

       a. Examples: acebutolol, pindolol

          • These agents have partial agonist activity.

       b. Uses

           (1) Preferred in patients with moderate heart block

           (2) May have an advantage in the treatment of patients with asthma, diabetes, and hyperlipidemias

Muscle Relaxants

I. Spasmolytics
- Certain chronic diseases (e.g., cerebral palsy, multiple sclerosis) are associated with abnormally high reflex activity in neuronal pathways controlling skeletal muscles, resulting in painful spasms or spasticity.
  A. Goals of spasmolytic therapy
  1. Reduction of excessive muscle tone without reduction in strength
  2. Reduction in spasm, which reduces pain and improves mobility
  B. γ-Aminobutyric acid (GABA)–mimetics (Box 6-1)
  1. Baclofen (GABA$_B$ agonist)
     a. Mechanism of action: interferes with release of excitatory transmitters in the brain and spinal cord
     b. Uses: spasticity in patients with central nervous system (CNS) disorders, such as multiple sclerosis, spinal cord injuries, and stroke
     c. Adverse effects: sedation, hypotension, muscle weakness
  2. Diazepam
     a. Benzodiazepine, which acts on the GABA$_A$ receptor
     b. Facilitates GABA-mediated presynaptic inhibition in the brain and spinal cord (see Chapter 7)
  C. Other relaxants (see Box 6-1)
  1. Botulinum toxin
     a. Type A toxin blocks neuromuscular conduction by binding to receptor sites on motor nerve terminals, entering nerve terminals, and inhibiting the release of acetylcholine.
     b. Uses:
        (1) Spasticity associated with cerebral palsy (pediatrics) or stroke (adults)
        (2) Sialorrhea (excessive drooling)
        (3) Facial wrinkles
        (4) Cervical dystonia

> Diazepam acts on GABA$_A$; baclofen acts on GABA$_B$ receptors.

BOX 6-1

SPASMOLYTICS

GABA-Mimetics
Baclofen
Diazepam

Other Relaxants
Botulinum toxin
Cyclobenzaprine
Dantrolene
Tizanidine

---

        (5) Strabismus
        (6) Hyperhydrosis
   2. Cyclobenzaprine
     a. Relieves local skeletal muscle spasms, associated with acute, painful musculoskeletal conditions, through central action, probably at the brainstem level
     b. Ineffective in spasticity caused by central nervous system (CNS) disorders, such as multiple schlerosis, spinal cord injuries, and stroke
     c. Sedating
   3. Dantrolene
     a. Mechanism of action: decreases the release of intracellular calcium from the sarcoplasmic reticulum, "uncoupling" the excitation-contraction process
     b. Uses
       (1) Spasticity from CNS disorders such as cerebral palsy or spinal cord injury
       (2) Malignant hyperthermia after halothane/succinylcholine exposure
       (3) Neuroleptic malignant syndrome caused by antipsychotics
     c. Adverse effects: hepatotoxicity, significant muscle weakness
   4. Tizanidine
     a. Mechanism of action
       (1) Stimulates presynaptic α_2 adrenoreceptors
       (2) Inhibits spinal interneuron firing
     b. Use: spasticity associated with conditions such as cerebral palsy and spinal cord injury
     c. Adverse effects: sedation, hypotension, muscle weakness (less than with baclofen)

II. Nicotinic Receptor Antagonists
  • Nicotinic receptor antagonists include ganglionic blockers (see Chapter 4) and neuromuscular blockers (Box 6-2).
  • Neuromuscular blockers may be classified as either depolarizing or nondepolarizing (Table 6-1).

Tizanidine is similar to clonidine with fewer peripheral effects.

BOX 6-2

NEUROMUSCULAR BLOCKERS

Nondepolarizing Drugs
Atracurium
Mivacurium
Pancuronium
Rocuronium
Tubocurarine
Vecuronium

Depolarizing Drugs
Succinylcholine

TABLE 6-1:
Comparison of Nondepolarizing and Depolarizing Neuromuscular Blockers

Effect	Competitive	Depolarizing
Action at receptor	Antagonist	Agonist
Effect on motor end plate depolarization	None	Partial persistent depolarization
Initial effect on striated muscle	None	Fasciculation
Muscles affected first	Small muscles	Skeletal muscle
Muscles affected last	Respiratory	Respiratory
Effect of AChE inhibitors	Reversal	No effect or increased duration
Effect of ACh agonists	Reversal	No effect
Effect on previously administered D-tubocurarine	Additive	Antagonism
Effect on previously administered succinylcholine	No effect of antagonism	Tachyphylaxis or no effect
Effect of halothane	Increase potency	Decrease potency
Effect of antibiotics	Increase potency	Decrease potency
Effect of calcium channel blockers	Increase potency	Increase potency

ACh, acetylcholine; AChE, acetylcholinesterase.

A. Nondepolarizing neuromuscular blockers
  • Also known as curariform drugs, of which tubocurarine is the prototype
  1. Mechanism of action
    • These drugs compete with acetylcholine (ACh) at nicotinic receptors at the neuromuscular junction, producing muscle relaxation and paralysis.
  2. Uses
    a. Induction of muscle relaxation during surgery
    b. Facilitation of intubation
    c. Adjunct to electroconvulsive therapy for prevention of injury

3. Drug interactions
   a. Muscle relaxation is reversed by acetylcholinesterase (AChE) inhibitors such as neostigmine.
   b. Use with inhaled anesthetics (isoflurane) or aminoglycoside antibiotics (gentamicin) may potentiate or prolong blockade.
4. Adverse effects
   a. Respiratory paralysis: can be reversed with neostigmine
   b. Blockade of autonomic ganglia: produce hypotension
   c. Histamine release (most profound with tubocurarine): flushing, hypotension, urticaria, pruritus, erythema, bronchospasms

B. Depolarizing neuromuscular blockers (succinylcholine)
1. Mechanism of action
   a. These drugs bind to nicotinic receptors in skeletal muscle, causing persistent depolarization of the neuromuscular junction.
   b. This action initially produces an agonist-like stimulation of skeletal muscles (fasciculations) followed by sustained muscle paralysis.
   c. The response changes over time.
      (1) Phase I: continuous depolarization at end plate
         • Cholinesterase inhibitors prolong paralysis at this phase.
      (2) Phase II: resistance to depolarization
         • Cholinesterase inhibitors may reverse paralysis at this phase.
2. Use: production of muscle relaxation during surgery or electroconvulsive therapy
3. Adverse effects: hyperkalemia, muscle pain, malignant hyperthermia
4. Precaution
   • Blockade may be prolonged if the patient has a genetic variant of plasma cholinesterase that metabolizes the drug very slowly.

Nondepolarizing neuromuscular blockers are reversed by AChE inhibitors.

Tubocurarine is noted for histamine release.

Depolarizing neuromuscular blockers may be potentiated by AChE inhibitors.

Succinylcholine may cause malignant hyperthermia.

7 **CHAPTER**

Sedative-Hypnotic and Anxiolytic Drugs

I. Basic Properties
- Sedative-hypnotics and anxiolytics are used to reduce anxiety or to induce sleep (Box 7-1).
- These agents, especially the barbiturates, produce central nervous system (CNS) depression at the level of the brain, spinal cord, and brainstem.
- These agents cause tolerance and physical dependence (withdrawal) if used for long periods.
- Barbiturates and other older sedative-hypnotics cause complete CNS depression, whereas benzodiazepines do not (Fig. 7-1).
A. Pharmacokinetics
  1. Metabolism primarily occurs by the microsomal system in the liver.
  2. Duration of action is variable.
     - The half-life ($t_{1/2}$) of these drugs ranges from minutes to days.
     - Many benzodiazepine metabolites are active, thus increasing the duration of action of the parent drug.
B. Mechanism of action
  - Sedative-hypnotics facilitate chloride flux through the γ-aminobutyric acid (GABA) receptor chloride channel complex, which hyperpolarizes the neuron (Fig. 7-2).
C. Uses: sedation, hypnosis, or anesthesia, depending on dose
  1. Sleep induction (hypnosis)
  2. Anxiety relief (anxiolytic)
  3. Sedation

Benzodiazepines increase the frequency of chloride channel opening.

Barbiturates increase the length of time that the chloride channel remains open.

BOX 7-1

SEDATIVE-HYPNOTICS AND ANXIOLYTICS

Benzodiazepines
Alprazolam
Chlordiazepoxide
Clorazepate
Diazepam
Estazolam
Flurazepam
Lorazepam
Midazolam
Oxazepam
Prazepam
Quazepam
Temazepam
Triazolam
Barbiturates
Pentobarbital
Phenobarbital
Secobarbital
Thiopental

Other Sedative-Hypnotics
Chloral hydrate
Diphenhydramine
Esopiclone
Meprobamate
Paraldehyde
Propranolol
Zaleplon
Zolpidem

Nonsedating Anxiolytic
Buspirone

Benzodiazepine Antagonist
Flumazenil

---

4. Preanesthesia (see Chapter 8)
5. Anticonvulsant properties (see Chapter 9)
   - Phenobarbital, clonazepam, and diazepam are used clinically.
6. Central-acting muscle relaxants (see Chapter 6)

D. Adverse effects
   - Chronic use may lead to toxicity.
   1. General effects
      a. Drowsiness
      b. Impaired performance and judgment
      c. "Hangover"
      d. Risk of drug abuse and addiction
      e. Withdrawal syndrome (most frequently seen with short-acting sedative-hypnotics that are used for long periods)
   2. Overdose results in severe CNS depression, which may manifest as coma, hypotension, and respiratory cessation, especially when agents are given in combination.
   3. Treatment of overdose
      a. Observe continuously
      b. Prevent absorption of ingested drug (charcoal, lavage)

Sedative-hypnotic drugs should *not* be used in combination with alcohol.

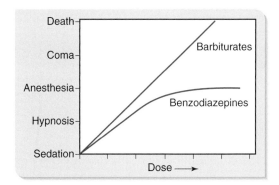

7-1: Dose-response curves for barbiturates and for benzodiazepines. Barbiturates produce complete central nervous system depression leading to anesthesia, coma, and death, even when given orally. Benzodiazepines may cause anesthesia and respiratory depression with intravenous, but not oral, administration.

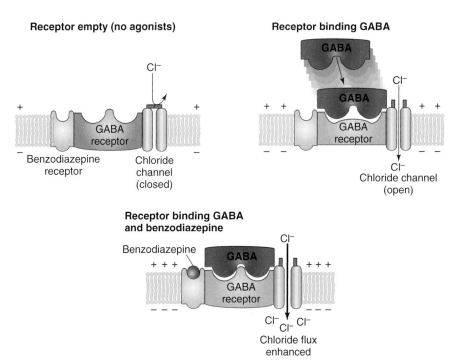

7-2: Benzodiazepine-GABA-chloride ionophore complex. Benzodiazepines increase the frequency of channel opening. Barbiturates increase the length of time that the channels remain open.

       c. Support respiration

       d. Prevent or treat hypotension or shock

       e. Maintain renal function

       f. Increase rate of drug excretion

         (1) Alkaline diuresis

           • Useful for some barbiturates, such as phenobarbital

         (2) Peritoneal dialysis

         (3) Hemodialysis

  E. Precautions

    1. Porphyria or a family history of porphyria may be a problem.

      • Barbiturates may increase porphyrin synthesis.

    2. Hepatic or renal insufficiency requires a reduced dose.

    3. Additive effect of drugs in combination may have serious consequences.

II. Benzodiazepines (see Box 7-1)

  • These anxiolytic drugs are associated with a reduced risk of respiratory depression and coma, which gives them a major advantage over the barbiturates (see Fig. 7-1).

  • The incidence of dependence is probably lower with benzodiazepines than with barbiturates.

  A. Pharmacokinetics

    1. Enterohepatic circulation with many agents

    2. Variable duration of action

      • Most agents accumulate with multiple dosing as a result of long plasma half-lives.

      a. Short-acting agents: triazolam. midazolam

      b. Intermediate-acting agents: alprazolam, estazolam, lorazepam, oxazepam, temazepam

      c. Long-acting agents: chlordiazepoxide, clorazepate, diazepam, flurazepam, prazepam, quazepam

  B. Mechanism of action (see Fig. 7-1)

    1. Benzodiazepines bind to specific receptors on the $GABA_A$ receptor–ionophore complex.

      • Alcohols, as well as barbiturates, interact at these receptors.

    2. Benzodiazepines potentiate the activity of GABA on chloride ion influx by increasing the frequency of the openings of the chloride channels.

  C. Uses

    • All of the general uses listed in Section IC, plus the following indications:

    1. Alcohol withdrawal

    2. Status epilepticus (intravenous diazepam or lorazepam)

  D. Adverse effects

    1. Ataxia, retrograde amnesia

    2. Moderate addictive potential

      a. Physical dependence when used in high doses for several months

      b. Withdrawal symptoms: anxiety, agitation, depression, "rebound" insomnia

Triazolam is noted for causing traveler's amnesia.

E. Benzodiazepine antagonist
- Flumazenil, a benzodiazepine antagonist, stops action or reverses toxicity.

F. BZ_1 benzodiazepine agonists
- These drugs act on the BZ_1 subset of benzodiazepine receptors.
- Unlike the benzodiazepines, these drugs produce muscle relaxation and anticonvulsant effects only at doses much higher than the hypnotic dose.
- Effects are reversed by flumazenil

1. Zolpidem is a short-acting, nonbenzodiazepine sedative-hypnotic for the short-term treatment of insomnia.
2. Zaleplon is also a short-acting, nonbenzodiazepine sedative-hypnotic for the short-term treatment of insomnia; zaleplon has a faster onset of action and a shorter terminal elimination half-life than zolpidem.
3. Eszopiclone is a longer acting nonbenzodiazepine sedative-hypnotic; it was the first agent indicated for chronic treatment of insomnia; it has properties similar to the BZ_1 agonists but is nonselective (agonist at BZ_1 and BZ_2).

III. Barbiturates
A. Pharmacokinetics
1. Elimination occurs by metabolism in the liver and excretion of the parent compound or its metabolites in the urine.
   a. Phenobarbital is a weak organic acid, whose excretion is enhanced by alkalinization of urine.
   b. The effects of thiopental are terminated by redistribution.
2. Duration of action
   a. Ultrashort-acting: thiopental
   b. Intermediate-acting: pentobarbital, secobarbital
   c. Long-acting: phenobarbital
B. Mechanism of action
1. Barbiturates facilitate the actions of GABA.
   - Unlike benzodiazepines, these agents increase the length of time that the GABA-gated chloride channel remains open.
2. The multiplicity of barbiturate binding sites is the basis of the ability to induce full surgical anesthesia (see Fig. 7-1).
C. Effects
1. Low doses: depression of sensory function, sedation without analgesia, drowsiness
2. High doses: depression of motor function, depression of medullary centers of brain (circulatory and respiratory depression), marked sedation, sleep, anesthesia
3. Induce cytochrome P-450 metabolizing enzymes; many drug-drug interactions

IV. Other Sedative-Hypnotics
- Some of these agents are structurally related to the barbiturates and have similar properties.
A. Diphenhydramine: antihistamine found in over-the-counter (OTC) "sleep aids"

It is possible to reduce rebound effects by slowly reducing the dose of longer-acting benzodiazepines.

Adverse effects of barbiturates: ataxia, retrograde amnesia, impaired performance, dependence, withdrawal symptoms

B. Buspirone
  1. Mechanism of action: partial agonist at 5-hydroxytryptamine (5-HT$_{1A}$) serotonin receptors in the brain
  2. Uses
    a. Antianxiety (several days of use required for the drug to become effective)
    b. No hypnotic, anticonvulsant, or muscle relaxant properties
  3. Adverse effects
    a. Some sedation but less than most benzodiazepines
    b. No evidence of tolerance, rebound anxiety on withdrawal of drug, cross-tolerance to benzodiazepines, drug abuse, or additive effects
C. Chloral hydrate
  • Structurally related to alcohol, with trichloroethanol as active metabolite
  • Paraldehyde is a short-acting congener.
  1. Use
    a. Very rapid-acting hypnotic, which was often used in children
    b. Low incidence of abuse
  2. Adverse effect: bad taste and smell
D. Meprobamate: an oral anxiolytic; use replaced by benzodiazepines
E. Propranolol: used to treat performance anxiety

V. Alcohols
  A. Ethanol
    1. Pharmacokinetics
      a. Rapid, complete absorption
        • Conversion to acetate by two enzymes: alcohol dehydrogenase and acetaldehyde dehydrogenase
      b. Zero-order kinetics

Ethanol eliminated by zero-order kinetics

    2. Mechanism of action: potentiates actions at the GABA receptor
      a. CNS depressant with synergistic effects with many other CNS depressants
      b. Cross-tolerant with other sedative-hypnotic drugs
    3. Adverse effects
      a. Liver: hepatic failure and cirrhosis
      b. Gastrointestinal: nutritional deficiencies (malabsorption) and bleeding
      c. Nervous system

Avoid alcohol during pregnancy

        (1) Peripheral neuropathy ("stocking glove" pattern)
        (2) Wernicke-Korsakoff syndrome: thiamine deficiency; ataxia, confusion, ophthalmoplegia
      d. Endocrine: gynecomastia, testicular atrophy
      e. Fetal alcohol syndrome: teratogenic effects when used during pregnancy
        • Mental retardation, growth deficiency, microcephaly, wide-spaced eyes
      f. Alcoholism
        (1) Withdrawal syndrome
          (a) Insomnia

        (b) Tremor, anxiety, seizures, hallucinations (delirium tremens)

        (c) Diarrhea, nausea

    (2) Management: benzodiazepines (only in abstinent patients), antihypertensives

  4. Drug interactions: drugs that inhibit acetaldehyde dehydrogenase

    a. Disulfiram, which is used in the treatment of alcoholism

    b. Metronidazole (has disulfiram-like effect)

    c. Oral hypoglycemic agents (chlorpropamide)

B. Other alcohols

  1. Methanol

    a. Conversion to formic acid can lead to blindness and severe anion gap metabolic acidosis.

    b. Intoxicated patients are treated with ethanol or fomepizole.

      • Ethanol competes with methanol for the dehydrogenase enzymes.

  2. Ethylene glycol

    • Antifreeze

    • Adverse effects: severe anion gap metabolic acidosis, hypocalcemia, renal damage

    • Intoxicated patients are treated with ethanol or fomepizole.

> Disulfiram use leads to nausea, hypotension, headache, and flushing when patients drink alcohol; thus, it is used to help patients stop drinking.

Anesthetics

I. General Anesthetics
   A. Goals of balanced anesthesia
      1. Analgesia: elimination of perception and reaction to pain
      2. Amnesia: loss of memory, which is not essential but desirable during most surgical procedures
      3. Loss of consciousness: essential for many surgical procedures (e.g., cardiac, orthopedic)
      4. Muscle relaxation
         a. Occurs in varying degrees
         b. Usually has to be further supplied by neuromuscular relaxants
      5. Suppression of autonomic and sensory reflexes: requires use of additional medications to suppress the enhanced autonomic and sensory reactions that occur during surgical procedures
   B. Inhalation anesthetics (Box 8-1 and Table 8-1)
      1. General considerations
         a. Depth of anesthesia directly relates to the partial pressure of the anesthetic in the brain.
         b. Anesthetic potency is expressed as the minimum alveolar concentration (MAC).
            - MAC is the concentration in inspired air at which 50% of patients have no response to a skin incision.
            - The higher the lipid solubility, the greater the potency.
         c. Speed of induction is influenced by several factors.
            (1) Higher inspired concentration = more rapid induction
            (2) Lower solubility in blood = more rapid induction
            (3) Higher ventilation rate = more rapid induction
            (4) Lower pulmonary blood flow = more rapid induction
         d. The lower the blood-gas partition coefficient, the more rapid is the onset and recovery from anesthesia.

Nitrous oxide (0.47) and desflurane (0.42) = rapid onset and recovery

The use of halothane may lead to hepatotoxicity and malignant hyperthermia.

BOX 8-1

GENERAL ANESTHETICS

Inhalation Anesthetics

Desflurane
Enflurane
Halothane
Isoflurane
Nitrous oxide
Sevoflurane

Parenteral Anesthetics

Alfentanil
Etomidate
Fentanyl
Ketamine
Lorazepam
Midazolam
Propofol
Sufentanil
Thiopental

TABLE 8-1:
Properties of Inhalation Anesthetics

Agent	MAC (% vol/vol)	Blood:Gas Partition Coefficient	Rate of Induction and Emergence	Amount Metabolized	Skeletal Muscle Relaxation	Effect on Cardiovascular System	Effect on Liver and Kidney
Nonhalo-genated (Gaseous)							
Nitrous oxide	>100	0.47	Rapid	None	None	↓ Heart rate No arrhythmias	None
Halo-genated (Volatile)							
Desflurane	6.0	0.42	Rapid	<2%	Medium	↑ Heart rate and blood pressure (transient)	None
Enflurane	1.7	1.9	Medium	5% (fluoride)	Medium	↓ Heart rate No arrhythmias; does not sensitize heart to catecholamines	Hepatotoxic
Halothane	0.75	2.3	Slow	20%	Low	Sensitizes heart to catecholamines	Hepatotoxic
Isoflurane	1.3	1.4	Medium	<2% (fluoride)	Medium	↓ Heart rate No arrhythmias; does not sensitize heart to catecholamines	None
Sevoflurane	1.9	0.65	Rapid	<2%	Medium	None	Nephrotoxic (rare)

MAC, minimum alveolar concentration.

2. Nitrous oxide (N_2O)
   - Gaseous anesthetic
   a. Characteristics
      (1) Cannot produce surgical anesthesia by itself
         - To produce unconsciousness, N_2O must be used with other anesthetics.
      (2) Significantly reduces the MAC for halogenated anesthetics when used as an adjunct to anesthesia
   b. Pharmacokinetics: extremely fast absorption and elimination, resulting in rapid induction and recovery from anesthesia
   c. Uses: has good analgesic properties
      - Analgesia in obstetrics and procedures that do not require unconsciousness, such as dental procedures
   d. Contraindications: head injury, preexisting increased intracranial pressure, tumor
      - N_2O can raise intracranial pressure.

N_2O has excellent analgesic properties.

3. Volatile halogenated hydrocarbons (see Box 8-1 and Table 8-1)
   - These agents are of variable potency (MAC) and blood solubility; they may sensitize the heart to the arrhythmogenic effects of catecholamines.

C. Parenteral anesthetics (see Box 8-1)
   - These anesthetics are useful for procedures of short duration, induction for inhalation anesthesia (wide use), and supplementation of weak inhalation agents such as N_2O.
   1. Ultrashort-acting barbiturates (thiopental, methohexital): poor analgesia
      a. Pharmacokinetics
         (1) Extremely rapid onset and action due to high lipid solubility
         (2) Brief duration of action due to redistribution from brain to other tissues
      b. Primary uses
         (1) Induction of anesthesia
         (2) Procedures of short duration
   2. Propofol

Patients ambulate more rapidly after propofol than after thiopental.

   a. Preferred for 1-day surgical procedures because patients can ambulate sooner and recover from the effects of anesthesia more rapidly
   b. May cause hypotension
   3. Dissociative anesthetics
      - Example: ketamine
      - During induction, patients feel dissociated from the environment (i.e., in trancelike states).

Like phencyclidine, ketamine is also used for recreational purposes.

   a. Mechanism of action: blocks the *N*-methyl-D-aspartate (NMDA) receptor
   b. Uses
      (1) Allows patients, particularly children, to be awake and respond to commands yet endure painful stimuli
      (2) Example: changing painful burn dressings

c. Adverse effects
  (1) Increased heart rate, cardiac output, and arterial blood pressure
  (2) Postoperative psychotic phenomena (hallucinations)
    • Rarely used in adults because of this effect
4. High-potency opioid anesthetics
  • Examples: fentanyl, alfentanil, sufentanil
  • Used in cardiothoracic surgery to avoid the cardiac effects of many inhalation agents (see Chapter 19)
5. Midazolam or lorazepam: used for procedures that require consciousness
6. Etomidate
  • A short-acting, intravenous general anesthetic
  • Minimal cardiovascular effects
  • No histamine release
  • Useful for patients with compromised cardiopulmonary function
D. Preanesthetic medications (Table 8-2)
  1. Increase analgesia, muscle relaxation
  2. Decrease vagal reflexes, postoperative nausea and vomiting

II. Local Anesthetics (Box 8-2)
  • Local anesthetics reversibly abolish sensory perception, especially pain, in restricted areas of the body.
  A. Pharmacokinetics
    • During administration, the vasoconstrictors norepinephrine and epinephrine are often added to localize the anesthetic to the injection site, prolong the anesthetic effect, and slow absorption, thus minimizing systemic toxicity.

Norepinephrine and epinephrine often localize anesthetics to the injection site, prolong the anesthetic effect, and slow absorption.

TABLE 8-2: Preanesthetic Drugs

Drug Class	Specific Agent	Effect(s)
Opioids	Morphine Meperidine Fentanyl	Sedation to decrease tension and anxiety Analgesia
Barbiturates	Pentobarbital Secobarbital Thiopental	Decreased apprehension Sedation Rapid induction
Benzodiazepines	Diazepam Lorazepam	Decreased apprehension Sedation Rapid induction
Phenothiazines	Prochlorperazine Promethazine	Antiemetic Antihistaminic effect Antiemetic Decreased motor activity
Anticholinergic drugs	Atropine Scopolamine Glycopyrrolate	Inhibition of secretions, vomiting, and laryngospasms
Antiemetics	Droperidol Hydroxyzine Benzquinamide	Prevention of postoperative vomiting

> **BOX 8-2**
>
> ## LOCAL ANESTHETICS
>
> **Esters**
> Benzocaine
> Cocaine
> Procaine
> Tetracaine
>
> **Amides**
> Bupivacaine
> Lidocaine
> Mepivacaine
> Prilocaine

Ester local anesthetics are more allergenic than amides.

1. Route of administration: topical application or local injection
2. Metabolism
   a. Esters are metabolized by plasma pseudocholinesterases.
      - Therefore, many have a shorter duration of action (minutes).
      - All ester-type local anesthetics, except cocaine, are metabolized to *p*-aminobenzoic acid derivatives; these metabolites are allergenic.
   b. Amides are metabolized by cytochrome P-450s or amidases in the liver.
      - Therefore, many have a longer duration of action (hours).

The names of all amides contain two "i"s (e.g., lidocaine).

B. Mechanism of action
   - Local anesthetics cause reversible blockade of nerve conduction.
   1. Decrease the nerve membrane permeability to sodium by binding to open or inactivated sodium channels
   2. Diffuse across the nerve membrane in the nonionized form and then block the channel in the ionized form from the inside of the nerve membrane
   3. Reduce the rate of membrane depolarization
   4. Raise the threshold of electrical excitability
   5. Affect pain fibers first because they are small and unmyelinated
C. Adverse effects
   1. Central nervous system (CNS): seizures, lightheadedness, sedation
   2. Cardiovascular system: myocardial depression, hypotension, cardiac arrest
      - Some agents, such as lidocaine, have antiarrhythmic effects.

With local anesthetics, loss of sensation occurs in the following sequence: pain, temperature, touch, movement.

D. Specific local anesthetics
   1. Esters
      - Examples: procaine, tetracaine, benzocaine, cocaine
      a. Uses: topical, infiltration, nerve block, spinal anesthesia
         - Cocaine is also a vasoconstrictor because it blocks norepinephrine uptake.

   b. Adverse effects: CNS stimulation, higher incidence of seizures
2. Amides
   • Examples: lidocaine, bupivacaine, mepivacaine, prilocaine
   • These agents are preferred for all types of infiltration, nerve blocks, and spinal anesthesia because of their slower metabolism and longer half-life ($t_{1/2}$).

Use of cocaine on the mucosa of the nose and paranasal sinuses causes shrinkage and minimizes bleeding.

9 Anticonvulsant Drugs

TARGET TOPICS

- Treatment of generalized tonic-clonic seizures
- Treatment of partial seizures
- Treatment of absence seizures
- Treatment of status epilepticus

Many patients receive two anticonvulsant drugs, because decreased doses of each individual drug can be given, minimizing adverse effects.

I. Anticonvulsant Therapy
- Seizures are episodes of abnormal electrical activity in the brain that may lead to involuntary movements and sensations, which are accompanied by characteristic changes on electroencephalography (EEG).
  A. Classification of seizures (Table 9-1)
  B. Drugs used in the treatment of seizures (Table 9-2)

II. Drugs Used in the Treatment of Partial Seizures and Generalized Tonic-Clonic Seizures (Box 9-1; see also Table 9-2)
  A. Phenytoin and fosphenytoin
    1. Pharmacokinetics: exhibit high plasma protein-binding, which can affect drug levels and activity
      a. Both zero-order (high blood levels) and first-order kinetics (low blood levels)
      b. Metabolism in the liver
    2. Mechanism of action: block voltage-sensitive sodium channels in the neuronal membrane
    3. Uses (see Table 9-2)
    4. Adverse effects
      a. Sedation
      b. Cerebellar ataxia, nystagmus, diplopia
      c. Induction of liver enzymes, which leads to vitamin D deficiency
        - Affects the epiphyseal plate and results in osteomalacia
      d. Gingival hyperplasia
      e. Hirsutism
      f. Folate deficiency, leading to megaloblastic anemia
      g. Teratogenic ability (fetal hydantoin syndrome)
  B. Phenobarbital (see Chapter 7)

Anticonvulsants that block sodium channels: phenytoin, carbamazepine, lamotrigine, felbamate, valproic acid, topiramate, zonisamide

TABLE 9-1:
**International
Classification of
Partial and
Generalized
Seizures**

Classification	Origin and Features
Partial (Focal) Seizures	Arising in one cerebral hemisphere
Simple partial seizure	No alteration of consciousness
Complex partial seizure	Altered consciousness, automatisms, and behavioral changes
Secondarily generalized seizure	Focal seizure becoming generalized and accompanied by loss of consciousness
Generalized Seizures	Arising in both cerebral hemispheres and accompanied by loss of consciousness
Tonic-clonic (grand mal) seizure	Increased muscle tone followed by spasms of muscle contraction and relaxation
Tonic seizure	Increased muscle tone
Clonic seizure	Spasms of muscle contraction and relaxation
Myoclonic seizure	Rhythmic, jerking spasms
Atonic seizure	Sudden loss of all muscle tone
Absence (petit mal) seizure	Brief loss of consciousness, with minor muscle twitches and eye blinking

TABLE 9-2:
**Choice of
Antiepileptic Drugs
for Seizure
Disorders**

Drug	Partial Seizures	GENERALIZED SEIZURES Tonic-Clonic	Absence	Myoclonic	Atonic	Status Epilepticus
Carbamazepine	1	1	W	—	—	—
Phenytoin	1	1	W	—	—	2
Phenobarbital	2	2	—	—	—	3
Primidone	2	2	—	—	—	—
Gabapentin	A	—	—	—	A	—
Lamotrigine	A	A	A	—	A	—
Topiramate	A	—	—	—	—	—
Ethosuximide	—	—	1*	—	—	—
Valproate	2	1	2*	1	1	—
Clonazepam	—	W	3	2	1	—
Diazepam	—	—	—	—	—	1
Lorazepam	—	—	—	—	—	1

*For absence seizures in children, ethosuximide is the drug of first choice and valproate is the drug of second choice. For absence seizures in adults, valproate is probably the drug of first choice.
1, Drugs of first choice; 2, drug of second choice; 3, drug of third choice; A, drug for adjunct use with other drugs; W, drug that may worsen seizure.

1. Mechanism of action: enhances the inhibitory action of the γ-aminobutyric acid (GABA) receptor by increasing the time that the chloride channel remains open
2. Adverse effects
   a. Induction of liver enzymes
   b. Sedation
   c. Increase in irritability and hyperactivity in children (paradoxical effect)
   d. Agitation and confusion in the elderly

Anticonvulsants that potentiate GABA mechanisms: barbiturates, primidone, benzodiazepines, vigabatrin, gabapentin, tiagabine, valproic acid

BOX 9-1

ANTICONVULSANTS

Drugs Used to Treat Partial and Generalized Tonic-Clonic Seizures

Carbamazepine
Phenobarbital
Phenytoin/fosphenytoin
Primidone
Valproate

Adjunct Drugs Used to Treat Partial Seizures

Clorazepate
Felbamate
Gabapentin
Lamotrigine
Levetiracetam
Tiagabine
Topiramate
Vigabatrin
Zonisamide

Drugs Used to Treat Absence, Myoclonic, or Atonic Seizures

Clonazepam
Ethosuximide
Lamotrigine
Valproate

Drugs Used to Treat Status Epilepticus

Diazepam
Lorazepam
Phenobarbital
Phenytoin

C. Carbamazepine
- Structurally related to imipramine and other tricyclic antidepressants
1. Mechanism of action: blocks voltage-sensitive sodium channels, inhibiting sustained, repetitive firing
2. Uses
   a. Drug of choice for partial seizures
      - Often used first if the patient also has generalized tonic-clonic seizures
   b. Trigeminal neuralgia and neuropathic pain
   c. Bipolar affective disorder (alternative to lithium)

Many anticonvulsants are used to treat neuropathic pain.

3. Adverse effects
   a. Diplopia and ataxia (most common)
   b. Induction of liver microsomal enzymes
      • Carbamazepine accelerates its own metabolism and the metabolism of other drugs.
   c. Aplastic anemia and agranulocytosis
      • Requires monitoring with complete blood count (CBC)

D. Valproate (valproic acid)
   1. Mechanism of action
      a. Increases concentrations of GABA in the brain
      b. Suppresses repetitive neuronal firing through inhibition of voltage-sensitive sodium channels
      c. Blocks T-type calcium current
   2. Uses
      a. Absence seizures
         • Valproate is the preferred agent if the patient also has generalized tonic-clonic seizures.
      b. Complex partial seizures and myoclonic seizures
   3. Adverse effects
      a. The most serious adverse reaction is liver failure.
      b. The incidence of central nervous system (CNS) and gastrointestinal (GI) effects is high.
      c. Valproate inhibits its own metabolism as well as the metabolism of other drugs.

E. Primidone
   1. The action of primidone is due both to the parent compound and to its metabolites, phenobarbital and phenylethylmalonamide (PEMA).
   2. This drug is frequently added to the regimen when satisfactory seizure control is not achieved with phenytoin or carbamazepine.

F. Vigabatrin
   1. Mechanism of action: potentiates GABA by irreversibly inhibiting GABA-transaminase
   2. Use: most effective in the management of partial seizures

G. Gabapentin
   1. Mechanism of action: may alter GABA metabolism or its nonsynaptic release
   2. Uses
      a. Adjunctive management of partial seizures with or without secondary generalized tonic-clonic seizures
      b. Neuropathic pain

H. Lamotrigine
   1. Mechanism of action: acts at voltage-sensitive sodium channels to stabilize neuronal membranes
   2. Use: adjunctive management for refractory partial seizures with or without secondary generalized tonic-clonic seizures

I. Tiagabine
   1. Mechanism of action: inhibits neuronal and glial uptake of GABA

Carbamazepine interacts with phenobarbital, phenytoin, primidone, and valproic acid, reducing their therapeutic effect.

Valproate inhibits the metabolism of phenytoin, phenobarbital, and carbamazepine, increasing the toxicity of these drugs.

      2. Use: adjunctive treatment of partial seizures
- J. Felbamate
  1. Mechanism of action: blocks the increase in the frequency of NMDA receptor-mediated channel openings
  2. Use: approved for the management of partial seizures in adults and Lennox-Gastaut syndrome in children and adults; due to the occurrence of aplastic anemia and acute hepatic failure, use is limited to management of seizures refractory to other agents
- K. Levetiracetam
  1. Mechanism of action: alters inhibitory and excitatory neurotransmission
  2. Uses: adjunctive therapy in the management of partial seizures with or without secondary generalization
- L. Zonisamide
  1. Mechanism of action: acts at sodium and calcium channels
     - Stops the spread of seizures
     - Suppresses the seizure focus
  2. Use: approved for adjunctive management of partial seizures in adults 16 years and older with epilepsy
- M. Topiramate
  1. Mechanism of action
     - Reduces voltage-gated sodium currents
     - Activates a hyperpolarizing potassium current
     - Enhances postsynaptic $GABA_A$ receptor currents
  2. Uses
     - Refractory partial seizures and refractory generalized tonic-clonic seizures
     - Migraine prophylaxis
  3. Adverse effects
     - Drowsiness, dizziness, ataxia

III. Absence (Petit Mal) Seizures and Drugs Used in Their Treatment (see Box 9-1 and Table 9-2)
- Absence seizures are primarily a childhood disorder.
- A. Features
  1. Brief lapses of consciousness
  2. Characteristic spike-and-wave pattern on EEG (3/sec)
- B. Therapeutic drugs
  1. Ethosuximide: effective in a high percentage of cases
     a. Mechanism of action: reduces current in T-type calcium channel found on primary afferent neurons
     b. Adverse effects: GI upset, drowsiness
  2. Valproate (used for both tonic-clonic and absence seizures)
  3. Clonazepam
     - Tolerance develops within a few months, making the drug inappropriate for long-term therapy (see Chapter 7).

IV. Status Epilepticus and Drugs Used in Its Treatment (see Box 9-1 and Table 9-2)
- Status epilepticus is a life-threatening emergency involving repeated seizures.

Anticonvulsants that reduce T-type calcium currents: ethosuximide, valproic acid, lamotrigine, zonisamide

A. Treatment of choice
   1. Diazepam (intravenous)
   2. Lorazepam (intravenous)
B. Other therapeutic drugs
   1. Phenytoin (intravenous) given by loading dose over 20 to 30 minutes
   2. General anesthetics (intravenous thiopental)

Most anticonvulsants are relatively contraindicated during pregnancy.

10

Psychotherapeutic Drugs

TARGET TOPICS

- Antipsychotic drugs
- Antidepressants
- Mood stabilizers
- Attention-deficit hyperactivity disorder drugs

I. Antipsychotic Drugs (Box 10-1)
- Neuroleptics are useful in the treatment of schizophrenia.
- These drugs reduce positive symptoms (e.g., paranoia, hallucinations, delusions) more than negative symptoms (e.g., emotional blunting, poor socialization, cognitive deficit) in patients with schizophrenia.
- The newer "atypical" antipsychotics are more effective, especially against negative symptoms, and less toxic than the older but less expensive traditional antipsychotics.
- Late in 2003, the Food and Drug Administration requested all manufacturers to include product label warnings about the potential for an increased risk of hyperglycemia and diabetes with the use of "atypical" antipsychotics.

A. Pharmacokinetics
- Most antipsychotics are metabolized to active and inactive metabolites.
1. Immediate onset after intramuscular or intravenous injection
2. Slow and variable absorption after oral administration

B. Mechanism of action (Table 10-1)
1. Blockade of dopamine D_2 receptor correlates best with antipsychotic activity.
2. Blockade of dopamine D_3 and D_4 receptors may also contribute to therapeutic effects.
3. Blockade of serotonin receptors may contribute to benefits against negative symptoms.
4. Blockade of other receptors also occurs (see Table 10-1).

C. Uses
1. Schizophrenic reactions, mania, psychosis
- The actions of the neuroleptic agents in the mesolimbic and mesocortical pathways are most important for their antipsychotic effects.
2. Nausea (antiemetic): prochlorperazine, benzquinamide

"Atypical drugs" may cause hyperglycemia.

Antipsychotic effects of neuroleptic agents are related to blockade of dopamine receptors.

BOX 10-1

ANTIPSYCHOTIC DRUGS

Phenothiazines

Chlorpromazine
Fluphenazine
Thioridazine
Trifluoperazine

Thioxanthenes

Thiothixene

Butyrophenones

Droperidol
Haloperidol

Azepines ("Atypical")

Clozapine
Olanzapine
Quetiapine

Other Drugs ("Atypical")

Aripiprazole
Risperidone
Ziprasidone

**TABLE 10-1:
Mechanisms and
Effects of
Neuroleptic Agents**

Mechanism	Action
Blockade of dopamine D_1 and D_2 receptors	Antipsychotic, extrapyramidal, and endocrine effects
Blockade of α-adrenergic receptors	Hypotension
Blockade of histamine H_1 receptors	Sedation
Blockade of muscarinic receptors	Anticholinergic effects (e.g., dry mouth, urinary retention)
Blockade of serotonin receptors	Antipsychotic effects

    3. Intractable hiccoughs: chlorpromazine
    4. Antipruritic: promethazine
  D. Adverse effects
    • Neuroleptics cause unpleasant effects.
    1. Behavioral effects, such as "pseudodepression"
    2. Neurologic effects
      a. Extrapyramidal effects and iatrogenic parkinsonism
      b. Dystonic reactions and akathisia

- The best treatment is diphenhydramine or benztropine (antimuscarinic action).
  (1) Acute dystonic reactions (1–5 days): involvement of neck and head muscles
  (2) Akathisia (5–60 days): restlessness and agitation seen as continuous movement
  (3) Parkinsonian syndrome (5–30 days): extrapyramidal effects; tremors, rigidity, shuffling gait, postural abnormalities
  (4) Neuroleptic malignant syndrome (weeks): catatonia, stupor, fever, unstable blood pressure (autonomic instability); may be fatal
    - Treatment involves stopping the neuroleptic drug and using dantrolene or bromocriptine.
  (5) Perioral tremor (months or years): "rabbit syndrome" (involuntary movement of the lips)
    - Treatment involves the use of anticholinergic agents.
  (6) Tardive dyskinesia (months or years): stereotypical involuntary movements
    (a) Frequently irreversible
    (b) Results from effects on dopamine D_2 receptors
    (c) Treatment involves clozapine or diazepam
  c. Decrease in seizure threshold
    - Use caution when giving neuroleptics to individuals with epilepsy.
    - Avoid giving these drugs to patients who are undergoing withdrawal from central nervous system (CNS) depressants.
E. Specific drugs (Table 10-2)
  1. Aliphatic phenothiazines: chlorpromazine
    - Least potent phenothiazine
  2. Piperidine phenothiazines: thioridazine
    a. Generally low incidence of acute extrapyramidal effects
    b. Requires regular eye examinations because of retinitis pigmentosa
  3. Piperazine phenothiazines: fluphenazine
    - Generally high incidence of acute extrapyramidal effects
  4. Butyrophenones: haloperidol, droperidol
    a. Additional uses for haloperidol: treatment of Tourette's syndrome and acute psychosis
    b. Extremely high incidence of acute extrapyramidal effects
  5. Azepines ("atypical" agents)
    a. Clozapine
      (1) Mechanism of action: blocks serotonin and dopamine, primarily the dopamine D_1 and D_4 receptors, with a greater effect on the serotonin receptors
        (a) Has less effect on dopamine D_2 receptors than traditional antipsychotics
        (b) Has a greater effect on negative symptoms of schizophrenia than the older traditional antipsychotics
      (2) Adverse effects
        (a) Low incidence of extrapyramidal effects

Tardive dyskinesia is associated with prolonged use of traditional neuroleptics.

Use of neuroleptics leads to hyperprolactinemia, which results in amenorrhea-galactorrhea syndrome and infertility in women and loss of libido, impotence, and infertility in men.

Clozapine is associated with agranulocytosis.

TABLE 10-2:
Effects of Antipsychotic Drugs

Drug	Relative Potency*	Extrapyramidal Effects	Sedative Action	Hypotensive Actions	Anticholinergic Effects
Phenothiazines					
Chlorpromazine (aliphatic)	Low	Medium	High	High	Medium
Fluphenazine (piperazine)	High	High	Low	Very low	Low
Thioridazine (piperidine)	Low	Low	High	High	Very high
Trifluoperazine (piperazine)	High	High	Low	Low	Medium
Thioxanthenes					
Thiothixene	High	Medium-high	Low	Medium	Very low
Butyrophenones					
Haloperidol	High	Very high	Low	Very low	Very low
"Atypicals"					
Aripiprazole	High	Very low	Very low	Low	Very low
Clozapine	Medium	Very low	High	Medium	High
Olanzapine	High	Very low	Low	Low	Medium
Risperidone	High	Low	Low	Low	Very low
Ziprasidone	Medium	Very low	Low	Very low	Very low

*Potency: low = 50–2000 mg/d; medium = 20–250 mg/d; high = 1–100 mg/d.

    (b) High incidence of agranulocytosis (1–2%), which necessitates regular complete blood counts (CBCs)
  b. Olanzapine: newer clozapine-like agent with no notable incidence of agranulocytosis
  c. Quetiapine: a newer "atypical" antipsychotic agent structurally similar to clozapine, a dibenzodiazepine structure
6. Benzisoxazoles ("atypical"; risperidone): monoaminergic antagonist with a high affinity for both serotonin 5-HT$_2$ (5-hydroxytryptamine) and dopamine D$_2$ receptors
  a. Widely used for long-term therapy
  b. Associated with fewer extrapyramidal symptoms
7. Dihydroindolone ("atypical"; ziprasidone): an atypical antipsychotic, pharmacologically distinct from traditional agents such as the phenothiazines or haloperidol
  a. This drug offers advantages over others by causing less weight gain and greater effects against depressive symptoms in patients with schizophrenia or schizoaffective disorders.
  b. A serious side effect of ziprasidone is QTc interval prolongation.

Ziprasidone is associated with prolonged QTc intervals.

8. Dihydrocarbostyril ("atypical"; aripiprazole): a new class of atypical antipsychotic drugs known as dopamine system stabilizers (i.e., partial agonist); approved for several treatments:
   a. Schizophrenia
   b. Mania
   c. Bipolar disorders

Avipiprazole is a partial dopamine agonist.

II. Antidepressants and Mood Stabilizers (Box 10-2)
   • Depression can be classified as reactive (i.e., response to grief or illness); endogenous (i.e., genetically determined biochemical condition); or bipolar affective (i.e., manic-depressive disorder).

BOX 10-2

ANTIDEPRESSANTS

Tricyclic Antidepressants
Amitriptyline
Clomipramine
Desipramine
Imipramine
Nortriptyline

SSRIs
Citalopram
Escitalopram
Fluoxetine
Fluvoxamine
Paroxetine
Sertraline

MAO Inhibitors
Phenelzine
Tranylcypromine

Other Antidepressants
Amoxapine
Bupropion
Duloxetine
Maprotiline
Mirtazapine
Nefazodone
Trazodone
Venlafaxine

- Antidepressant drugs are used to treat endogenous and bipolar affective forms of depression.
- Late in 2004, the Food and Drug Administration directed manufacturers of all antidepressants to include a Black Box warning, regarding the increased risk of suicidal thinking in children and adolescents treated with these agents.

Antidepressants may increase suicide risk.

A. Tricyclic antidepressants (TCAs) (see Box 10-2)
  1. Pharmacokinetics
    - Clinical improvement requires use for 2 to 3 weeks, thus reducing compliance.
  2. Mechanism of action
    - Most TCAs block the reuptake of serotonin and norepinephrine, causing accumulation of these monoamines in the synaptic cleft.
    - Accumulation of monoamines in the synaptic cleft produces multiple adaptations in receptor and transport systems.
  3. Uses
    a. Depression
    b. Chronic pain (amitriptyline)
    c. Insomnia (trazodone)
    d. Enuresis (imipramine)
    e. Obsessive-compulsive disorder (clomipramine)
  4. Adverse effects
    a. Sedation, which is due to blockade of histamine H_1 receptors
    b. Full range of anticholinergic effects, such as dry mouth, because agents are potent anticholinergics
    c. Full range of phenothiazine-like effects, especially orthostatic hypotension, resulting from α_1-receptor blockade
    d. Rare acute extrapyramidal signs, because these agents are not potent dopamine blockers
    e. Overdose: electrical cardiac conduction problems (correct with sodium bicarbonate) and convulsions (treat with diazepam)

TCAs produce conduction abnormalities: ECG is needed prior to therapy to rule out atrioventricular (AV) block or other abnormalities.

B. Selective serotonin reuptake inhibitors (SSRIs) (Table 10-3; see also Box 10-2)
  1. Mechanism of action
    a. Highly specific serotonin reuptake blockade at the neuronal membrane
    b. Dramatically decreased binding to histamine, acetylcholine, and norepinephrine receptors, which leads to less sedative, anticholinergic, and cardiovascular effects when compared with TCAs
  2. Uses
    a. Depression
    b. Obsessive-compulsive disorder
    c. Panic disorders
    d. Premenstrual dysphoric disorders (PMDD)
    e. Bulimia nervosa
  3. Adverse effects: nausea, nervousness, insomnia, headache, sexual dysfunction

SSRIs do not cause weight gain as do TCAs.

TABLE 10-3
Pharmacologic Profile of Antidepressants

Drug	Antimuscarinic Effects	Sedative Effects	AMINE PUMP BLOCKADE		
			Serotonin	Norepinephrine	Dopamine
Tricyclic Antidepressants					
Amitriptyline	+++	+++	+++	++	0
Clomipramine	++	+++	+++	+	0
Desipramine	+	+	0	+++	0
Imipramine	++	++	+++	++	0
Nortriptyline	++	++	+++	++	0
Selective Serotonin Reuptake Inhibitors (SSRI)					
Citalopram	0	0	+++	0	0
Escitalopram	0	0	+++	0	0
Fluoxetine	+	+	+++	0, +	0, +
Fluvoxamine	0	0	+++	0	0
Paroxetine	0	0	+++	0	0
Sertraline	+	0	+++	0	0
Other Antidepressants					
Amoxapine	++	++	+	++	+
Atomoxetine (SNRI)	0	0	0	+++	0
Bupropion	0	0	+, 0	+, 0	+
Duloxetine (dual inhibitor)	0	0	+++	++	0, +
Maprotiline (SNRI)	++	++	0	+++	0
Mirtazapine*	0	+++	0	0	0
Nefazodone	+++	++	+, 0	0	0
Trazodone	0	+++	++	0	0
Venlafaxine (dual inhibitor)	0	0	+++	++	0, +

*Blocks α_2-adrenoreceptors and 5-HT$_2$ serotonin receptors.
0, None; +, slight; ++, moderate; +++, extensive.
SNRI, selective norepinephrine reuptake inhibitor.

C. Other antidepressants (see Box 10-2)
  1. Mechanism of action: greater selectivity than TCAs for either norepinephrine or serotonin
  2. Adverse effects: less cardiotoxicity and anticholinergic activity than TCAs
  3. Selected antidepressants
    a. Amoxapine
      • Use: depression in psychotic patients
      • Also has antipsychotic activity
    b. Bupropion
      • Structurally similar to amphetamine; inhibits dopamine reuptake
      (1) Uses: depression, smoking cessation, attention-deficit hyperactivity disorders
      (2) Adverse effects: seizures, anorexia, aggravation of psychosis
    c. Maprotiline: selective norepinephrine reuptake inhibitor (SNRI)

Bupropion is used for smoking cessation.

d. Mirtazapine
  (1) Mechanism of action: blockade of 5-HT$_2$ serotonin and α_2-adrenergic presynaptic receptors on adrenergic and serotonergic neurons
  (2) Use: treat depression in patients who do not tolerate SSRIs; useful in treating depression with coexisting anxiety disorder
  (3) Adverse effects (reputed): weight gain, sedation

Mirtazapine noted for causing weight gain.

e. Trazodone
  (1) Mechanism of action
    (a) Inhibits serotonin reuptake into the presynaptic neurons
    (b) Has no anticholinergic activity
  (2) Uses
    (a) Depression
    (b) Insomnia (low doses), which causes sedation

Trazodone may cause priapism (prolonged, painful erection of the penis), which can lead to impotence.

f. Nefazodone: less sedating than trazodone
g. Venlafaxine and duloxetine:
  (1) Mechanism of action: similar mechanism of action to the TCAs ("dual inhibitors") but a better side-effect profile, because they do not block α_1-adrenergic, histamine H$_1$, or muscarinic receptors
  (2) Uses: depression; duloxetine is useful for painful physical symptoms (e.g., back pain, shoulder pain) associated with depression

D. Monoamine oxidase (MAO) inhibitors
  1. Pharmacokinetics
    a. Long-lasting effects due to irreversible inhibition of the enzyme
    b. Therapeutic effect develops after 2 to 4 weeks of treatment.
  2. Mechanism of action: inhibition of MAO, thus increasing concentration of norepinephrine and serotonin in the brain
  3. Uses
    a. "Atypical" depression, characterized by attendant anxiety and phobic features
    b. Depression in patients refractory to TCAs
  4. Adverse effects
    a. Postural hypotension
    b. CNS effects, such as restlessness and insomnia
    c. Hepatotoxicity
    d. Possible hypertensive crisis

Ingestion of tyramine-containing foods (e.g., certain cheeses, wines, preserved meats) while taking MAO inhibitors may precipitate a hypertensive crisis.

  5. Drug interactions: meperidine, TCAs, SSRIs
    • Due to "serotonin syndrome" (marked increase in synaptic serotonin)
    • Possible severe reactions, characterized by excitation, sweating, rigidity, hypertension, severe respiratory depression, coma, and vascular collapse, possibly resulting in death

Patients who are taking MAO inhibitors should not take meperidine, TCAs, or SSRIs.

E. Mood stabilizers
  1. Lithium: used in the treatment of bipolar disorders because it decreases the severity of the manic phase and lengthens the time between manic phases

a. Pharmacokinetics
  (1) Narrow range of therapeutic serum levels
  (2) Delayed onset of action (6–10 days)
b. Mechanism of action: unknown, but known to modify ion fluxes, neurotransmitter synthesis, turnover rates, and second messenger systems, particularly the inositol phosphate (IP_3) pathway
c. Uses
  (1) Bipolar disorders
  (2) Nonpsychiatric uses
    (a) Neutropenia, thyrotoxic crisis, migraine and cluster headaches
    (b) Considered a last choice for syndrome of inappropriate antidiuretic hormone (SIADH) secretion
d. Adverse effects: evident at therapeutic serum concentrations
  (1) Symptoms and signs
    (a) Fine hand tremor, dry mouth, weight gain
    (b) Mild nausea and vomiting, diarrhea
    (c) Polydipsia, polyuria, impotence, decreased libido, nephrotic syndrome
  (2) Electrocardiogram
    • Flattened or inverted T waves produced by the inhibition of potassium cellular reuptake, leading to intracellular hypokalemia
2. Alternatives to lithium use in bipolar disorders
  • Carbamazepine, clonazepam, valproic acid, olanzapine

III. Attention-deficit Hyperactivity Disorder Drugs (Box 10-3)
  A. Amphetamine: a CNS-stimulant used for the treatment of attention-deficit disorders, narcolepsy, and exogenous obesity
  B. Methylphenidate: a CNS stimulant similar to the amphetamines used in the treatment of narcolepsy and as adjunctive treatment in children with attention-deficit hyperactivity disorders (ADHD)
  C. Bupropion: an antidepressant that selectively inhibits dopamine reuptake and is used off-label for the treatment of ADHD and neuropathic pain
  D. Atomoxetine: a selective norepinephrine reuptake inhibitor (SNRI) that is the first nonstimulant drug approved for ADHD

> Frequent adverse effect of lithium is tremor; treated with propranolol.
>
> Use of lithium causes nephrogenic diabetes insipidus and hypothyroidism.

BOX 10-3

ATTENTION-DEFICIT HYPERACTIVITY DISORDER DRUGS

Amphetamine
Bupropion
Methylphenidate
Atomoxetine

Drugs Used in the Treatment of Parkinson's Disease

TARGET TOPICS

- Pathogenesis of Parkinson's disease
- L-Dopa–carbidopa
- Dopamine agonists
- Amantadine, entacapone, tolcapone, and selegiline
- Anticholinergics

I. General Considerations
  A. Parkinsonism is associated with lesions in the basal ganglia, especially the substantia nigra and the globus pallidus.
  B. There is a reduction in the number of cells in the substantia nigra and a decrease in the dopamine content.
  C. The lesions result in increased and improper modulation of motor activity by the extrapyramidal system, leading to a resting tremor, rigidity, and bradykinesia.
  D. Therapy aims to increase the dopamine content through "replacement therapy" or reducing acetylcholine (ACh) activity, because proper function depends on the balance between the inhibitory neurotransmitter dopamine and the excitatory neurotransmitter ACh.

II. Drugs Used to Treat Parkinson's Disease (Box 11-1 and Fig. 11-1)
  A. Levodopa (L-dopa)
    1. Pharmacokinetics
      a. L-Dopa has the ability to cross the blood-brain barrier.
        • Dopamine cannot be used to treat Parkinson's disease, because this agent does not readily enter the brain after systemic administration.
      b. L-Dopa is rapidly metabolized, predominantly by decarboxylation to dopamine, and excreted into the urine.
      c. L-Dopa is always given in combination with carbidopa, a peripheral dopa decarboxylase inhibitor.
    2. Mechanism of action

BOX 11-1

DRUGS USED TO TREAT PARKINSON'S DISEASE

Dopaminergic Drugs

Amantadine
Carbidopa
Entacapone
L-Dopa
Selegiline
Tolcapone

Dopamine Receptor Agonists

Bromocriptine
Pergolide
Pramipexole
Ropinirole

Anticholinergics

Benztropine
Trihexyphenidyl

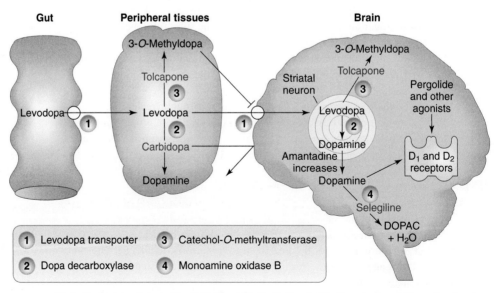

11-1: *Mechanisms of dopaminergic drugs used in the treatment of Parkinson's disease. Dopa decarboxylase is inhibited by carbidopa in the peripheral tissues but not in the brain, because carbidopa does not cross the blood-brain barrier. Catechol-O-methyltransferase is inhibited by tolcapone in both the peripheral tissues and the brain. Monoamine oxidase B is inhibited by selegiline. DOPAC, dihydroxyphenylacetic acid; D_1 and D_2, dopamine receptor subtypes.*

- L-Dopa enters the brain and is converted to dopamine, which reacts with dopamine receptors in the central nervous system (CNS).

3. Adverse effects
   a. Severe gastrointestinal problems: nausea, vomiting, anorexia, peptic ulcer
   b. Postural hypotension
   c. Dyskinesia: development of abnormal involuntary movements
      - Choreoathetosis, the most common presentation, involves the face and limbs.
      - Effects resemble tardive dyskinesia induced by phenothiazines.
   d. Arrhythmias
   e. Hypersexuality

B. Other drugs used to treat Parkinson's disease
   1. Bromocriptine
      a. Mechanism of action: direct dopamine agonist that enters the CNS
      b. Uses
         - Lack of response to L-dopa or an unstable reaction to L-dopa
         - "On-off" symptoms, in which improved motility alternates with marked akinesia
   2. Pergolide
      a. Mechanism of action: potent dopamine agonist that acts at the dopamine D_1 and D_2 receptors
      b. Use: "on-off" symptoms
   3. Pramipexole
      a. Mechanism of action: dopamine agonist that binds to both the dopamine D_2 and D_3 receptors in the striatum and substantia nigra
      b. Uses: can delay the need for L-dopa and reduce the "off" symptoms
   4. Ropinirole
      a. Mechanism of action: agonist that acts at both the dopamine D_2 and D_3 receptors
      b. Uses: can delay the need for L-dopa and reduce the "off" symptoms
   5. Amantadine
      a. Mechanism of action: antiviral agent that releases dopamine and may block dopamine reuptake
      b. Uses: early treatment of tremor, bradykinesia, rigidity associated with Parkinson's disease.
   6. Selegiline
      a. Mechanism of action: indirect dopamine agonist that selectively inhibits monoamine oxidase B, an enzyme that inactivates dopamine
      b. Use: most commonly given in conjunction with L-dopa, but may be effective by itself as a "neuroprotectant" due to its antioxidant and antiapoptotic effects
   7. Tolcapone
      a. Mechanism of action: catechol-*O*-methyltransferase (COMT) inhibitor that decreases the inactivation of L-dopa, and thus increases dopamine levels in the brain
      b. Use: adjunct to L-dopa–carbidopa

Use of carbidopa with L-dopa allows more L-dopa to enter the brain.

Pramipexole is now used as monotherapy for mild Parkinson's disease.

Ropinirole is now used as monotherapy for mild Parkinson's disease.

Dopamine is metabolized by MAO-B; norepinephrine and serotonin are metabolized by MAO-A.

Selegiline, a selective MAO-B inhibitor, produces less interaction with tyramine than the nonselective MAO inhibitors.

Tolcapone causes hepatotoxicity.

8. Entacapone
   a. A reversible inhibitor of peripheral catechol-O-methyltransferase (COMT)
   b. Used as an adjunct to L-dopa–carbidopa therapy in the treatment of Parkinson's disease
   c. Preferred over tolcapone because of lower hepatotoxicity
9. Anticholinergic drugs
   • Examples: benztropine, trihexyphenidyl
   a. Only those agents with anticholinergic activity that enter the CNS are prescribed.
   b. These drugs also decrease the tremor and symptoms produced by a dopamine D_2 receptor antagonist such as haloperidol.

12 CHAPTER

Antiarrhythmic Drugs

TARGET TOPICS

- Electrophysiology of the heart
- Class I antiarrhythmic drugs (sodium channel blockers)
- Class II antiarrhythmic drugs (β-blockers)
- Class III antiarrhythmic drugs (potassium channel blockers)
- Class IV antiarrhythmic drugs (calcium channel blockers)
- Miscellaneous antiarrhythmic drugs (adenosine, digoxin, magnesium, potassium)

I. General Considerations
   A. Cardiac contraction (Fig. 12-1): five-step process
      1. Spontaneous development of the action potential in the sinoatrial (SA) node
      2. Spread of the impulse through the atrium
      3. Temporary delay of the impulse at the atrioventricular (AV) node
      4. Rapid spread of the impulse along the two branches of the bundle of His and the Purkinje fibers
      5. Spread of the impulse along the cardiac muscle fibers of the ventricles
   B. Electrophysiology of the heart
      1. Action potential (Fig. 12-2)
         a. The action potential is the resting membrane potential of the myocardium (approximately -90 mV).
         b. It results from an unequal distribution of ions (high Na^+ outside, high K^+ inside).
      2. Five phases of the action potential
         a. Rapid depolarization (phase 0)
            (1) Rapid inward movement of Na^+ due to the opening of voltage-gated sodium channels
            (2) Variation in resting membrane potential: -90 mV $\rightarrow$ $+15$ mV
         b. Initial rapid repolarization (phase 1)
            • Inactivation of sodium channels and influx of Cl^-

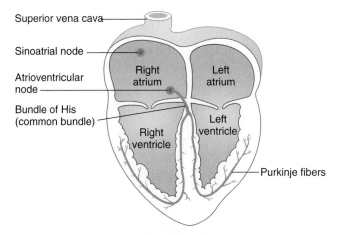

12-1: *Schematic drawing of the heart.*

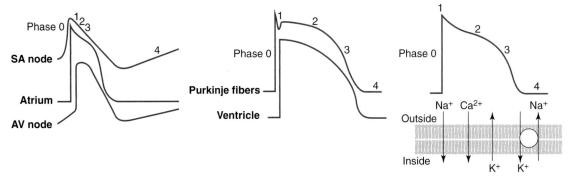

12-2: *Schematic representation of cardiac electrical activity in the sinoatrial (SA) node and Purkinje fibers as well as ion permeability changes and transport processes that occur during an action potential. AV, atrioventricular.*

    c. Plateau phase (phase 2)
       • Slow but prolonged opening of voltage-gated calcium channels
    d. Repolarization (phase 3)
       (1) Closure of calcium channels and K^+ efflux through potassium channels
       (2) Return of inactivated sodium channels to resting phase
    e. Diastole (phase 4)
       • Restoration of ionic concentrations by Na^+/K^+-activated ATPase (adenosine triphosphatase) and restoration of resting potential
3. Important electrocardiographic (ECG) parameters (Fig. 12-3)
    a. P wave = atrial depolarization
    b. PR interval = delay of conduction through the AV node
    c. QRS complex = ventricular depolarization
    d. T wave = ventricular repolarization
    e. QT interval = duration of action potential in the ventricles

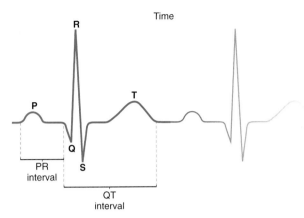

12-3: *Schematic electrocardiogram (ECG) showing depolarization and repolarization of the heart. The P wave is produced by atrial depolarization, the QRS complex by ventricular polarization, and the T wave by ventricular repolarization. The PR interval measures the conduction time from atrium to ventricle, and the QT interval measures the duration of the ventricular action potential. The QRS complex measures the intraventricular conduction time.*

TABLE 12-1: Effects of Antiarrhythmic Drugs on the Electrophysiology of the Heart

Drug (Class)	SA Node Rate	AV Node Refractory Period	PR Interval	QRS Duration	QT Interval
Quinidine (IA)	↑↓	↑↓	↑↓	↑↑↑	↑↑
Lidocaine (IB)	N	N	N	N	N
Propranolol (II)	↓↓	↑↑	↑↑	N	N
Sotalol (III)	↓↓	↑↑	↑↑	N	↑↑↑
Verapamil (IV)	↓↓	↑↑	↑↑	N	N

AV, atrioventricular; N, no major effect; SA, sinoatrial.

II. Arrhythmias and Their Treatment
- Arrhythmias are irregularities in heart rhythm that result from disturbances in pulse formation, impulse conduction, or both.
  A. Antiarrhythmic drugs produce effects by altering one or more of the following factors:
    1. Automaticity
    2. Conduction velocity
    3. Refractory period
    4. Membrane responsiveness
  B. These agents have varying effects on the electrophysiology of the heart (Table 12-1).

III. Antiarrhythmic Drugs (Box 12-1)
  A. Class I drugs: sodium channel blockers
    - All class I agents, which are generally local anesthetics, bind to open and inactivated sodium channels, thus inhibiting phase 0 depolarization of the action potential (Fig. 12-4).

BOX 12-1

ANTIARRHYTHMIC DRUGS

Sodium Channel Blockers

Class IA
Disopyramide
Procainamide
Quinidine

Class IB
Lidocaine
Mexiletine
Tocainide

Class IC
Flecainide
Propafenone

Other Antiarrhythmic Drugs

Class II
Esmolol
Metoprolol
Propranolol

Class III
Amiodarone
Dofetilide
Ibutilide
Sotalol

Class IV
Diltiazem
Verapamil

Miscellaneous Antiarrhythmic Agents

Adenosine
Digoxin
Magnesium
Potassium

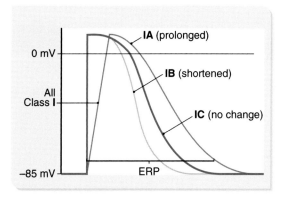 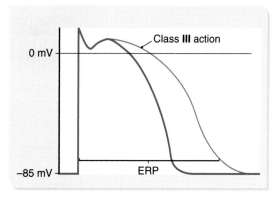

12-4: *Effects of class I and class III antiarrhythmics on the action potential and the electrocardiogram (ECG). ERP, effective refractory period.*

- Lidocaine is more effective in the treatment of ventricular arrhythmias, whereas quinidine and procainamide are more effective in the treatment of atrial arrhythmias.
1. Class IA drugs: also block potassium channel; thus prolong action potential
   - Examples: quinidine, procainamide
   a. Quinidine
      (1) Mechanism of action
          (a) Inhibition of sodium channels, extending the effective refractory period (ERP) of the myocardial cell membrane, thereby decreasing myocardial conduction velocity, excitability, and contractility
          (b) Blockade of α-adrenergic receptors, leading to a reflex increase in the SA node rate and producing vasodilation
          (c) Blockade of I_K channel, prolonging duration of action potential
          (d) Blockade of muscarinic receptors, thereby enhancing conduction through AV node
      (2) Uses
          (a) Conversion to or maintenance of sinus rhythm in patients with atrial fibrillation, flutter, or ventricular tachycardia
          (b) Treatment of paroxysmal supraventricular tachycardia (PSVT)
          (c) Prevention of PSVT in patients with reentrant tachycardias, including Wolff-Parkinson-White syndrome
      (3) Adverse effects
          (a) Torsades de pointes
          (b) ECG changes: prolonged QRS complex, giant U wave, ST-segment depression, flattened T wave
          (c) Diarrhea
          (d) Cinchonism: giddiness, lightheadedness, ringing in the ears, impaired hearing, blurred vision

Quinidine and procainamide are effective against both atrial and ventricular arrhythmias.

Class I drugs and ERP: class IA, prolong ERP; class IB, reduce ERP; class IC, no change

Quinidine may cause cinchonism.

About one third of patients who receive long-term procainamide therapy develop reversible lupus-related symptoms.

b. Procainamide
- This local anesthetic is equivalent to quinidine as an antiarrhythmic agent and has similar cardiac and toxic effects.
- Additional adverse effect: induces systemic lupus erythematosus
- The 2000 guidelines added intravenous procainamide to the cardiopulmonary resuscitation algorithm for refractory ventricular fibrillation/pulseless ventricular tachycardia.

2. Class IB drugs
- Examples: lidocaine, tocainide, mexiletine
- Class IB drugs decrease the duration of the action potential.

Lidocaine has a high "first pass" effect.

a. Lidocaine (see Chapter 8)
(1) Pharmacokinetics
(a) Short-acting because of rapid hepatic metabolism
(b) Loading dose should be followed by continuous intravenous infusion.
(2) Mechanism of action
(a) Acts primarily on the Purkinje fibers, depressing automaticity and shortening the refractory period
(b) Has a higher affinity for ischemic tissue, suppressing spontaneous depolarizations in the ventricles by inhibiting reentry mechanisms
(3) Use: suppression of ventricular tachycardia; the 2000 guidelines now consider lidocaine a second choice behind other alternative agents for the treatment of ventricular arrhythmias associated with cardiopulmonary resuscitation.
(4) Adverse effects: seizures (in elderly patients)
b. Tocainide and mexiletine: orally effective congeners of lidocaine
(1) Pharmacokinetics
(a) Resistant to first-pass hepatic metabolism
(b) Half-life ($t_{1/2}$): 8 to 20 hours
(2) Use (oral administration): ventricular arrhythmias
(3) Adverse effects: dizziness, vertigo, nausea, vomiting, arrhythmias

B. Class II drugs: β-adrenergic receptor antagonists (see Chapter 5)
- Examples: propranolol, metoprolol, esmolol
- Class II drugs slow phase 4 depolarization in the SA node.
1. Mechanism of action: blockade of β_1-receptors
a. Reduce heart rate
b. Reduce myocardial contractility
c. Prolong AV conduction
d. Prolong the AV refractory period
2. Propranolol
a. Uses
(1) Treatment and prophylaxis of PSVT and atrial fibrillation (orally effective)
(2) Possible prevention of recurrent infarction in patients recovering from myocardial infarction (MI)

   b. Adverse effects: sedation, sleep disturbance, sexual dysfunction, cardiac
      disturbance, asthma
3. Esmolol
   a. Pharmacokinetics
      (1) Very short-acting ($t_{1/2}$ = 9 min)
      (2) Administered by intravenous infusion
   b. Uses
      (1) Short-term control of supraventricular tachyarrhythmias, including
          sinus tachycardia and PSVT
      (2) Emergency control of ventricular rate in patients with atrial
          fibrillation or atrial flutter
   c. Adverse effects: AV block, cardiac arrest

C. Class III: potassium channel blockers
   • Examples: sotalol, amiodarone, ibutilide, dofetilide
   • Class III drugs increase the duration of the action potential (see Fig. 12-4).
   1. Mechanism of action
      a. Prolong repolarization
      b. Increase the ERP
   2. Amiodarone
      a. Pharmacokinetics
         (1) Long $t_{1/2}$ (13–103 days)
         (2) Time required to achieve steady-state therapeutic levels: 15 to
             30 days
      b. Use: approved for atrial and ventricular arrhythmias; the 2000
         guidelines recommend that intravenous amiodarone be used prior to
         lidocaine in patients receiving life support for ventricular
         fibrillation/pulseless ventricular tachycardia.
         • Amiodarone is very effective against both supraventricular and
           ventricular arrhythmias (atrial fibrillation or flutter, supraventricular
           tachycardia), but its toxicity is worthy of consideration.
      c. Adverse effects
         (1) Cardiovascular effects: torsades de pointes, ECG changes
             (prolonged QT interval and QRS complex)
         (2) Other effects
             • Pulmonary reactions such as pneumonitis, fibrosis (most severe)
             • Photodermatitis, paresthesias, tremor, ataxia, thyroid dysfunction,
               constipation
   3. Sotalol
      • This drug is an oral, nonselective β-adrenergic receptor antagonist that
        also blocks potassium channels.
      a. Uses: life-threatening sustained ventricular tachycardia, atrial fibrillation
      b. Adverse effects: prolonged QT interval, torsades de pointes
   4. Ibutilide
      a. Mechanism of action: blocks delayed rectifier potassium current and
         promotes the influx of sodium through slow inward sodium channels;
         it converts atrial fibrillation or flutter to normal sinus rhythm without
         altering blood pressure, heart rate, QRS duration, or PR interval.

Esmolol for emergency
treatment; propranolol for
prophylactic treatment of
supraventricular
arrhythmias

Class IA and class III are
most likely to cause
torsades de pointes.

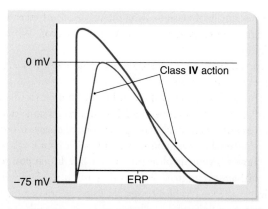

12-5: *Effects of class II and class IV antiarrhythmics on the action potential. ERP, effective refractory period.*

  b. Use: it is an intravenous Class III antiarrhythmic agent recommended for rapid conversion of atrial fibrillation or atrial flutter to normal sinus rhythm.
 5. Dofetilide: a class III antiarrhythmic used for the conversion and maintenance of normal sinus rhythm in atrial fibrillation/flutter in highly symptomatic patients
D. Class IV: calcium channel blockers (Fig. 12-5)
 • Examples: verapamil, diltiazem
 • Class IV drugs slow phase 4 depolarization in the SA node and decrease the heart rate.
 1. Mechanism of action: blockade of calcium uptake via a voltage-sensitive channel (L-type), thereby reducing inward flow of calcium into myocardial cells
 2. Effects on the myocardium
  a. Reduce the rate of SA node discharge
  b. Slow conduction through the AV node
  c. Prolong the AV node refractory period (prolong the PR interval)
  d. Decrease myocardial contractility
 3. Vasodilation
 4. Uses
  a. Treatment of PSVT
  b. Control of ventricular rate in atrial flutter or atrial fibrillation
   • Verapamil is more effective than digoxin.
 5. Adverse effects: hypotension, dizziness, constipation, edema, AV block
E. Miscellaneous antiarrhythmic drugs
 1. Adenosine
  a. Pharmacokinetics
   (1) In blood, $t_{1/2}$ about 10 seconds
   (2) Route of administration: intravenous
  b. Mechanism of action: enhanced potassium conductance with inhibition of cyclic adenosine monophosphate (cAMP)–dependent calcium influx

Verapamil has the strongest cardiac effects among the calcium channel blockers.

Verapamil is often used to control the ventricular rate of patients with atrial fibrillation.

   c. Uses: the drug of choice in the management of reentrant PSVTs including those associated with Wolff-Parkinson-White syndrome
2. Digoxin (see Chapter 14)
   • Uses: atrial fibrillation (decreases AV conduction), heart failure
3. Magnesium (intravenous)
   a. Mechanism of action: unknown but likely an anti-calcium effect
   b. Uses: torsades de pointes; the 2000 guidelines conclude that intravenous magnesium during cardiopulmonary resuscitation is only effective for the treatment of patients with hypomagnesemic states or polymorphic ventricular tachycardia (torsades de pointes); digitalis-induced arrhythmias in patients that are in the hypomagnesemic state
4. Potassium (intravenous): treatment of hypokalemia or digoxin toxicity (arrhythmias or ECG changes) associated with hypokalemia

Adenosine is the drug of choice for prompt conversion of PSVT to sinus rhythm.

Digoxin is now used more to control ventricular rate than treat congestive heart failure.

Magnesium treats torsades de pointes.

Antihypertensive Drugs

I. General Considerations
- The diagnosis of hypertension in adults is confirmed when, on two subsequent visits, the average diastolic blood pressure exceeds 90 mm Hg or the average systolic blood pressure exceeds 140 mm Hg.
  A. Treatment rationale
  - Sustained hypertension leads to cardiovascular and renal damage, especially myocardial infarction (MI) and stroke.
  - Reducing blood pressure decreases risks of morbidity and death.
  B. Treatment methods
  1. First-line treatment: diet and lifestyle changes
  2. Second-line treatment: pharmacologic intervention (Box 13-1)
     - Selection of pharmacologic treatment is based on concomitant conditions (Table 13-1).

II. Diuretics (see Chapter 15)
- Diuretics decrease filling pressure of the heart and reduce peripheral resistance.
- Thiazides and thiazide-related diuretics are most often used because they have vasodilatory properties in addition to diuretic effects.
  A. Use: hypertension (first-line therapy)
  - Thiazides are administered alone or in combination with other drugs.
  B. Adverse effects: hypokalemia (except with potassium-sparing diuretics), hyperuricemia, sexual dysfunction, hyperglycemia, hyperlipidemia

BOX 13-1

ANTIHYPERTENSIVE DRUGS

Diuretics

Loop diuretics
Potassium-sparing diuretics
Thiazide diuretics

Sympatholytics

β-Receptor Antagonists
Atenolol
Metoprolol
Propranolol

α_1-Receptor Antagonists
Doxazosin
Prazosin
Terazosin

α_2-Receptor Agonists
Clonidine
Methyldopa

Vasodilators

Calcium channel blockers
Hydralazine
Minoxidil
Sodium nitroprusside
Fenoldopam

Angiotensin Inhibitors

Angiotensin-converting Enzyme (ACE) Inhibitors
Captopril
Enalapril
Lisinopril

Angiotensin Receptor Blockers
Losartan
Valsartan

III. Sympatholytic Drugs
   A. β-Adrenergic receptor antagonists (see Chapter 5)
      1. Pharmacologic properties
         a. Mechanism of action: blockade of β receptors
            (1) Decrease heart rate and contractility
            (2) Decrease blood pressure
            (3) Decrease renin release
            (4) Decrease sympathetic outflow from the brain
         b. Use: first-line drug therapy for hypertension, especially in patients with heart failure and previous MI
         c. Adverse effects: central nervous system (CNS) depression, increased serum lipids, exacerbate asthma, cardiac disturbances, sexual dysfunction

Abrupt withdrawal of beta blockers or clonidine leads to rebound hypertension.

TABLE 13-1:
Selection of Antihypertensive Drugs

Patient Characteristic	Most Preferred Drugs	Least Preferred Drugs
Demographic Traits		
African heritage	Calcium channel blocker, thiazide diuretic	—
Pregnancy	Methyldopa, hydralazine	ACE inhibitor, angiotensin receptor antagonist (ARB)
Lifestyle Traits		
Physically active	ACE inhibitor, calcium channel blocker, alpha blocker	Beta blocker
Noncompliance	Drug with once-daily dosage regimen; transdermal clonidine	Oral centrally acting α-adrenoceptor agonist
Concomitant Conditions		
Angina pectoris	Beta blocker, diltiazem, verapamil	Hydralazine, minoxidil
Asthma, COPD	Calcium channel blocker, ACE inhibitor	Beta blocker
Benign prostatic hyperplasia	Alpha blocker	—
Collagen disease	ACE inhibitor (but not captopril), calcium channel blocker	Hydralazine, methyldopa
Depression	ACE inhibitor, calcium channel blocker	Centrally acting α-adrenoceptor agonist, beta blocker, reserpine
Diabetes mellitus	ACE inhibitor, calcium channel blocker, angiotensin receptor antagonist	Beta blocker, diuretic
Gout	—	Diuretic
Heart failure	ACE inhibitor, diuretic, hydralazine	Calcium channel blocker
Hypercholesterolemia	Alpha blocker, ACE inhibitor, calcium channel blocker	Beta blocker, thiazide
Migraine	Beta blocker, calcium channel blocker	—
Myocardial infarction	Beta blocker, ACE inhibitor	—
Osteoporosis	Thiazide	—
Peripheral vascular disease	ACE inhibitor, calcium channel blocker, α-blocker	Beta blocker

ACE, angiotensin-converting enzyme; COPD, chronic obstructive pulmonary disease.

2. Selected drugs
   a. Propranolol (nonselective): inhibitor of both β_1 and β_2 receptors
   b. Metoprolol (selective): β_1-selective, half-life ($t_{1/2}$) 3 to 4 hours
   c. Atenolol (selective): β_1-selective, with a longer half-life ($t_{1/2}$) of 6 to 9 hours
      (1) Better tolerated than propranolol in patients with asthma
      (2) Fewer CNS-related adverse effects than other β-adrenergic receptor antagonists (less lipid-soluble)

B. α_2-Adrenergic receptor agonists
   1. Methyldopa
      a. Mechanism of action
         • This centrally acting agent is converted to α-methylnorepinephrine, which stimulates α_2-adrenergic receptors in the CNS to decrease sympathetic outflow.
      b. Adverse effects: sedation, dry mouth, postural hypotension, failure of ejaculation, anemia
         • Methyldopa, which triggers antibody production (positive Coombs' test), causes autoimmune hemolytic anemia.
   2. Clonidine
      a. Mechanism of action: direct stimulation of central α_2-receptors, decreasing sympathetic and increasing parasympathetic tone to reduce both blood pressure and heart rate
      b. Adverse effects: dry mouth, sedation, postural hypotension
         • Withdrawal from high-dose therapy may result in life-threatening hypertensive crises due to increased sympathetic activity.

C. α_1-Adrenergic receptor antagonists
   • Examples: prazosin, doxazosin, terazosin (see Chapter 5)
   1. Mechanism of action
      • α_1-Adrenergic receptor antagonists block α_1-receptors selectively on arterioles and venules, thus decreasing peripheral vascular resistance.
      • These drugs relax the bladder neck and the prostate by blocking the α_1-adrenergic receptors located in smooth muscle.
   2. Uses: hypertension, benign prostatic hyperplasia (BPH)
   3. Adverse effects: postural hypotension, dizziness

IV. Vasodilators
   • Directly relax vascular smooth muscles (Fig. 13-1)
   A. Hydralazine
      1. Pharmacokinetics
         • Oral bioavailability is dependent on the acetylation phenotype (N-acetyltransferase) of patients.
         • About 50% of patients are "slow" acetylators and 50% are "fast" acetylators.

Beta blockers all end in -olol (e.g., propranolol) except those that also block α receptors: labetalol, carvedilol.

Methyldopa is the preferred antihypertensive during pregnancy.

Patients receiving methyldopa may have a positive Coombs' test.

Clonidine is the only antihypertensive agent available as a transdermal patch.

Clonidine causes dry mouth.

Withdrawal from clonidine should occur slowly (over 1 week) to avoid a hypertensive crisis.

All α_1-adrenergic receptor antagonists end in -zosin.

Terazosin is recommended for the treatment of BPH.

Tamsulosin and alfuzosin, selective for α_1-receptors in prostrate, treat BPH without producing orthostatic hypotension; end in -sin.

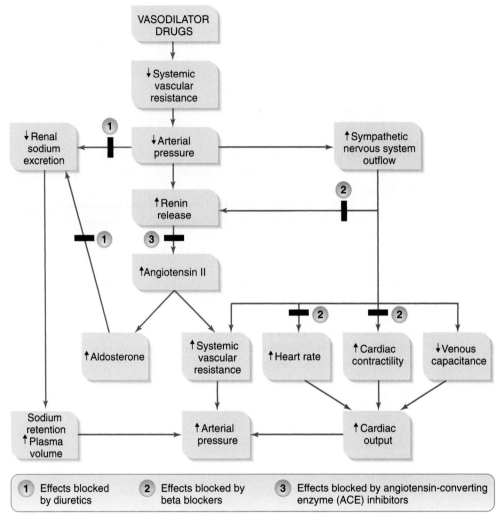

13-1: *Compensatory response to vasodilators when used to treat hypertension.*

The diagram shows:

VASODILATOR DRUGS → ↓Systemic vascular resistance → ↓Arterial pressure

↓Arterial pressure → ↓Renal sodium excretion (blocked by 1)
↓Arterial pressure → ↑Sympathetic nervous system outflow
↓Arterial pressure → ↑Renin release

↑Sympathetic nervous system outflow → ↑Renin release (blocked by 2)

↑Renin release → ↑Angiotensin II (blocked by 3)

↑Angiotensin II → ↑Aldosterone, ↑Systemic vascular resistance
↑Aldosterone → ↓Renal sodium excretion (blocked by 1)

↑Sympathetic nervous system outflow → ↑Systemic vascular resistance, ↑Heart rate (blocked by 2), ↑Cardiac contractility (blocked by 2), ↓Venous capacitance

↓Renal sodium excretion → Sodium retention ↑Plasma volume → ↑Arterial pressure
↑Systemic vascular resistance → ↑Arterial pressure
↑Heart rate, ↑Cardiac contractility, ↓Venous capacitance → ↑Cardiac output → ↑Arterial pressure

Legend:
1. Effects blocked by diuretics
2. Effects blocked by beta blockers
3. Effects blocked by angiotensin-converting enzyme (ACE) inhibitors

The combination therapy with isosorbide dinitrate and hydralazine is specially effective in the African-American population.

Hydralazine and procainamide cause lupus-like adverse effects.

2. Mechanism of action
   • Relaxation of the vascular smooth muscle of the arterioles causes reflex tachycardia and increased renin secretion, which may be blocked by propranolol (or by centrally acting agents).
3. Uses: heart failure (with nitrates), hypertension (safe in pregnancy)
4. Adverse effects
   a. Drug-induced systemic lupus erythematosus–like syndrome, which is reversible on drug withdrawal (10–20%)
   b. Peripheral neuritis with paresthesias (numbness, pain, and tingling in the hands and feet)
      • This effect can be prevented by the administration of pyridoxine.

B. Minoxidil: potent arteriolar dilator
   1. Mechanism of action
      - Induction of delay in the hydrolysis of cyclic adenosine monophosphate (cAMP) via inhibition of phosphodiesterase may contribute to vasodilatory action.
   2. Uses: hypertension, facilitation of hair growth (topically)
   3. Adverse effects: tachyphylaxis, palpitations
C. Sodium nitroprusside
   1. Pharmacokinetics
      - Metabolic conversion to cyanide and thiocyanate may cause severe toxic reactions if the infusion of sodium nitroprusside is continued for several days.
      - Arterial pressure may be titrated by intravenous administration because of its rapid action and short (minutes) half-life ($t_{1/2}$).
   2. Mechanism of action
      a. Occurs via the release of nitric oxide
      b. Involves relaxation of smooth muscle in arterioles and venules
      c. Decreases both preload and afterload
   3. Uses: hypertensive emergencies, acute MI, aortic dissection
   4. Adverse effects: hypotension, tachycardia, cyanide toxicity
D. Calcium channel blockers (see Chapter 12)
   - Examples: nifedipine, diltiazem, verapamil (slow-release or long-acting preparations)
   1. Uses: control of elevated blood pressure by relaxation of smooth muscles
   2. Adverse effects: edema
E. Fenoldopam: an intravenous dopamine DA_1 agonist used for the acute treatment of severe hypertension

V. Drugs That Affect the Renin Angiotensin System (RAS)
   A. Angiotensin-converting enzyme (ACE) inhibitors
      - Examples: captopril, enalapril
      1. Mechanism of action: blockade of conversion of angiotensin I to angiotensin II by inhibiting ACE
         a. Inhibition of inactivation of bradykinin (cough, angioedema)
         b. Increased plasma renin due to decrease in angiotensin II and aldosterone
         c. Decrease both preload and afterload
      2. Uses: hypertension, diabetic nephropathy, heart failure, post-MI
      3. Adverse effects: proteinuria, acute renal failure in patients with renal artery stenosis
      4. Contraindication: pregnancy
   B. Angiotensin receptor blockers (ARBs)
      - Examples: losartan, valsartan
      1. Mechanism of action: blockade of angiotensin II type 1 (AT_1) receptors
         - More complete inhibition of angiotensin effects than ACE inhibitors
         - No effect on bradykinin metabolism

All dihydropyridine calcium channel blockers end in -dipine: amlodipine, felodipine, isradipine, nicardipine, nisoldipine, nifedipine, nimodipine.

Relative efficacy of calcium channel blockers as vasodilators: nifedipine > diltiazem > verapamil

Relative efficacy of calcium channel blockers in control of heart rate: verapamil > diltiazem > nifedipine

All ACE inhibitors end in -pril: benazepril, captopril, enalapril, fosinopril, lisinopril, moexipril, perindopril, quinapril, ramipril, trandolapril.

Hyperkalemia, dry cough, and angioedema often occur in patients taking ACE inhibitors.

All angiotensin receptor blockers end in -sartan: candesartan, eprosartan, irbesartan, losartan, olmisartan, telmisartan, valsartan

ACE inhibitors and ARBs are contraindicated in pregnancy and lactation.

2. Uses: hypertension, heart failure, diabetic nephropathy
3. Adverse effects: similar to those of the ACE inhibitors, but no cough and angioedema; also contraindicated during pregnancy; hyperkalemia

VI. Drugs Used in the Emergency Treatment of Hypertension (Box 13-2)

BOX 13-2

DRUGS USED IN THE EMERGENCY TREATMENT OF HYPERTENSION

Diazoxide
Fenoldopam
Hydralazine
Labetalol

Methyldopa
Nitroglycerin, intravenous
Sodium nitroprusside

14

Other Cardiovascular Drugs

TARGET TOPICS

- Drugs used to treat angina
- Drugs used to lower lipid levels
- Drugs used to treat heart failure

I. General Considerations
   A. The goal of antianginal therapy is to decrease oxygen demand of myocardial tissue or increase oxygen supply (Fig. 14-1).
   B. Antianginal drugs are used to treat angina pectoris caused by myocardial ischemia (Box 14-1).
   C. Coronary blood flow depends on aortic diastolic pressure, duration of diastole, and resistance of the coronary vascular bed.
   D. Antianginal drugs have vasodilator action on the coronary, cerebral, and peripheral vascular beds.

> Objective of antianginal therapy: to balance O_2 demand with O_2 supply in myocardial tissue

II. Antianginal Drugs
   A. Nitrites and nitrates
      1. Pharmacokinetics
         - Classification is primarily based on duration of action.
         a. Rapid-acting agents: amyl nitrite (inhalation); nitroglycerin (intravenous, sublingual)
         b. Long-acting agents: isosorbide dinitrate (regular oral, sustained-release oral, sublingual); nitroglycerin (transdermal, ointment, sustained-release oral)
      2. Mechanism of action
         - Release of the nitrite ion, which is metabolized to nitric oxide, activates guanylyl cyclase, increasing cyclic guanosine monophosphate (cGMP) levels, which in turn relaxes vascular smooth muscle.
         a. Nitrates do *not* increase total coronary blood flow in patients with ischemia, but they redistribute blood to ischemic areas, thus correcting the myocardial oxygen imbalance (see Fig. 14-1).
         b. Nitrate-induced vasodilation increases venous capacitance and decreases arteriole resistance, thereby reducing preload and afterload and lowering oxygen demand; preload is affected greater than afterload.

> Nitrate-induced vasodilation results in lower cardiac oxygen demand.

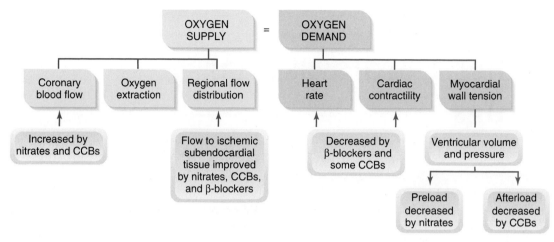

14-1: *Effects of nitrates, calcium channel blockers (CCBs), and beta blockers on myocardial oxygen supply and demand.*

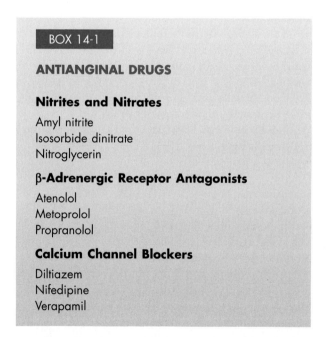

BOX 14-1

ANTIANGINAL DRUGS

Nitrites and Nitrates

Amyl nitrite
Isosorbide dinitrate
Nitroglycerin

β-Adrenergic Receptor Antagonists

Atenolol
Metoprolol
Propranolol

Calcium Channel Blockers

Diltiazem
Nifedipine
Verapamil

3. Uses
   a. Treatment of acute angina pectoris, prophylaxis of angina attacks
   b. Treatment of heart failure (with hydralazine)
   c. Treatment of hypertensive emergencies, control of perioperative hypertension
4. Adverse effects
   a. Headaches (usually transient), dizziness, hypotension, flushing

  b. Reflex tachycardia
  c. Methemoglobinemia (nitrites)
5. Tolerance
  a. Develops and disappears rapidly (2–3 days)
     • Headaches disappear as tolerance develops.
  b. Limits the usefulness of nitrates in continuous prophylaxis
     • To counter tolerance, patches are usually removed between 10:00 PM and 6 AM.
B. β-Adrenergic receptor antagonists (see Chapter 5)
  1. Mechanism of action
     • β-Adrenergic receptor antagonists inhibit the reflex tachycardia produced by nitrates.
     • Subsequent reductions in heart rate, myocardial contractility, and blood pressure decrease myocardial oxygen requirements.
  2. Use: angina (in combination with other drugs, such as nitrates)
C. Calcium channel blockers (see Chapter 12)
  1. Mechanism of action
     a. Block calcium movement into cells, inhibiting excitation-contraction coupling in myocardial and smooth muscle cells
     b. Reduce heart rate, blood pressure, and contractility
  2. Uses: coronary artery disease and Prinzmetal's or variant angina; also used to treat hypertension and arrhythmias
  3. Adverse effects: flushing, edema, dizziness, constipation

III. Drugs That Affect Cholesterol and Lipid Metabolism
  A. General considerations
    1. Hyperlipidemia is defined as high levels of serum lipids.
      a. Primary hyperlipidemia is caused by genetic predisposition.
      b. Secondary hyperlipidemia arises as a complication of disease states, such as diabetes, hypothyroidism, Cushing's disease, and acromegaly.
    2. Atherosclerosis may result from high levels of plasma lipids, although the exact pathogenesis remains unknown.
    3. Therapy
      a. First-line treatment: control by diet and lifestyle modifications
      b. Second-line treatment: pharmacologic intervention
      (Table 14-1)
        • The metabolism of lipoproteins and the mechanism of action of some antihyperlipidemic drugs are summarized in Figure 14-2.
  B. Bile acid–binding resins (Box 14-2)
    • Examples: cholestyramine, colestipol, colesevelam
    1. Mechanism of action
      a. Resins bind bile acids in the intestine to form an insoluble, nonabsorbable complex that is excreted in the feces along with the unchanged resin.
      b. This action causes an increase in the conversion of plasma cholesterol to bile acids, thus decreasing plasma cholesterol levels.

"Monday disease": Industrial workers had severe headaches on Monday from organic nitrates in the workplace; each day the headache was less due to tolerance. The tolerance was reversed over the weekend and the cycle started again on Monday.

Beta blockers are not effective in treating Prinzmetal's angina.

Beta blockers reduce heart rate and blood pressure, leading to relief of angina and improved exercise tolerance in patents with severe angina.

Calcium channel blockers are effective in the treatment of Prinzmetal's angina.

TABLE 14-1:
Effects of Drug Therapy on Serum Lipid Concentrations

Drug or Class	LDL Concentration (%)	HDL Concentration (%)	Total Decrease in Triglyceride Concentration (%)	Other Effects
HMG-CoA reductase inhibitors	↓ 10–15	↑ 10	↓ 10–20	Increase in hepatic LDL receptors
Bile acid-binding resins	↓ 20–40	↑ 0–2	↑ 0–5	Increase in hepatic LDL receptors
Gemfibrozil	↓ 10	↑ 10–25	↓ 40–50	Activation of lipoprotein lipase
Niacin	↓ 10–15	↑ 10	↓ 20–80	Decrease in lipolysis and lipoprotein levels

HDL, high-density lipoprotein; LDL, low-density lipoprotein.

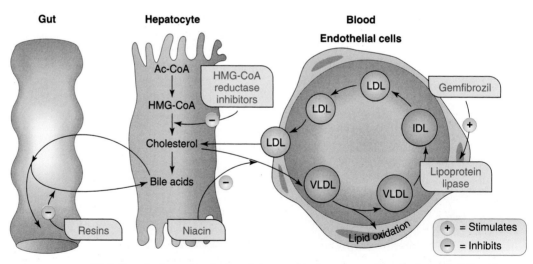

14-2: Sites of action and mechanisms of drugs used in the treatment of hyperlipidemia. The bile acid resins decrease the reabsorption of bile acids from the gut. The HMG-CoA (3-hydroxy-3-methylglutaryl coenzyme A) reductase inhibitors block the rate-limiting step of cholesterol synthesis. Niacin affects lipid metabolism, transport, and clearance. Gemfibrozil stimulates lipoprotein lipase. IDL, intermediate-density lipoproteins; LDL, low-density lipoproteins; VLDL, very low density lipoproteins; Ac-CoA, acetyl-CoA.

2. Uses
   a. Elevated low-density lipoprotein (LDL) level (in combination with other drugs); heterozygous familial hypercholesterolemia
   b. Reduction of itching in cholestasis

BOX 14-2

DRUGS USED IN THE TREATMENT OF HYPERCHOLESTEROLEMIA

Bile Acid–Binding Resins

Cholestyramine
Colestipol
Colesevelam

HMG-CoA Reductase Inhibitors

Atorvastatin
Fluvastatin
Lovastatin
Pravastatin
Simvastatin

Lipoprotein Lipase Stimulators

Gemfibrozil
Fenofibrate
Niacin

Inhibitors of Cholesterol Absorption

Ezetimibe

---

3. Adverse effects
    a. Nausea, malabsorption of fat-soluble vitamins (e.g., vitamin K) and other drugs such as digoxin, iron salts, tetracycline, and warfarin in the intestine due to the binding of these drugs to the resin
    b. Constipation
C. HMG-CoA (3-hydroxy-3-methylglutaryl coenzyme A) reductase inhibitors
    • Examples: atorvastatin, lovastatin, pravastatin ("statins")
    1. Mechanism of action
        a. The "statins" inhibit HMG-CoA reductase (the rate-limiting step in cholesterol synthesis), thereby decreasing cholesterol levels.
        b. The resulting increase in synthesis of LDL cholesterol receptors in cell walls decreases plasma cholesterol.
    2. Use: elevated LDL plasma levels
    3. Adverse effects
        a. Elevated hepatic enzymes
        b. Skeletal muscle toxicity (elevated creatine kinase), myositis
D. Lipoprotein lipase stimulators
    1. Fibric acid derivatives (gemfibrozil and fenofibrate)
        a. Mechanism of action

All these drug names end in -statin: atorvastatin, fluvastatin, lovastatin, pravastatin, rosuvastatin, simvastatin.

Monitor liver functional enzymes (LFE) and muscle enzymes (creatine kinase) with -statins.

(1) Ligands for the peroxisome proliferators-activated receptor-alpha (PPARα) protein, a receptor that regulates transcription of genes involved in lipid metabolism

(2) Activates lipoprotein lipase, promoting delivery of triglycerides to adipose tissue

(3) Decreases hepatic triglyceride production

(4) Interferes with the formation of very low density lipoprotein (VLDL) in the liver

b. Uses: hypertriglyceridemia, hyperlipoproteinemia

c. Adverse effects: myalgias, cholelithiasis; counter indicated in patients with pre-existing gallbladder disease

2. Niacin (nicotinic acid)

a. Mechanism of action

(1) Reduces hepatic VLDL secretion (like gemfibrozil)

(2) Enhances VLDL clearance by activating lipoprotein lipase (like gemfibrozil)

(3) Decreases LDL and triglycerides and increases high-density lipoproteins (HDLs)

b. Uses: almost all types of hyperlipidemia, especially those that are genetically induced

• Used in combination with bile acid resins

c. Adverse effects

(1) Generalized pruritus as a result of peripheral vasodilation, characterized by flushing, warmth, and burning or tingling of the skin, especially of the face or neck

(2) Increased hepatic enzymes

E. Drugs that prevent cholesterol absorption

1. Ezetimibe

a. Selectively blocks the intestinal absorption of cholesterol and phytosterols

b. Used as monotherapy or in combination with HMG-CoA reductase inhibitors (-statins) for the treatment of hypercholesterolemia

IV. Inotropic Agents and Treatment of Heart Failure (Box 14-3)

• Drugs that should be considered in the treatment of heart failure include inotropes (digoxin, dobutamine, inamrinone), β-adrenergic receptor antagonists, vasodilators (nitrates, hydralazine, nesiritide, bosentan), diuretics (especially loops), angiotensin receptor blockers (ARBs), and ACE (angiotensin-converting enzyme) inhibitors (Fig. 14-3).

A. Digoxin (see Chapter 12)

• Digoxin has a positive inotropic and various electrophysiologic effects on the heart (see Fig. 14-3).

• It is derived from the leaves of the plant *Digitalis purpurea* (foxglove) or *D. lanata*.

1. Pharmacokinetics (Table 14-2)

2. Mechanism of action

a. Inhibition of Na^+/K^+-activated ATPase, thus increasing the force of myocardial contraction by increasing available intracellular calcium

---

Fibric acid drugs may aggravate gallbladder disease.

Peripheral vasodilation occurs frequently with niacin; pretreatment with aspirin prevents this development.

Quinidine increases digoxin levels by interfering with tissue protein binding and renal excretion of digoxin.

BOX 14-3

DRUGS USED IN THE TREATMENT OF HEART FAILURE

Digitalis Glycosides

Digoxin

Other Inotropic Agents

β-Adrenergics
Dobutamine
Dopamine

Phosphodiesterase Inhibitors
Inamrinone
Milrinone

Vasodilators

Bosentan
Hydralazine
Nesiritide
Nitrates
Sodium nitroprusside

Diuretics

Loop
Furosemide

Potassium-sparing
Eplerenone
Spironolactone

Thiazide
Hydrochlorothiazide

Angiotensin-converting Enzyme (ACE) Inhibitors

Captopril
Enalapril
Lisinopril

Angiotensin Receptor Blockers (ARBs)

Losartan
Valsartan

β-Adrenergic Receptor Antagonists

Atenolol
Carvedilol
Metoprolol

    b. Increase vagal stimulation, leading to decreased heart rate
    c. Slow conduction through the atrioventricular (AV) node
  3. Uses: treatment of heart failure (today used late in therapy) and control of ventricular rate in the management of atrial fibrillation
  4. Adverse effects
    a. Toxicity
      (1) Nausea and vomiting (earliest signs of intoxication)
      (2) Mental status changes
      (3) Changes in color vision (green or yellow halos)
      (4) Changes on electrocardiogram: decreased QT interval, increased PR interval, ST-segment depression, all types of arrhythmias (most serious signs of intoxication)

> Digoxin has a low therapeutic index.

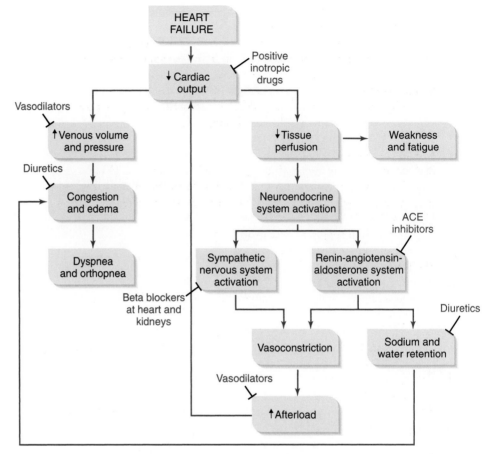

14-3: *Algorithm of the pathogenesis and treatment of heart failure, indicating the sites where certain drugs may interfere with the development of heart failure. ACE, angiotensin-converting enzyme.*

TABLE 14-2:
Pharmacokinetic Parameters of Digitalis Glycosides

Parameter	Digoxin
Route of administration	Oral, intravenous
Oral bioavailability (%)	75
Time to peak effect (hr)	3–6
Volume of distribution (L/kg)	6.3*
Plasma protein binding (%)	20–40
Half-life (hr)	40
Elimination	Renal

*The large volume of distribution of digoxin is due to tissue protein binding; it is displaced by quinidine.

  b. Treatment of toxicity
   (1) Discontinue medication
   (2) Correct either potassium or magnesium deficiency
   (3) Give digoxin antibody (digoxin immune Fab, or Digibind) for severe toxicity
 5. Precautions
  - The hypokalemia that often occurs with diuretic therapy increases the toxicity associated with digoxin therapy.
B. Diuretics (see Chapter 15)
 1. Decrease edema
 2. Loop diuretics are preferred for congestive heart failure (CHF) or pulmonary edema; thiazide diuretics are preferred for hypertension.
C. Angiotensin-converting enzyme (ACE) inhibitors and angiotensin receptor blockers (ARBs) (see Chapter 13)
 1. Decrease peripheral resistance
 2. Decrease salt and water retention
 3. Decrease tissue remodeling
D. β-Adrenergic receptor antagonists (see Chapter 5)
 1. Increase life expectancy in patients with mild and moderate congestive heart failure
 2. Decrease workload on heart and accompanying remodeling
 3. Alpha and beta blockers (carvedilol) also effective in extending the life expectancy of CHF patients
E. Beta agonists in severe heart failure (dobutamine and dopamine)
 1. Stimulate β_1 receptors in heart
 2. Positive inotropic agents that should be used for acute treatment only
F. Phosphodiesterase inhibitors
 1. Examples: inamrinone, milrinone
 2. Cyclic AMP–dependent inotropes and vasodilators, which are given intravenously for the short-term management of congestive heart failure
 3. Long-term use is associated with increased morbidity and mortality rates.
G. Vasodilators
 1. Hydralazine and organic nitrates (see Chapter 13)
  a. Decrease preload and/or afterload
 2. Nesiritide
  a. An intravenous recombinant form of a human brain natriuretic peptide (BNP), a naturally occurring hormone produced in the ventricles of the heart
  b. Indicated for the acute treatment of decompensated congestive heart failure (CHF)
 3. Bosentan: an endothelin-receptor antagonist; indicated for use in primary pulmonary hypertension

Potassium wasting diuretics increase the toxicity of digoxin.

ACE inhibitors all end in -pril.

ARBs all end in -sartan.

Diuretics

TARGET TOPICS

- Carbonic anhydrase inhibitors
- Loop diuretics
- Thiazide diuretics
- Potassium-sparing diuretics
- Osmotic diuretics
- Drugs that affect water excretion

I. General Considerations
  A. Role of the kidney
    1. The kidney is the most important organ in maintaining body fluid composition.
    2. It is the chief means of excreting most drugs and nonvolatile metabolic waste products.
    3. It plays a fundamental role in maintaining pH, controlling levels of electrolytes and water, and conserving substances such as glucose and amino acids.
  B. Functions of the renal nephrons
    1. Glomerular filtration
      a. Blood is forced into the glomerulus and filtered through capillaries into the glomerular capsule.
        • The glomerular filtration rate (GFR) is 120 mL/min.
      b. Plasma filtrate is composed of fluids and soluble constituents.
      c. Substances normally *not* filtered include cells, plasma proteins and substances bound to them, lipids, and other macromolecules.
        • Approximately 99% of the filtrate is reabsorbed.
    2. Tubular secretion
      a. This process involves the movement of substances from the blood into the renal tubular lumen.
      b. Many drugs (e.g., penicillins, glucuronide conjugates of drugs) are actively secreted by anion or cation transport systems.

II. Diuretics
  • Classification is based on sites (Fig. 15-1) and mechanisms of action (Table 15-1).
  A. Carbonic anhydrase inhibitors (Box 15-1)
    • Examples: acetazolamide, dorzolamide

GFR = 120 mL/min

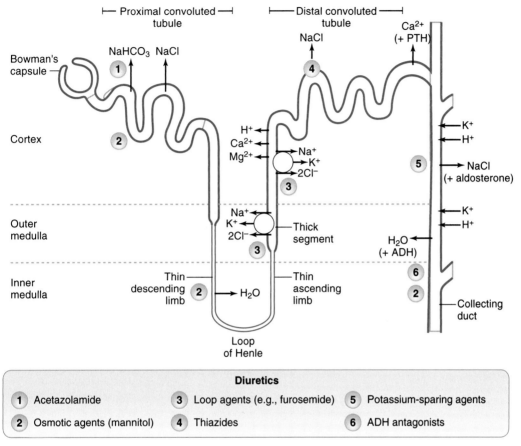

15-1: *Tubule transport systems and sites of action of diuretics. ADH, antidiuretic hormone; PTH, parathyroid hormone.*

1. Carbonic anhydrase inhibitors act in the proximal renal tubules, changing the composition of urine by increasing bicarbonate, sodium, and potassium excretion.
2. This effect lasts only 3 to 4 days.
   - Uses: glaucoma, acute mountain sickness, petit mal seizures, to produce urinary alkalosis and treat metabolic alkalosis
   - Contraindications: hepatic cirrhosis (decreased ammonia excretion)
B. Loop (high-ceiling) diuretics
   - Examples: ethacrynic acid, furosemide
   - Loop diuretics cause a profound diuresis (much greater than that produced by thiazides) and a decreased preload to the heart.
   - These drugs are useful in patients with renal impairment because they retain their effectiveness when creatinine clearance is less than 30 mL/min (normal = 120 mL/min).
   - Loop diuretics upregulate cyclooxygenase activity, thereby increasing PGE_2 and PGI_2 activity, resulting in increased renal blood flow.

TABLE 15-1:
Mechanisms, Uses, and Adverse Effects of Different Diuretics

Drug Class (Agent)	Mechanism	Uses	Adverse Effects
Carbonic anhydrase inhibitors (acetazolamide)	Inhibit carbonic anhydrase in proximal tubule, changing composition of urine	Glaucoma Urinary alkalinization Acute mountain sickness Pseudotumor cerebri	Hyperchloremic Metabolic acidosis
Loop diuretics (furosemide)	Inhibit $Na^+/K^+/2Cl^-$ symport along thick ascending limb of loop of Henle	Acute pulmonary edema Refractory edema Hypertension Hyperkalemia Ascites	Hyperglycemia Hyperuricemia Hypocalcemia Hypomagnesium Dehydration Hypokalemia Metabolic alkalosis
Loop diuretics (ethacrynic acid)	Inhibit sulfhydryl-catalyzed enzyme systems responsible for reabsorption of sodium and chloride in proximal and distal tubules	Edema Sulfonamide sensitivity	Ototoxicity
Thiazide diuretics (hydrochlorothiazide)	Inhibit Na^+/Cl^- symport in distal convoluted tubule	Hypertension Heart failure Nephrolithiasis Nephrogenic diabetes insipidus	Hypokalemic metabolic alkalosis Hypomagnesemia Hypercalcemia Hyperlipidemia Hyperglycemia Hyperuricemia
Potassium-sparing diuretics (triamterene)	Inhibit Na^+/K^+ ion exchange in distal tubule and collecting duct	Adjunctive treatment of edema hypertension in combination with thiazides or loop diuretics Antagonize potassium loss associated with other diuretics	Cardiac arrhythmias from hyperkalemia Hyperchlorenic metabolic acidosis
Potassium-sparing diuretics (spironolactone)	Block binding of aldosterone to receptors in cells of distal renal tubules	Diagnose primary hyperaldosteronism Treat polycystic ovary syndrome, hirsutism, ascites, and heart failure	Gynecomastia
Osmotic diuretics (mannitol)	Increase osmotic gradient between blood and tissues and remove water because diuretic is filtered and not reabsorbed	Maintain urine flow in acute renal failure Treat acute oliguria Reduce intracranial pressure and cerebral edema Treat acute glaucoma	Electrolyte imbalances Expansion of extracellular fluid

1. Ethacrynic acid
   a. Mechanism of action: inhibition of sulfhydryl-catalyzed enzyme systems, which is responsible for reabsorption of sodium and chloride in the proximal and distal tubules

BOX 15-1

DIURETICS

Carbonic Anhydrase Inhibitors
Acetazolamide
Dorzolamide

Loop Diuretics
Bumetanide
Ethacrynic acid
Furosemide
Torsemide

Thiazide and Thiazide-like Diuretics
Chlorthalidone
Hydrochlorothiazide
Indapamide
Metolazone
Quinethazone

Potassium-sparing Diuretics
Aldosterone antagonists
Eplerenone
Spironolactone

Sodium-Potassium Exchange Inhibitors
Amiloride
Triamterene

Osmotic Diuretics
Glycerol
Mannitol

    b. Uses
      (1) In patients who are hypersensitive to sulfonamide drugs such as thiazides and furosemide (the most commonly used loop diuretic)
      (2) Edema related to heart failure or cirrhosis
    c. Adverse effects: ototoxicity, leading to hearing loss and tinnitus
  2. Furosemide
    • This drug is structurally related to thiazides and has many of the properties of those diuretics.
    a. Mechanism of action: inhibition of reabsorption of sodium and chloride by blocking $Na^+/K^+/2Cl^-$ symport in the ascending limb of the loop of Henle

Loop diuretics and thiazides cause hypokalemia; administer them in combination with a potassium-sparing diuretic.

Thiazide-like diuretics: chlorthalidone, indapamide, metolazone, quinethazone

Use thiazide diuretics in patients who form calcium calculi because these drugs decrease calcium excretion, thus preventing calculi formation.

Use thiazide diuretics cautiously in patients with diabetes mellitus, gout, and hyperlipidemia, as well as those who are receiving digitalis glycosides.

Renin-angiotensin system inhibitors may increase hyperkalemia when using potassium-sparing diuretics.

Osmotic diuretics are absolutely contraindicated in pulmonary edema or CHF.

     b. Uses: hypertension, heart failure, ascites, hypercalcemia, pulmonary edema
     c. Adverse effects: dehydration, hyperglycemia, hypokalemia, hypomagnesemia, hypercalcemia, hyperuricemia, metabolic alkalosis

C. Thiazide diuretics
- These diuretics differ from each other only in potency and duration of action.
- The most commonly used thiazide diuretic is hydrochlorothiazide.
  1. Mechanism of action: reduction in plasma volume, which increases plasma renin activity and aldosterone excretion, resulting in a decrease in renal blood flow and GFR
  2. Uses: hypertension, heart failure, edema, renal calculi (decreased calcium excretion), nephrogenic diabetes insipidus
  3. Adverse effects: hypokalemia, metabolic alkalosis, hyperlipidemia, hyperuricemia, hypomagnesemia, decreased glucose tolerance

D. Potassium-sparing diuretics
- These drugs are used in combination with other diuretics to protect against hypokalemia.
  1. Aldosterone antagonists
     - Example: spironolactone, eplerenone
     a. Mechanism of action: competitive inhibition of the aldosterone receptor, eplerenone is more specific
     b. Uses
        (1) Diagnosis of primary hyperaldosteronism
        (2) Treatment of heart failure
        (3) Adjunct with thiazides or loop diuretics to prevent hypokalemia
        (4) Hypertrichosis (spironolactone)
     c. Adverse effects: antiandrogenic effects, such as impotence, gynecomastia, and hyperkalemia
  2. Sodium-potassium ion exchange inhibitors
     - Examples: triamterene, amiloride
     a. When potassium loss is minimal, sodium-potassium ion exchange inhibition causes only a slight reduction in potassium excretion.
     b. When potassium renal clearance is increased by loop diuretics or mineralocorticoids, these drugs cause a significant decrease in potassium excretion.

E. Osmotic diuretics
- Examples: mannitol, glycerol
- Any agent that is filtered and not completely reabsorbed
  1. Mechanism of action: rise in blood osmolality
     - This action increases the osmotic gradient between blood and tissues.
     - It facilitates the flow of fluid out of the tissues (including the brain and the eye) and into the interstitial fluid.
  2. Uses: increased intracranial pressure, glaucoma, removal of water-soluble toxins
  3. Adverse effects: circulatory overload, pulmonary edema

III. Agents That Affect Water Excretion
   A. Vasopressin (antidiuretic hormone, or ADH)
      • ADH is a peptide hormone synthesized in and secreted by the hypothalamus and stored in and released from the posterior pituitary.
      • Its antidiuretic effects are due to increased reabsorption of water at the renal collecting ducts.
      1. Mechanism of action: stimulation of adenylyl cyclase activity, which leads to:
         a. Increased cyclic adenosine monophosphate (cAMP) in the distal convoluted tubule and collecting duct
         b. Increased reabsorption of water and decreased urine flow
         c. Increased urine osmolality, with maintenance of serum osmolality within an acceptable physiologic range (280–307 mOsm/kg)
      2. Uses
         a. Central (neurogenic) diabetes insipidus caused by a deficiency of pituitary vasopressin secretion
         b. Adjunct in treatment of esophageal varices, hemorrhage, upper gastrointestinal bleeding, variceal bleeding (vasoconstrictor effect)
      3. Adverse effect: water intoxication (overhydration)
   B. Desmopressin
      • Administered orally and intranasally
      • More potent and much longer acting than vasopressin
      1. Mechanism of action: structural analogue of vasopressin
         • 4000 : 1 antidiuretic-to-vasopressor activity
      2. Uses
         a. Usual agent for central (neurogenic) diabetes insipidus
         b. Nocturnal enuresis, hemophilia A, von Willebrand's disease
      3. Adverse effects: water intoxication (overhydration)
   C. ADH antagonists
      • ADH antagonists inhibit effects of ADH at the collecting tubule.
      1. Lithium salts
         a. Mechanism of action: reduction in vasopressin (V_2) receptor–mediated stimulation of adenylyl cyclase in the medullary collecting tubule of the nephron, thus increasing renal sodium and potassium clearance
         b. Use: syndrome of inappropriate ADH (SIADH) secretion
            • Last choice for treatment
         c. Adverse effects: polyuria that is usually, but not always, reversible
      2. Demeclocycline
         • Attenuates antidiuretic effects of vasopressin
         a. Mechanism of action: reduced formation of cAMP, limiting the actions of ADH in the distal portion of the convoluted tubules and collecting ducts of the kidneys
         b. Use: SIADH secretion
         c. Adverse effects: nephrogenic diabetes insipidus (treated with thiazide diuretics or amiloride), renal failure

Neurogenic diabetes insipidus: treat with desmopressin

Nephrogenic diabetes insipidus: treat with a thiazide diuretic

Drugs Used in the Treatment of Coagulation Disorders

TARGET TOPICS

- Antithrombotic drugs
- Heparins
- Oral anticoagulants
- Fibrinolytic drugs
- Hemostatic drugs

I. General Considerations
   A. Clot formation at the tissue level results from complex interactions (Fig. 16-1).
      - Enzymatic pathway for clot formation (Fig. 16-2)
   B. Hematologic drugs
      - These agents have various clinical indications (Table 16-1).
      1. Drugs used to reduce thrombi
         a. Antithrombotic drugs
         b. Anticoagulant drugs
         c. Fibrinolytic drugs
      2. Hemostatic drugs, which prevent bleeding

II. Antithrombotic Drugs (Antiplatelet Drugs)
    - Antithrombotic drugs interfere with platelet adhesion, aggregation, or synthesis (Box 16-1; see also Fig. 16-2).
    A. Aspirin
       - This nonsteroidal anti-inflammatory drug (NSAID) is also used as an analgesic and as an antipyretic (see Chapter 18).
       1. Mechanism of action
          a. Aspirin inhibits synthesis of thromboxane A_2 (TXA_2), a potent platelet aggregator, by irreversible acetylation of cyclooxygenase (COX-1) in platelets.
          b. TXA_2 increases the PIP_2 pathway in platelets, causing aggregation (reduced by aspirin).
          c. Low-dose aspirin therapy inhibits cyclooxygenase to prevent synthesis of TXA_2 without decreasing the synthesis of prostacyclin (PGI_2) in

COX-1 is in platelets and is inhibited by low-dose aspirin.

COX-2 is in endothelial cells and is inhibited by high-dose aspirin and selective COX-2 inhibitors (celecoxib, rofecoxib).

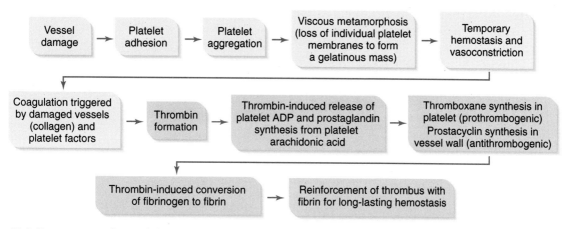

16-1: *Events occurring after vessel damage that lead to the formation of fibrin clots. Note the involvement of both platelets and the coagulation pathway. ADP, adenosine diphosphate.*

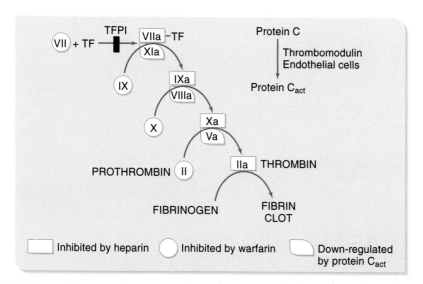

16-2: *Intrinsic and extrinsic pathways of coagulation. Tissue factor is generated by the extrinsic pathway and is important in maintaining the velocity of the intrinsic pathway. Warfarin inhibits the hepatic synthesis of factors VII, IX, X, and II. Heparins accelerate the destruction of activated factors by antithrombin III. Unfractionated heparins have their greatest effect on factor IIa, whereas low-molecular-weight heparins have their greatest effect on factor Xa. Protein C_{act}, activated protein C; TF, tissue factor; TFPI, tissue factor pathway inhibitor.*

endothelial cells, which inhibits platelet aggregation.

   d. Higher doses of aspirin inhibit synthesis of both TXA_2 and PGI_2.

2. Uses (see Table 16-1)

3. Adverse effects

   a. Gastrointestinal (GI) irritation and bleeding

TXA_2 causes platelet aggregation and vasoconstriction.

PGI_2 inhibits platelet aggregation and causes vasodilation.

TABLE 16-1:
Clinical Uses of Anticoagulant, Antiplatelet, and Fibrinolytic Drugs

Clinical Use	Primary Drug*	Secondary Drug*
Acute thrombotic stroke	Fibrinolytic drug	—
Artificial heart valve	Warfarin or aspirin	Dipyridamole
Atrial fibrillation	Heparin, warfarin, or LMWH	Aspirin
Deep vein thrombosis		
Treatment	Heparin, warfarin, or LMWH	—
Surgical prophylaxis	LMWH	Heparin
Heparin-induced thrombocytopenia (HIT)	Rudins	Argatroban
Myocardial infarction		
Treatment	Fibrinolytic drug, heparin, aspirin, or abciximab	—
Prevention	Aspirin	Clopidogrel
Percutaneous transluminal coronary angioplasty	Abciximab, heparin, aspirin, or clopidogrel	—
Pulmonary embolism	Fibrinolytic drug, heparin, warfarin, or LMWH	—
Stroke	Aspirin, clopidogrel, or warfarin	—
Transient ischemic attacks	Aspirin	Warfarin
Unstable angina	Aspirin, abciximab, heparin, or LMWH	—

*If aspirin is contraindicated or not tolerated, ticlopidine may be used. If warfarin is contraindicated or not tolerated, another oral anticoagulant may be used.
LMWH, low-molecular-weight heparin.

BOX 16-1

ANTITHROMBOTIC DRUGS

Platelet Inhibitors

Aspirin
Anagrelide
Cilostazol
Clopidogrel
Dipyridamole
Ticlopidine

Platelet-Receptor Glycoprotein Inhibitors

Abciximab
Eptifibatide
Tirofiban

   b. Tinnitus, respiratory alkalosis followed by metabolic acidosis (high doses)
B. Platelet aggregation inhibitors
   1. Ticlopidine and clopidogrel
      a. Mechanism of action
         (1) Interferes with adenosine diphosphate (ADP)–induced binding of fibrinogen to platelet membrane at specific receptor sites
         (2) Inhibits platelet aggregation and platelet-platelet interactions
      b. Uses
         (1) Prevents thrombotic stroke (initial or recurrent) in patients who are intolerant or unresponsive to aspirin
         (2) Prevents thrombus formation in patients with cardiac stents and in treatment of acute coronary syndromes (in combination with aspirin)
      c. Adverse effects
         • Clopidogrel is associated with a lower incidence of adverse cutaneous, GI, and hematologic reactions than ticlopidine.
         (1) Severe bone marrow toxicity, including agranulocytosis, aplastic anemia, pancytopenia (rare); mostly with ticlopidine
         (2) Thrombotic thrombocytopenic purpura
         (3) Clopidogrel causes many drug-drug interactions: fluvastatin, phenytoin, tamoxifen, tolbutamide, warfarin.
   2. Dipyridamole (vasodilator)
      a. Mechanism of action
         (1) Decreases platelet adhesion
         (2) Potentiates action of prostacyclin, which is coupled to a cyclic adenosine monophosphate (cAMP)–generating system in platelets and vasculature, causing vasodilation
      b. Uses
         (1) Prevention of thrombotic stroke (in combination with aspirin)
         (2) As vasodilator during myocardial perfusion scans (cardiac stress test)
C. Abciximab (Fig. 16-3): platelet-receptor glycoprotein inhibitor
   • Newer glycoprotein IIb and IIIa inhibitors include eptifibatide and tirofiban.
   1. Mechanism of action: binds to the glycoprotein receptors IIb and IIIa on activated platelets
      • Abciximab prevents binding of fibrinogen, von Willebrand factor, and other adhesive molecules to the glycoprotein receptor.
      • When given intravenously, the drug produces rapid inhibition of platelet aggregation.
   2. Uses: acute coronary syndromes, percutaneous transluminal coronary angioplasty
   3. Adverse effects: bleeding, thrombocytopenia
D. Cilostazol
   • Antithrombotic, antiplatelet and vasodilatory action

Use low-dose aspirin to prevent thrombus formation.

Ticlopidine is more toxic than clopidogrel.

Clopidogrel causes more drug-drug interactions than ticlopidine.

Because of the risk of bone marrow toxicity, patients who are receiving ticlopidine must have frequent complete blood counts (CBCs) with white blood cell differential count.

Cilostazol for treatment of intermittent claudication

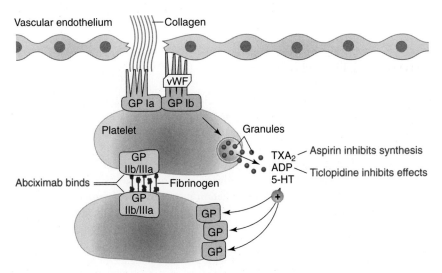

16-3: *Platelet aggregation and sites of drug action. ADP, adenosine diphosphate; GP, glycoprotein; 5-HT, 5-hydroxytryptamine; TXA₂, thromboxane A₂; vWF, von Willebrand's factor.*

- Inhibits phosphodiesterase type III, and thereby, increases cAMP levels
- Uses: intermittent claudication and peripheral vascular disease

E. Anagrelide

- Reduces elevated platelet counts in patients with essential thrombosis (too many platelets)
- Inhibits megakaryocyte development in late postmitotic stage

Anagrelide for treatment of too many platelets

- Used for treatment of thrombocytosis secondary to myeloproliferative disorders

III. Anticoagulants (Box 16-2)

- Pharmacologic properties of most common used agents (Tables 16-2 and 16-3).

A. Standard unfractionated heparin (UFH)

1. Mechanism of action
   - Heparin accelerates the action of antithrombin III (ATIII) to neutralize thrombin (factor IIa) and to a lesser extent other clotting factors

Activated PTT (1.5–2 times control): basis for calculation of the heparin dose

2. Uses (see Table 16-1)
3. Adverse effects: bleeding, hyperkalemia, thrombocytopenia

B. Low-molecular-weight heparins (LMWHs)

- Examples: enoxaparin, dalteparin, tinzaparin

1. Mechanism of action: antifactor Xa (mostly) and antifactor IIa activity
2. Uses
   a. Primary prevention of deep vein thrombosis after hip replacement
   b. Other thrombolytic diseases (see Table 16-1)
   c. LMWHs have pharmacokinetic, pharmacodynamic, and safety advantages over UFH
   d. Not readily reversed with protamine sulfate
3. Adverse effects: bleeding, allergic reactions

BOX 16-2

ANTICOAGULANTS

Heparin-Related Compounds

Fondaparinux
Heparin (UFH)
Low-molecular-weight heparins (LMWHs): enoxaparin, dalteparin, tinzaparin

Direct Thrombin Inhibitors

The rudins: hirudin, bivalirudin, desirudin, lepirudin
Argatroban

Oral Anticoagulants

Warfarin

Property	Heparin	Warfarin
Route of administration	Parenteral/subcutaneous	Oral
Site of action	Blood (in vivo and in vitro)	Liver
Onset of action	Immediate	Delayed; depends on half-lives of factors being replaced
Duration of action	4 hours	2–5 days
Mechanism of action	Accelerates action of antithrombin III to neutralize thrombin	Interferes with hepatic synthesis of vitamin K–dependent clotting factors
Laboratory control of dose	PTT	PT, INR
Antidote	Protamine sulfate	Vitamin K (phytonadione), fresh frozen plasma
Safety in pregnancy	Yes	No (fetal warfarin syndrome)

TABLE 16-2: Comparison of the Properties of Heparin and Warfarin

INR, international normalized ratio; PT, prothrombin time; PTT, partial thromboplastin time.

Property	Heparin	LMWH
Anti-Xa versus anti-IIa activity	1 : 1	2 : 1–4 : 1
PTT monitoring	Required	Not required
Inhibition of platelet function	++++	++
Endothelial cell protein binding	Extensive	Minimal
Dose-dependent clearance	Yes	No
Elimination half-life	Short (50–90 min)	Long (2–5 times longer)

TABLE 16-3: Comparison Between Unfractionated Heparin and Low-Molecular-Weight Heparins

LMWH, low-molecular-weight heparin; PTT, partial thromboplastin time.

TABLE 16-4:
Drugs That Interact
with Warfarin

Drug	Mechanism of Interaction
Enhanced Response	
Allopurinol	Inhibits metabolism
Cimetidine	Inhibits metabolism
Ciprofloxacin	Inhibits metabolism
Co-trimoxazole	Inhibits metabolism
Erythromycin	Inhibits metabolism
Fluconazole	Inhibits metabolism
Metronidazole	Inhibits metabolism
Broad-spectrum antibiotics	Reduce availability of vitamin K
Sulfonamides	Displace from plasma albumin
Diminished Response	
Barbiturates	Induces hepatic microsomal enzymes
Carbamazepine	Induces hepatic microsomal enzymes
Primidone	Induces hepatic microsomal enzymes
Rifampin	Induces hepatic microsomal enzymes
Cholestyramine	Inhibits absorption
Estrogens	Stimulates synthesis of clotting factors
Vitamin K	Competes with warfarin

C. Fondaparinux: a synthetic pentasaccharide anticoagulant
- Antithrombotic activity as a result of ATIII-mediated selective inhibition of factor Xa
- Elimination half-life of 18 hours; allows for once a day dosing
- Uses: venous thromboembolism prophylaxis following orthopedic surgery, pulmonary embolism (PE), deep vein thrombosis (DVT)

D. Direct thrombin inhibitors: most are derivatives of hirudin (referred to as rudin's) peptide found in leeches
- Examples: lepirudin, desirudin, bivalirudin, argatroban
- Used for anticoagulation in patients with heparin-induced thrombocytopenia (HIT)

E. Oral anticoagulants (warfarin)
- Structurally related to vitamin K
1. Mechanism of action: inhibits γ-carboxylation of functional vitamin K–dependent clotting factors in the liver
2. Uses (see Table 16-1)
3. Adverse effects: bleeding
4. Contraindications: pregnancy, bleeding disorders
5. Drug interactions (many)
- Most relate to the cytochrome P-450 system (Table 16-4).

IV. Fibrinolytic (Thrombolytic) Drugs (Box 16-3)
A. Basis of therapy
- When coagulation begins, plasminogen is converted to plasmin, a protease that limits the spread of new clots and dissolves the fibrin in established clots (Fig. 16-4).

PT (1.5 times control) and INR (2–3 times control): basis for calculation of the warfarin dose

Warfarin can cause fetal hemorrhage and skeletal malformations (fetal warfarin syndrome).

BOX 16-3

FIBRINOLYTIC DRUGS

Forms of Recombinant Tissue Plasminogen Activator (tPA)
Alteplase
Reteplase
Tenecteplase

Other Fibrinolytic Agents
Anistreplase
Streptokinase
Urokinase

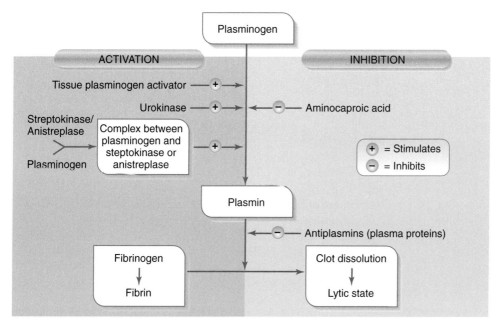

16-4: Site of action of drugs acting on the fibrinolytic system. Fibrinolytic drugs accelerate the conversion of plasminogen to plasmin, which is a protease that breaks down fibrinogen and fibrin to degradation products.

1. Mechanism of action: dissolution of clots by catalyzing formation of plasmin from its precursor, plasminogen
2. Uses (see Table 16-1)
   • Thrombolytic drugs must be given within 6 to 12 hours of a myocardial infarction (MI) to limit cardiac damage and within 3 hours of a stroke.
B. Drugs used in thrombolytic therapy
   1. Alteplase, reteplase, and tenecteplase: recombinant forms of human tissue plasminogen activator (tPA)

Administer alteplase within 3 hours of symptoms of ischemic stroke.

a. Mechanism of action: direct cleavage of the bond in plasminogen
- These thrombolytic drugs selectively work within the thrombi.

b. Uses
- In the United States, these agents are the most commonly used drugs for thrombolysis in acute MI, pulmonary embolism, and acute stroke.

2. Streptokinase: nonenzymatic protein isolated from streptococci

a. Mechanism of action
- Streptokinase acts indirectly by forming an activator complex with plasminogen to form plasmin.
- Action occurs both within thrombi and in circulating blood, leading to lysis of both normal and pathologic thrombi.

b. Antidote: aminocaproic acid or tranexamic acid

3. Urokinase: enzyme derived from cultured human kidney cells

4. Anistreplase
- Acetylated complex containing a combination of streptokinase and human plasminogen
- Preferentially works within the thrombi rather than converting free plasminogen to plasmin

V. Hemostatic Drugs (Box 16-4)

A. Vitamin K
- This fat-soluble vitamin is found in leafy green vegetables.
- It is produced by bacteria that colonize the human intestine and needs bile salts for absorption.
- It is required for γ-carboxylation of glutamate residues in prothrombin (factor II) and factors XII, IX, and X.

1. Uses

a. Prevention of hemorrhagic disease of the newborn (intramuscular or subcutaneous)

b. Treatment of dietary vitamin K deficiencies and reversal of the effect of warfarin (oral or parenteral)

BOX 16-4

HEMOSTATIC DRUGS

Fibrinolytic inhibitors
    Aminocaproic acid
Plasma fractions
Heparin antagonist
    Protamine sulfate
Vitamin K
    Phytonadione

      2. Adverse effects
- Hemolysis, jaundice, and hyperbilirubinemia occasionally occur in newborns.

B. Plasma fractions
- Available as factor VIII concentrate and factor IX concentrate, either from pooled human plasma or as recombinant antihemophilic factor
1. Uses: hemophilias A and B marked by deficiencies of factor VIII and factor IX
2. Adverse effects: risk of acquired immunodeficiency syndrome (AIDS) and hepatitis transmission from concentrated plasma fractions

C. Fibrinolytic inhibitor (aminocaproic acid)
- Use: systemic or urinary hyperfibrinolysis (as in aplastic anemia, abruptio placentae, hepatic cirrhosis)

D. Protamine sulfate
1. Mechanism of action: chemical antagonist of heparin; less effective against LMWHs
2. Use: hemorrhage associated with heparin overdose

Hematopoietic Drugs

TARGET TOPICS

- Treatment of iron deficiency anemia
- Treatment of folate and vitamin B_{12} deficiency anemia
- Treatment of deficiencies in hematopoietic factors

I. General Considerations
   A. Causes of anemia
      1. Failure to produce sufficient red blood cells (RBCs)
      2. Inadequate synthesis of hemoglobin
      3. Destruction of RBCs
   B. Classification of types of anemia by mean corpuscular volume (MCV)
      - Different conditions may lead to the development of the various types of anemia (Table 17-1).
      1. Microcytic: smaller than normal RBCs and decreased MCV ($<80\ \mu m^3$)
         - Iron deficiency results in small RBCs with insufficient hemoglobin (microcytic hypochromic anemia).
      2. Macrocytic: larger than normal RBCs and increased MCV ($>100\ \mu m^3$)
         - Both folic acid deficiency and vitamin B_{12} deficiency cause impaired production and maturation of erythroid precursors (macrocytic hyperchromic or megaloblastic anemia).
      3. Normocytic: normal-sized RBCs and normal MCV ($80–100\ \mu m^3$)
         - Erythropoietin deficiency results in normocytic anemia.
   C. Agents used to treat anemia (Box 17-1)

II. Minerals: Iron
   A. Role of iron
      1. Requirement for the synthesis of hemoglobin and myoglobin
      2. Cofactor in enzymes (cytochromes)
   B. Causes of iron deficiency (see Table 17-1)
   C. Clinical use: iron deficiency anemia
      - Drug of choice: ferrous sulfate
      - Iron dextran: when parenteral administration required

Microcytic anemia due to iron deficiency

Macrocytic anemia due to folic acide or vitamin B_{12} deficiency

Normocytic anemia due to erythropoietin deficiency

TABLE 17-1:
Etiology of Anemia

Types of Anemia	Specific Cause/Pathophysiology
Microcytic Anemia	
Iron deficiency anemia	Increased need (e.g., growth, pregnancy, menstruation) Blood loss (e.g., gastrointestinal bleeding) Inadequate dietary intake Malabsorption
Anemia of chronic disease	Chronic infection, cancer, or liver disease Failure of increase in red blood cell production due to sequestration of iron in reticuloendothelial system
Thalassemia	Hereditary disorder characterized by decreased globulin chain production
Megaloblastic Anemia	
Folic acid deficiency anemia	Inadequate dietary intake Increased need during pregnancy Interference with utilization by other drugs (phenytoin, primidone, and phenobarbital; oral contraceptives; isoniazid) Malabsorption syndromes (e.g., high rates of cell turnover as in hemolytic anemia or alcoholism, or poor liver function)
Vitamin B_{12} deficiency anemia	Pernicious anemia (lack of intrinsic factor [IF]), which may occur following gastrectomy Lack of receptors for IF-vitamin B_{12} complex in ileum Fish tapeworm infestations Crohn's disease/ileotomy
Normocytic Anemia	
Anemia due to bone marrow failure	Myelofibrosis and multiple myeloma: direct effects Myelosuppressive chemotherapy Deficiency of hematopoietic growth factors and hormones (as in chronic renal failure)

D. Adverse effects
   1. Acute toxicity (when given orally): constipation; gastrointestinal (GI) irritation; necrosis; nausea; hematemesis; green, tarry stools
      • In children, acute iron toxicity is seen as acute poisoning.
   2. Chronic toxicity: hemochromatosis

III. Vitamins
   • Both folic acid deficiency and vitamin B_{12} deficiency can lead to hematologic impairment and show hypersegmented polymorphonuclear neutrophils as well as anemia on blood smear.
   A. Folic acid
      1. Role of folic acid
         a. Folic acid is essential for normal DNA synthesis and normal mitosis of proliferating cells.

Acute iron toxicity requires treatment with deferoxamine, an iron chelating drug.

BOX 17-1

HEMATOPOIETIC DRUGS

Minerals

Ferrous sulfate
Iron dextran

Vitamins

Folic acid
Vitamin B_{12}

Hematopoietic Growth Factors

Epoetin alfa
Filgrastim
Oprelvekin
Sargramostim

---

      b. It is readily and completely absorbed from the small intestine by active transport.
  2. Causes of folic acid deficiency (see Table 17-1)
  3. Clinical use
      a. Treatment of folate deficiency
      b. Prophylaxis of neural tube defects (spina bifida) in pregnancy
B. Vitamin B_{12}
  1. Role of vitamin B_{12}
      a. Vitamin B_{12} is essential for normal DNA synthesis (hematopoiesis); it is required to convert 5-methyl THF (dietary form) to tetrahydrofolate (THF), the active folate used in hematopoiesis.

> Neurologic changes may result from vitamin B_{12} deficiency.

      b. It is essential for maintenance of myelin throughout the nervous system.
  2. Causes of vitamin B_{12} deficiency (see Table 17-1)
  3. Tests for vitamin B_{12} deficiency
      a. The Schilling test, which uses radioactive cobalt to test the body's ability to take up vitamin B_{12} from the GI tract
      b. The gastric acidity test and measurement of urinary methylmalonate levels
         • Achlorhydria (lack of gastric acidity) is associated with lack of intrinsic factor.
  4. Pharmacokinetics of vitamin B_{12}
      a. Absorption requires intrinsic factor, a glycoprotein synthesized by the parietal cells of the stomach.
         • Intrinsic factor binds vitamin B_{12}, and the intrinsic factor–vitamin B_{12} complex is absorbed in the ileum.

b. Metabolism involves enterohepatic circulation, and vitamin B_{12} is normally reabsorbed from the small intestine.
  - Depletion of the body's stores of vitamin B_{12} takes 3 to 6 years.
  c. Excretion occurs mainly in bile.
5. Use: vitamin B_{12} deficiency
  a. Vitamin B_{12} is given intramuscularly once a month to patients who cannot absorb it from their diet.
  b. Preferred agent for long-term use: cyanocobalamin

IV. Hematopoietic Growth Factors
  A. Role of hematopoietic growth factors
    - These growth factors control the proliferation and differentiation of pluripotent stem cells.
  B. Causes of bone marrow failure (see Table 17-1)
  C. Drugs used to treat bone marrow failure
    1. Epoetin alfa (erythropoietin)
      - Erythropoietin is a glycoprotein that stimulates RBC production.
      a. Used in patients with chronic renal failure, those with cancer who are receiving chemotherapy, and those with acquired immunodeficiency syndrome (AIDS)
      b. Used illegally by athletes for its performance-enhancing properties
    2. Sargramostim
      - Recombinant granulocyte-macrophage colony-stimulating factor (GM-CSF)
      a. Promotes myeloid recovery in patients with non-Hodgkin's lymphoma, acute lymphoblastic leukemia, and Hodgkin's disease who are undergoing bone marrow transplantation
      b. Promotes myeloid recovery after standard-dose chemotherapy
      c. Treats drug-induced bone marrow toxicity or neutropenia associated with AIDS
    3. Filgrastim
      - Granulocyte colony-stimulating factor (G-CSF)
      a. Prevents and treats chemotherapy-related febrile neutropenia
      b. Promotes myeloid recovery in patients undergoing bone marrow transplantation
    4. Oprelvekin
      - Recombinant human interleukin 11 (IL-11)
      a. Promotes the proliferation of hematopoietic stem cells and megakaryocyte progenitor cells; induces megakaryocyte maturation resulting in increased platelet production
      b. Prevents and treats chemotherapy-induced thrombocytopenia
      c. Reduce the need for platelet transfusions following myelosuppressive chemotherapy for nonmyeloid malignancies

18 CHAPTER

Nonsteroidal Anti-inflammatory Drugs and Other Nonopioid Analgesic-Antipyretic Drugs

TARGET TOPICS

- Aspirin
- Other NSAIDs
- COX-2 inhibitors
- Acetaminophen
- Migraine

I. General Considerations
  A. Nonsteroidal anti-inflammatory drugs (NSAIDs) inhibit the synthesis of eicosanoids from arachidonic acid (Fig. 18-1).
  B. These drugs primarily inhibit cyclooxygenase (COX), the enzyme responsible for the first step of prostaglandin synthesis.
    - COX-1 is constitutively expressed in many tissues, COX-2 is induced in inflammatory cells and is found in endothelial cells, and COX-3 is found in the brain.
    - Aspirin is the only irreversible inhibitor of COX.

II. NSAIDs (Box 18-1)
  A. Aspirin and other salicylates
    - Aspirin (acetylsalicylic acid), the prototype NSAID, is the standard against which all other NSAIDs are measured.
    1. Mechanism of action
      - Many effects of aspirin are due to irreversible inhibition of prostaglandin synthesis through acetylation of both COX-1 and COX-2.

Aspirin is an irreversible inhibitor of COX.

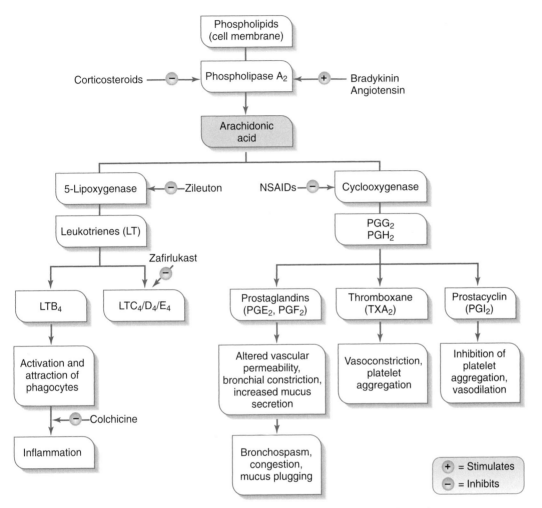

18-1: *Schematic representation of the arachidonic acid pathway, which depicts the mediators formed from arachidonic acid, their biologic function, and drugs that stimulate or inhibit their formation. NSAID, nonsteroidal anti-inflammatory drug.*

   a. Antiplatelet effect: prolonged bleeding time but no change in the other coagulation indicators (e.g., prothrombin time, partial thromboplastin time)
   b. Antithrombotic effect: inhibition of thromboxane synthesis (potent platelet aggregator and vasoconstrictor) via irreversible inhibition of platelet COX that lasts for the life span of platelets, or about 8 days (see Chapter 16)
2. Uses
   a. Fever, acute rheumatic fever, headache, mild pain, dysmenorrhea
   b. Inflammatory conditions such as osteoarthritis and rheumatoid arthritis
   c. Prevention of platelet aggregation in coronary artery disease, myocardial infarction, atrial fibrillation, postoperative deep vein thrombosis

Aspirin is the only NSAID without a BLACK BOX warning of increased cardiovascular events with prolonged use.

BOX 18-1

NONSTEROIDAL ANTI-INFLAMMATORY DRUGS (NSAIDS) AND OTHER NONOPIOID ANALGESICS

NSAIDs
Aspirin
Diclofenac
Ibuprofen
Indomethacin
Ketoprofen
Ketorolac (parenteral)
Naproxen
Oxaprozin
Piroxicam
Sulindac

COX-2 Inhibitors (Selective NSAIDs)
Celecoxib
Rofecoxib (removed from market)
Valdecoxib (removed from market)

Nonopioid and Non-NSAID Analgesics
Acetaminophen

---

3. Adverse effects
    a. Gastric irritation, gastrointestinal (GI) bleeding, peptic ulcer disease
        • Occurs to some degree with the use of all NSAIDs
    b. Salicylism (tinnitus, vertigo leading to deafness) with overdose (see Chapter 30)
        • Reversible with dosage reduction
    c. Respiratory alkalosis followed by an anion gap metabolic acidosis
    d. Renal failure
        • Possibly due to decrease in prostaglandin E_2 or I_2 production, which leads to acute tubular necrosis
4. Contraindications
    a. Hypersensitivity reactions
        • Occurrence in patients with aspirin-induced nasal polyps leads to urticaria and bronchoconstriction (aspirin-induced asthma); due to abnormal leukotriene production (treated with zafirlukast)
    b. Hemophilia
    c. Risk of Reye's syndrome
        • Aspirin should *not* be given to children with viral infections; use acetaminophen as an acceptable substitute.
B. Other nonselective NSAIDs
    • Examples: ibuprofen, naproxen, sulindac, piroxicam, indomethacin, ketorolac
    • The major differences among these agents involve duration of action and potency.
    • The Food and Drug Administration issued a warning that long-term use of a nonselective NSAID, such as naproxen and other NSAIDs, may be associated with an increased cardiovascular (CV) risk compared to placebo; likely due to effects on kidney, decreasing renal blood flow.

Patients with aspirin-induced nasal polyps or with allergic reactions (e.g., urticaria) to aspirin are at risk of developing bronchoconstriction or anaphylaxis and should not receive aspirin or other NSAIDs.

Drug of choice in children with fever: acetaminophen

1. Mechanism of action
   a. These NSAIDs reversibly bind to both COX-1 and COX-2, exhibiting antipyretic, analgesic, and anti-inflammatory effects that are similar to aspirin.
   b. Antipyretic effects involve blocking the production of prostaglandins in the central nervous system to reset the hypothalamic temperature control, facilitating heat dissipation by vasodilation.
2. Uses
   a. Mild to moderate pain, bone and joint trauma, inflammatory syndromes (e.g., rheumatoid arthritis, gout)
   b. Fever
   c. Closure of patent ductus arteriosus: indomethacin

   > Ketorolac is often used parenterally for postoperative pain.

3. Adverse effects
   a. Gastric upset and GI bleeding, due in part to inhibited synthesis of prostaglandins, which are protective in the GI tract
   b. Possibly decreased renal function, especially in patients with underlying renal disease, leading to renal failure (e.g., acute tubular necrosis)
   c. Risk of premature closure of patent ductus arteriosus in the fetus
      • Use after 20 weeks of pregnancy is *not* recommended.

C. COX-2 inhibitors
   • Examples: celecoxib, rofecoxib, valdecoxib
   • The Food and Drug Administration issued a warning in late 2004 that the COX-2 inhibitors may be associated with an increased risk of serious cardiovascular events (heart attack and stroke), especially when used chronically or in very high risk settings (e.g., after open heart surgery); rofecoxib and valdecoxib have been removed from the market.
   1. Mechanism of action: selective inhibition of COX-2
      • In contrast, most other NSAIDs are nonselective COX-1 and COX-2 inhibitors.

      > There is a lower incidence of life-threatening bleeds with the selective COX-2 inhibitors.

   2. Uses: rheumatic arthritis, osteoarthritis, acute pain, dysmenorrhea
   3. Adverse effects: GI bleeding, renal failure
      • Compared with other NSAIDs, COX-2 inhibitors have a lower incidence of gastrointestinal adverse effects.
      • Cyclooxygenase-2 (COX-2) is the isoform found in endothelial cells required for PGI_2 production; its inhibition is the likely cause of increased cardiovascular events.

      > The selective COX-2 inhibitors increase the TXA_2/PGI_2 ratio to an unfavorable balance.

III. Acetaminophen
   • Acetaminophen has no anti-inflammatory activity, although it has analgesic and antipyretic effects similar to those of aspirin.
   A. Mechanism of action: unknown but some evidence that it inhibits COX-3 in the brain
   B. Uses: osteoarthritis (pain), acute pain syndromes, fever
   C. Adverse effects
      • Acetaminophen neither produces gastric irritation nor affects platelet function.

      > Drug of choice for analgesic treatment of the elderly

---

BOX 18-2

DRUGS USED TO TREAT MIGRAINE HEADACHE

Treatment of an Acute Attack
Dihydroergotamine
Eletriptan
Ergotamine
Frovatriptan
Naratriptan
Rizatriptan
Sumatriptan
Zolmitriptan

Analgesics Used to Treat the Pain
Acetaminophen
Aspirin
Butorphanol (intranasally)
Codeine
Ibuprofen
Ketorolac
Naproxen

Drugs Used for Migraine Prophylaxis
Amitriptyline
Methysergide
Propranolol
Topiramate
Valproic acid
Verapamil

---

    1. Hepatic necrosis is the most serious result of acute overdose.
    2. Acetylcysteine is used to prevent hepatotoxicity after acute overdose (see Table 30-2).

IV. Drugs Used to Treat Migraine Headache (Box 18-2)
  A. Migraine has two phases:
    • First phase is vasoconstriction of intracranial arteries, associated with the prodrome of the attack (aura).
    • Second phase is vasodilation of the extracranial arteries during which headache occurs.
  B. Treatment of migraine
    1. Drugs for symptomatic treatment
      a. Sumatriptan is the prototype drug.
        (1) Mechanism of action

Note the common ending -triptan for $5\text{-}HT_{1D}$ agonists.

- Highly selective agonist of 5-HT$_{1D}$ (5-hydroxytryptamine) receptors
- The drug is not an analgesic; direct vasoconstriction is responsible for the decrease of pain.

(2) Adverse effects
- Coronary artery vasospasm, arrhythmias, cardiac arrest
- Cerebral vasospasm
- Peripheral vascular ischemia and bowel ischemia

(3) Contraindications
- Breastfeeding
- Cardiac disease
- Cerebrovascular disease
- Coronary artery disease
- Pregnancy
- Renal impairment
- Tobacco smoking

b. Ergotamine and dihydroergotamine
(1) Bind to 5-HT$_{1D}$ receptors, but not as specific as the -triptans
(2) Administered orally or by inhalation, sublingual, or by parenteral routes
(3) Adverse effects: due to vasoconstriction
(4) Contraindications: peripheral vascular disease, ischemic heart disease, peptic ulcers, pregnancy

c. Analgesics used to treat the pain (see Box 18-2)
d. Drugs for migraine prophylaxis (see Box 18-2)
- Decrease the occurrence of acute attacks
- No uniform medication for prophylaxis

(1) Beta blockers (see Chapter 5)
(2) Calcium channel blockers (see Chapter 12)
(3) Antidepressants (see Chapter 10)
(4) Anticonvulsants (see Chapter 9)
(5) Methysergide

All the other "triptans" are similar to sumatriptan, with slightly different pharmacokinetics and adverse effect profile.

Response to dihydroergotamine is diagnostic for migraine headache.

Opioid Analgesics and Antagonists

TARGET TOPICS

- Strong opioid agonists
- Moderate opioid agonists
- Mixed opioid agonists-antagonists
- Opioid antagonists

I. Opioid Agonists (Box 19-1)
- Opioid agonists are classified into three categories: strong, moderate, and weak.
  A. General features
   1. Mechanism of action
      - The effects of endogenous opioid peptides (endorphins and enkephalins) and exogenous opioids result from activation of specific opioid receptors (Table 19-1).
      - The major subtypes of opioid receptors—delta (δ), kappa (κ), and mu (μ)—have varying effects (Table 19-2).
   2. Pharmacologic actions of opioid agonists (Box 19-2)
   3. Uses
      a. Relief of severe pain
      b. Sedation and relief from anxiety (e.g., preoperatively)
      c. Cough suppression
      d. Diarrhea suppression
   4. Adverse effects (primarily extensions of pharmacologic actions)
      a. Respiratory depression and coma
      b. Sedation and central nervous system (CNS) depression
      c. Miosis
      d. Nausea and vomiting (stimulation of chemosensitive trigger zone, CTZ)
      e. Constipation
      f. Acute postural hypotension (histamine release)
      g. Miosis ("pinpoint pupil")
      h. Elevated intracranial pressure
         - Increased CO_2 → vasodilation → increased cerebral blood flow → increased intracranial pressure
      i. Abuse, physical and psychological dependence

Respiratory and CNS depression: most important adverse effects of opioid analgesics

Triad of respiratory depression, coma, and "pinpoint pupil" is classical sign of opioid overdose.

BOX 19-1

OPIOID AGONISTS

Strong Opioid Agonists

Fentanyl
Meperidine
Methadone
Morphine

Moderate Opioid Agonists

Codeine
Hydrocodone
Oxycodone

Weak Opioid Agonists

Dextromethorphan
Diphenoxylate
Loperamide
Propoxyphene
Tramadol

TABLE 19-1:
Effects of Representative Opioids on Opioid Receptor Subtypes

RECEPTOR SUBTYPE			
Opioid	Mu (μ)	Delta (δ)	Kappa (κ)
Buprenorphine	Partial agonist		Antagonist
Butorphanol	Partial agonist		Agonist
Codeine	Weak agonist	Weak agonist	Weak agnoist
Fentanyl	Agonist		Weak agnoist
Meperidine	Agonist		Strong agnoist
Morphine	Agonist	Weak agonist	Weak agonist
Nalbuphine	Antagonist		Agonist
Nalmefene	Antagonist	Antagonist	Antagonist
Naloxone	Antagonist	Antagonist	Antagonist
Naltrexone	Antagonist	Antagonist	Antagonist
Pentazocine	Partial agonist		Agonist

TABLE 19-2:
Opioid Receptors and Their Associated Effects

Receptor	Effects of Activation
Mu (μ) receptor	Analgesia, euphoria, respiratory depression, miosis, decreased gastrointestinal motility, and physical dependence
Kappa (κ) receptor	Analgesia, miosis, respiratory depression, dysphoria, and some psychomimetic effects
Delta (δ) receptor	Analgesia (spinal and supraspinal)

BOX 19-2

PHARMACOLOGIC ACTIONS OF OPIOID AGONISTS

Central Nervous System Effects

Analgesia
Euphoria or dysphoria
Inhibition of cough reflex
Miosis (pinpoint pupils)
Physical dependence
Respiratory depression (inhibit respiratory center in medulla)
Sedation

Cardiovascular Effects

Decreased myocardial oxygen demand
Vasodilation and orthostatic hypotension (histamine release)

Gastrointestinal and Biliary Effects

Decreased gastric motility and constipation (increased muscle tone leads to
 diminished propulsive peristalsis in colon)
Biliary colic from increased sphincter tone and pressure
Nausea and vomiting (from direct stimulation of chemoreceptor trigger zone)

Genitourinary Effects

Increased bladder sphincter tone
Increased urine retention

---

j. Abstinence syndrome on withdrawal of the drug
   • Symptoms and treatment of opioid overdose (see Chapter 30)
B. Specific opioid agonists
   1. Morphine
      • Morphine is the prototype opioid agonist, the standard against which all
        other analgesics are measured.
      a. Administration: intravenous, intramuscular, or buccal (the drug is less
         effective orally; oral-extended release products are used)
      b. Primary use: relief of severe pain associated with trauma, myocardial
         infarction (MI), or cancer
         • Other use: acute pulmonary edema to reduce perception of shortness
           of breath, anxiety, and cardiac preload and afterload
   2. Codeine
      a. Relative to morphine: less potent and less likely to cause physical
         dependence
      b. Codeine and codeine derivatives do not bind to μ receptors; They have
         to be metabolized to the corresponding morphine derivative.

Morphine: high first-pass
effect

Codeine is the most
constipating opioid.

c. Primary use: antitussive agent
- Other use: analgesic (mild to moderate pain; commonly given in combination with aspirin or acetaminophen)

3. Meperidine
    a. Uses
        (1) The Agency for Health Care Policy and Research Clinical Practice: Meperidine is recommended for use only in very brief courses in patients who are healthy or have problems with other opiate agonists; it is considered a second-line agent for the treatment of acute pain.
        (2) Obstetric analgesia (may prolong labor)
        (3) Acute pain syndromes, such as MI, neuralgia, painful procedures (short-term treatment)
        (4) Used to interrupt postoperative shivering and shaking chills caused by amphotericin B
    b. Specific adverse effect: anxiety and seizures due to accumulation of a metabolite (normeperidine)

4. Methadone
    a. Relative to morphine: longer duration of action and milder withdrawal symptoms
    b. Uses
        (1) Maintenance therapy for heroin addicts
        (2) Control of withdrawal symptoms from opioids
        (3) Neuropathic pain

5. Fentanyl and its derivatives
    - Available as long-acting transdermal patch for continuous pain relief
    a. Relative to morphine: less nausea
    b. Uses: Anesthesia, in some cases (cardiovascular surgery)
        - Other drugs for anesthesia: alfentanil and sufentanil

6. Tramadol
    a. Mechanism of action
        - Tramadol is a μ receptor partial agonist that also inhibits neuronal reuptake of norepinephrine and serotonin.
    b. Uses: acute and chronic pain syndromes
    c. Adverse effect: decreased seizure threshold

7. Loperamide and diphenoxylate
    - Drugs with minimal analgesic activity; used in the treatment of diarrhea

8. Dextromethorphan
    - Drug with minimal analgesic activity; used as an antitussive agent

9. Propoxyphene
    - Weak opioid agonist on the μ receptor, often combined with acetaminophen or aspirin

II. Mixed Opioid Agonists-Antagonists (Box 19-3)
    A. General considerations
        1. React with a particular receptor subtype (e.g., strong κ but weak μ agonist)

Fluoxetine and some other SSRIs inhibit CYP2D6 and prevent the bioactivation of codeine, hydrocodone, and oxycodone.

Use meperidine, rather than morphine, for pancreatitis; it produces less spasm of the sphincter of Oddi.

Meperidine is contraindicated to take with monoamine oxidase inhibitors (tranylcypromine, phenelzine).

Fentanyl is available as transdermal patches, lozenges, and lollipops.

Tramadol is used for neuropathic pain.

Atropine is added to diphenoxylate to deter abuse.

Propoxyphene is often overused in the geriatric population.

Partial agonists of the μ receptor may precipitate withdrawal reaction in opioid addicts.

> ### BOX 19-3
>
> **MIXED OPIOID AGONISTS-ANTAGONISTS**
>
> Buprenorphine
> Butorphanol
> Nalbuphine
> Pentazocine

> ### BOX 19-4
>
> **OPIOID ANTAGONISTS**
>
> Nalmefene
> Naloxone
> Naltrexone

    2. Effective analgesics
    3. Respiratory depressant effects do not rise proportionately with increasing doses.
    4. Associated with a much lower risk of drug dependence than morphine
  B. Buprenorphine (partial agonist on the μ receptor)
    1. Used for relief of moderate or severe pain
    2. Maintenance for opioid-dependent patients
  C. Butorphanol (κ agonist)
    • Uses: pain relief (parenterally), migraine headaches (nasal spray)
  D. Nalbuphine (κ agonist, μ antagonist)
    1. Used for relief of moderate to severe pain associated with acute and chronic disorders such as cancer, renal or biliary colic, and migraine or vascular headaches, as well as surgery
    2. Used as obstetric analgesia during labor and delivery
  E. Pentazocine (κ agonist): oldest mixed opioid agonist-antagonist
    1. Used for relief of moderate to severe pain
    2. CNS effects such as disorientation and hallucinations limit use.

III. Opioid Antagonists (Box 19-4)
  A. Mechanism of action: competition with opioid agonists for μ receptors to rapidly reverse the effects of morphine and other opioid agonists
  B. Uses
    1. Treatment of opioid overdose
    2. Precipitation of a withdrawal syndrome when given to chronic users of opioid drugs

20 **CHAPTER**

Drugs Used in the Treatment of Asthma and Chronic Obstructive Pulmonary Disease and Allergies

TARGET TOPICS

- Pharmacotherapy of asthma
- Use of anti-inflammatory drugs in the treatment of asthma and COPD
- Use of bronchodilators in the treatment of asthma and COPD
- Drugs used in the treatment of allergies

I. General Considerations
   A. Asthma
   - Asthma is an obstructive airway disorder resulting from smooth muscle hypertrophy, bronchospasm, increased mucus secretion, and mucosal edema.
   1. Both nonimmunogenic (Box 20-1) and immunogenic factors (Fig. 20-1) play a role in the pathogenesis of asthma.
      - Drug therapy, which includes anti-inflammatory agents and bronchodilators, affects these factors.
   2. Clinical symptoms include episodic bouts of coughing associated with dyspnea, wheezing, and chest tightness.
   3. A variety of drugs are used in the pharmacotherapy of asthma (Table 20-1).

BOX 20-1

FACTORS THAT MAY CAUSE ASTHMA

Viral infections
Environmental pollutants
  Ozone
  Nitrogen dioxide
Pharmacologic stimuli
  Aspirin
  β-Adrenergic receptor antagonists
  Dyes in food and medications

Occupational factors
  Metal salts
  Wood, animal, and insect dust
Exercise
Emotional stress
Immunogenic factors

TABLE 20-1: Asthma Pharmacotherapy

Drug Type	Example	Use
Daily Medications for Long-Term Control		
Inhaled corticosteroids	Beclomethasone	First-line treatment
Systemic corticosteroids	Betamethasone	Used to gain prompt control when initiating long-term inhaled corticosteroids
Mast cell stabilizers	Cromolyn	May be initial choice in children Also used as prevention before exercise or allergen exposure
Long-acting β_2-receptor agonist	Salmeterol	Given concomitantly with anti-inflammatory agents Not used for acute symptoms
Methylxanthines	Theophylline	Adjunct to inhaled corticosteroids
Leukotriene inhibitors	Zafirlukast	Prophylaxis and long-term management (alone or in combination)
"Rescue" Medications Useful in Acute Episode		
Short-acting β_2-receptor agonists	Albuterol	First choice for acute symptoms Prevention of exercise-induced bronchospasm Should be prescribed for all patients
Anticholinergic	Ipratropium	Additive benefit to inhaled β_2-receptor agonists in severe exacerbations Alternative for patients intolerant to β_2-receptor agonists

    B. Chronic obstructive pulmonary disease (COPD)
      • This progressive obstructive airway disorder, which usually results from smoking, is marked by airway reactivity.
      1. COPD involves chronic bronchitis and emphysema.
      2. Clinical symptoms include chronic cough with sputum production and dyspnea.

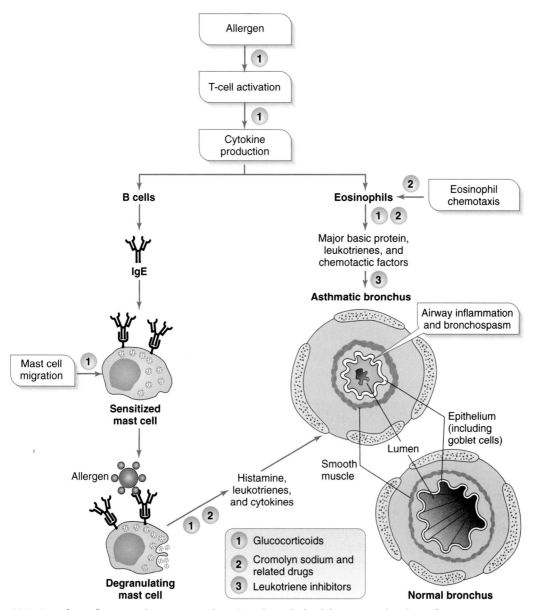

20-1: Sites of anti-inflammatory drug action in asthma. Cromolyn and related drugs prevent the release of mediators from mast cells and eosinophils. IgE, immunoglobin E.

II. Anti-inflammatory Agents Used to Treat Asthma (Box 20-2; see also Fig. 20-1)

   A. Corticosteroids

      1. Mechanism of action

         • Corticosteroids generally inhibit the inflammatory response, thereby preventing bronchoconstriction and producing smooth muscle relaxation.

BOX 20-2

ANTI-INFLAMMATORY AGENTS

Inhaled Corticosteroids

Beclomethasone
Budesonide
Flunisolide
Fluticasone
Triamcinolone

Oral Corticosteroids

Betamethasone
Methylprednisolone
Prednisone
Triamcinolone

Mast Cell Stabilizers

Cromolyn
Nedocromil

Leukotriene Inhibitors

Montelukast
Zafirlukast

Monoclonal Antibody

Omalizumab

---

a. Inhibition of the release of arachidonic acid by increasing the synthesis of lipocortin, which inhibits phospholipase A_2 activity

b. Decreased synthesis of cyclooxygenase-2 (COX-2), an inducible form of COX in inflammatory cells

c. Inhibition of the production of cytokines involved in the inflammatory cascade (interferon-γ, interleukin 1, interleukin 2)

d. Effect on the concentration, distribution, and function of peripheral leukocytes, increasing the concentration of neutrophils and decreasing the concentration of granulocytes, lymphocytes, and monocytes

2. Uses

a. Mild or moderate asthma or COPD (first-line therapy; maintenance therapy)
   • Inhaled steroids

b. Severe airway obstruction despite optimal bronchodilator therapy
   • Systemic (oral or intravenous) steroids

c. Asthma or COPD
   • Combination therapy with selective β_2-adrenergic receptor agonists such as salmeterol

d. Emergency treatment (parenteral) of severe asthma or COPD if bronchodilators do not resolve the airway obstruction
   • See Chapter 22 for the discussion of the use of these agents in rheumatic disorders.

3. Adverse effects: iatrogenic Cushing's syndrome, diabetes mellitus, hypertension, peptic ulcer disease, hypomania, psychosis, adrenal insufficiency on abrupt cessation of therapy (see Chapter 22)

Inhaled corticosteroids: fewer side effects than systemic corticosteroids

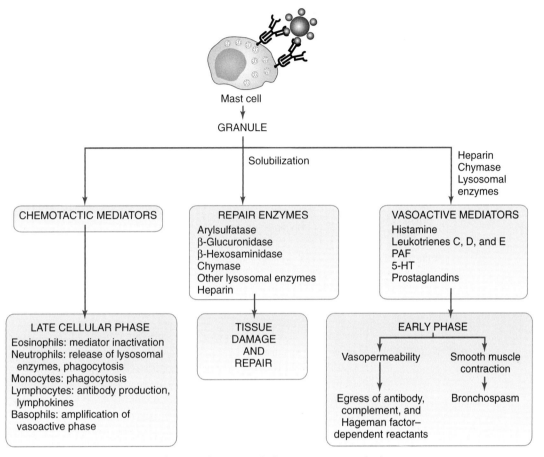

20-2: *Early-phase and late-phase responses in asthma. 5-HT, 5-hydroxytryptamine; PAF, platelet activating factor.*

- To prevent adrenal insufficiency, patients who have been receiving oral corticosteroid treatment for longer than 1 week should be given diminishing doses.

B. Mast cell stabilizers
  - Examples: cromolyn, nedocromil
  1. Pharmacokinetics
     - Administration in the form of an aerosol before exposure to agents that trigger asthma
  2. Mechanism of action (Fig. 20-2)
     a. Stabilize the plasma membranes of mast cells and eosinophils, preventing release of histamine, leukotrienes, and other mediators of airway inflammation
     b. Decrease activation of airway nerves (nedocromil)

Taper the dose of oral corticosteroids in patients who have been taking the drug for longer than 1 week.

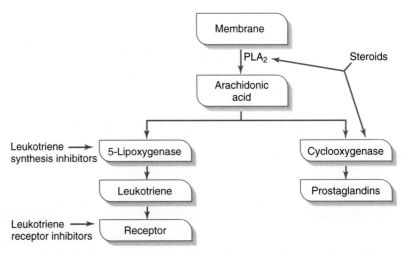

20-3: *Role of prostaglandins and leukotrienes in asthma. Zileuton is a leukotriene synthesis inhibitor. Zafirlukast is a leukotriene receptor inhibitor. PLA₂, Phospholipase A₂.*

3. Uses
   a. Prevention of asthmatic episodes, such as before exercise or in cold weather (primary use)
     • Less effective in reducing bronchial reactivity in acute settings
   b. Prevention of allergic rhinitis and seasonal conjunctivitis (*not* first-line agents)
4. Adverse effects: nausea, vomiting, dysgeusia (bad taste in mouth), cough
C. Leukotriene inhibitors
  1. Leukotriene synthesis inhibitor
   • Example: zileuton (discontinued)
   • Mechanism of action: selective inhibitor of 5-lipoxygenase, which catalyzes leukotriene formation (Fig. 20-3; see also Fig. 20-1)
  2. Leukotriene receptor antagonists
   • Examples: zafirlukast, montelukast
   a. Pharmacokinetics: oral administration
   b. Mechanism of action (see Figs. 20-1 and 20-3): selective inhibition of binding of leukotrienes to their receptors, reducing the airway inflammation that leads to edema, bronchoconstriction, and mucus secretion
   c. Uses
    (1) Control of chronic asthma
    (2) Not effective in acute bronchospasm
   d. Adverse effects: headache, gastritis, upper respiratory tract symptoms (e.g., flu-like symptoms)
   e. Drug interactions
    • Zafirlukast inhibits the activity of the cytochrome P-450 system.
D. Monoclonal antibody
  • Example: omalizumab

Note the common ending: -lukast

Leukotriene inhibitors are used prophylactically.

BOX 20-3

BRONCHODILATORS

Methylxanthines
Aminophylline
Theophylline

β₂-Adrenergic Receptor Agonists
Albuterol
Formoterol
Levalbuterol
Metaproterenol
Pirbuterol
Salmeterol
Terbutaline

Anticholinergic Drugs
Ipratropium
Tiotropium

- Pharmacokinetics: administered subcutaneously every 2 to 4 weeks
- Mechanism of action: binds to IgE's high affinity Fc receptor (FcεRI), on cells associated with the allergic response, lowering free serum IgE concentrations and preventing degranulation
- Uses: treatment of moderate to severe allergic asthma triggered by responses to allergens such as pollen, mold, dust mites, pet dander

III. Bronchodilators (Box 20-3)
    A. $β_2$-Adrenergic receptor agonists: general considerations (see Chapter 5)
        • Examples: albuterol, terbutaline, salmeterol
        1. Pharmacokinetics
          a. Administration: via a metered-dose inhaler or nebulizer, which has the greatest local effect on airway smooth muscle with the fewest systemic adverse effects
          b. Duration of action
            • Rapid-acting agents attain their maximal effect in 30 minutes.
            • Action persists for 3 to 4 hours.
        2. Mechanism of action (Fig. 20-4)
          • These potent bronchodilators (see Fig. 20-1) relax smooth muscle by activation of adenylyl cyclase, increasing cyclic adenosine monophosphate (cAMP) levels via β receptors.
        3. Uses
          a. Treatment of acute asthma attacks
          b. Prevention or treatment of bronchospasm caused by asthma or COPD

$β_2$-Receptor agonists: the only bronchodilators used to counteract acute asthma attacks

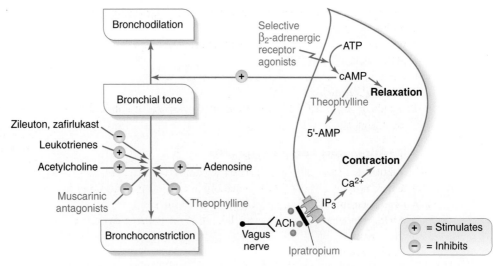

20-4: *Mechanism of action of bronchodilators. ACh, acetylcholine; 5'-AMP, 5'-adenosine monophosphate; ATP, adenosine triphosphate; cAMP, cyclic adenosine monophosphate; IP₃, inositol triphosphate.*

    c. Asthma prophylaxis (oral albuterol, metaproterenol)

    d. Emergency treatment of severe bronchospasm (subcutaneous terbutaline)

    e. Delay of premature labor (terbutaline; see Chapter 26)

  4. Adverse effects

    • Systemic adverse effects occur with overdose.

    • Many of these systemic effects are related to activation of the sympathetic nervous system, such as tachycardia, palpitations, anxiety, excitability, tremor, hyperglycemia, and hypokalemia.

B. β₂-Adrenergic receptor agonists: specific drugs

  1. Salmeterol: longer acting drug (12 hours)

    • Should *not* be used to treat acute asthma attacks

  2. Levalbuterol: R-isomer and active form of racemic albuterol

    • Inhalant with fewer central nervous system (CNS) and cardiac side effects

C. Epinephrine

  • Used in emergency settings as subcutaneous injection or microaerosol for rapid bronchodilation in severe airway obstruction (see Chapter 5)

D. Methylxanthines

  • Examples: theophylline, aminophylline

  1. Pharmacokinetics

    • Decreasing hepatic function and drugs that inhibit the cytochrome P-450 system (e.g., beta blockers, erythromycin, fluoroquinolones) increase the half-life ($t_{1/2}$) of theophylline.

    • Drugs that induce the cytochrome P-450 system (e.g., barbiturates, phenytoin, rifampin) hasten the elimination of theophylline.

  2. Mechanism of action (see Fig. 20-4)

Albuterol is a "rescue" medication.

The $t_{1/2}$ of theophylline is decreased in adults who smoke and in children.

      a. Antagonize adenosine receptors and affect intracellular calcium in smooth muscle cells

      b. Inhibit phosphodiesterase, an enzyme that catalyzes degradation of cAMP

         • The inhibition of phosphodiesterase probably causes bronchodilation.

      c. Other effects include CNS stimulation, cardiovascular action, and diuresis (slight).

   3. Uses

      a. Adjunctive treatment of acute asthma

      b. Prevention of bronchospasm associated with asthma or COPD

   4. Adverse effects: gastrointestinal (GI) irritation, headache, anxiety, diuresis, palpitations, premature ventricular contractions, seizures

   5. Precautions: patients with heart disease, liver disorders, seizure disorders, peptic ulcer disease

  E. Anticholinergic agents

    • Examples: ipratropium, tiotropium (muscarinic receptor antagonist; see Chapter 4)

   1. Pharmacokinetics

    • Administration via aerosol for local effects at muscarinic receptors in the airway

   2. Mechanism of action: blockade of the effects of vagus nerve stimulation

   3. Uses

      a. Prevention of bronchoconstriction in COPD (often given in combination with β_2-adrenergic receptor agonists)

      b. Treatment of asthma (less effective than β_2-adrenergic receptor agonists)

      c. Tiotropium can be given once a day for the maintenance treatment of COPD.

   4. Adverse effects: airway irritation, anticholinergic effects, GI upset, xerostomia, urinary retention, increased ocular pressure

IV. Antihistamines Used in the Treatment of Allergies (Box 20-4)

  A. H_1 antagonists

   1. Pharmacokinetics

      a. These antihistamines are available orally and topically and have short effective half-lives of 4 to 6 hours.

      b. First-generation antihistamines cross the blood-brain barrier and produce sedation.

      c. The second-generation antihistamines have less propensity to cross the blood-brain barrier and cause sedation.

   2. Pharmacodynamics

      a. Competitive blockers of H_1 receptors to reduce edema and itching

      b. No profound effect on gastric acid secretions in contrast to H_2 blockers

   3. Adverse effects

      a. CNS: sedation (first generation)

      b. GI: nausea, vomiting, constipation, diarrhea

      c. Atropine-like effects (first generation)

Theophylline has a narrow therapeutic index; levels need to be monitored closely when therapy is initiated.

First generation: diphenhydramine; dimenhydrinate; chlorpheniramine; tripelennamine; second generation: fexofenadine; loratadine; cetirizine, desloratadine

Second-generation antihistamines are often referred to as "nonsedating" antihistamines.

BOX 20-4

ANTIHISTAMINES USED IN THE TREATMENT OF ALLERGIES

First-Generation Antihistamines

Chlorpheniramine
Dimenhydrinate
Diphenhydramine
Hydroxyzine
Meclizine
Promethazine

Second-Generation Antihistamines

Cetirizine
Desloratadine
Fexofenadine
Loratadine

---

4. Uses
   a. Treatment of allergic reactions
   b. Motion sickness (dimenhydrinate, promethazine, meclizine, and hydroxyzine)
   c. Over-the-counter sleeping medications (diphenhydramine)
   d. Treatment of nausea and vomiting (promethazine)
5. Precautions
   a. Machine operation should be curtailed as drowsiness is common (first generation).
   b. Sedative effect is cumulative with other CNS sedative drugs (first generation).

Drugs Used in the Treatment of Gastrointestinal Disorders

TARGET TOPICS

- Treatment of peptic disorders
- Treatment of diarrhea
- Prokinetic drugs
- Treatment of nausea and vomiting
- Treatment of inflammatory bowel disease
- Treatment of constipation

I. Peptic Disorders
  - This group of disorders includes ulcers of the stomach, esophagus, and duodenum; Zollinger-Ellison syndrome; gastroesophageal reflux disease (GERD); gastritis; and esophagitis.
  - Physiologic stimulants of gastric acid secretion include gastrin, acetylcholine, and histamine acting on histamine H_2-receptors.

II. Drugs That Decrease Gastric Acidity (Box 21-1)
  A. Histamine H_2-receptor antagonists
    1. Cimetidine
      a. Mechanism of action
        (1) Blocks histamine action at the H_2-receptor site on parietal cells, thus inhibiting gastric acid secretion (Fig. 21-1)
        (2) Decreases production of pepsin
        (3) Inhibits postprandial and basal gastric acid secretion
      b. Uses
        (1) Healing of duodenal and gastric ulcers and prevention of their recurrence
          - Intractable peptic ulcers may require higher doses or combination therapy.
        (2) Control of secretory conditions such as Zollinger-Ellison syndrome and GERD
      c. Adverse effects: antiandrogenic effects (gynecomastia and male sexual dysfunction)

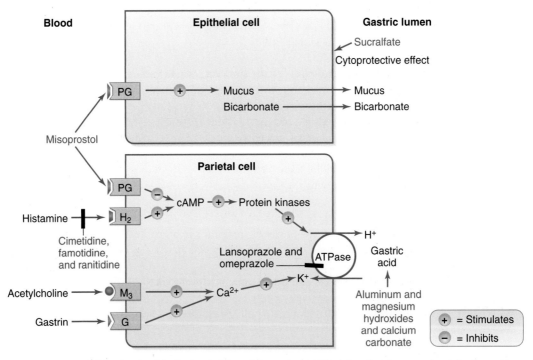

21-1: *Gastric acid secretion and sites of drug action. cAMP, cyclic adenosine monophosphate; G, gastrin receptor; H₂, histamine H₂-receptor; M₃, muscarinic M₃ receptor; PG, prostaglandin receptor.*

d. Drug interactions: inhibition of liver microsomal metabolism of many drugs that utilize the cytochrome P-450 system (e.g., beta blockers, benzodiazepines, calcium channel blockers, opioid agonists, tricyclic antidepressants)

2. Other H_2-receptor antagonists
   - Examples: ranitidine, famotidine, nizatidine
   - Therapeutic effects are similar to cimetidine.
   - Drug interactions and antiandrogenic effects occur less commonly than with cimetidine.
   a. All three are more potent than cimetidine.
      (1) Use: treatment of duodenal ulcers associated with *Helicobacter pylori* (given with a bismuth compound and an antibiotic)
      (2) Adverse effect: thrombocytopenia
   b. Famotidine: most potent H_2-receptor antagonist

B. Proton pump inhibitors (PPI) (see Box 21-1)
   - Examples: omeprazole, lansoprazole
   1. Mechanism of action
      a. Intragastric pH is higher and remains elevated longer than with H_2-receptor antagonist therapy.
      b. Proton pump inhibitors suppress gastric acid secretion by inhibiting the proton pump, $H^+/K^+/ATPase$, in parietal cells (see Fig. 21-1).
      c. After activation, omeprazole binds irreversibly to the proton pump on the secretory surface of parietal cells.
   2. Uses
      a. Drugs of choice for Zollinger-Ellison syndrome resulting from gastrin-secreting tumors
      b. Most effective agents for GERD
      c. Duodenal ulcer, esophagitis, and gastric ulcer
         (1) When used to treat peptic ulcer disease, these drugs promote healing, but relapse may occur.
         (2) Proton pump inhibitors must be given in combination with agents that eliminate *H. pylori*.

C. Antacids: weak bases
   - Examples: sodium bicarbonate, aluminum hydroxide, magnesium hydroxide, calcium carbonate
   1. Mechanism of action: neutralize gastric hydrochloric acid and generally raise stomach pH from 1 to 3.0 to 3.5
   2. Uses: symptomatic relief of acid indigestion, heartburn, GERD

III. Cytoprotective Agents (Box 21-2)
   A. Sucralfate
      1. Pharmacokinetics
         a. Poorly soluble molecule that polymerizes in acid environment
         b. No significant absorption and no systemic effect
      2. Mechanism of action
         a. Selectively binds to necrotic ulcer tissue and acts as barrier to acid, pepsin, and bile, allowing duodenal ulcers time to heal

---

Cimetidine extends the half-life ($t_{1/2}$) of many drugs that are metabolized in the liver.

Note common ending -tidine for all H_2-receptor antagonists

H_2-receptor blockade: over 90% reduction in basal, food-stimulated, and nocturnal gastric acid secretion

Note common ending -prazol to all PPIs

Proton pump inhibitors are more effective than H_2-receptor blockers for treatment of peptic ulcer disease and GERD.

Magnesium salts produce diarrhea while aluminum and calcium salts produce constipation.

Antacids affect the absorption of many drugs, such as fluoroquinolones and tetracycline.

BOX 21-2

CYTOPROTECTIVE DRUGS

Sucralfate

Prostaglandin analogues (e.g., misoprostol)

Colloidal bismuth compounds (e.g., bismuth subsalicylate)

Sucralfate requires acid pH for activation and should not be administered with antacids or H$_2$-receptor antagonists.

    b. Stimulates synthesis of prostaglandins, which have cytoprotective effects on the gastrointestinal tract

  3. Uses

    a. Treatment of active peptic ulcer disease

    b. Suppression of recurrence

B. Misoprostol: synthetic, oral prostaglandin E$_1$ analogue

  1. Mechanism of action

    a. Inhibits secretion of gastrin

    b. Promotes secretion of mucus and bicarbonate

  2. Use: prevention of nonsteroidal anti-inflammatory drug (NSAID) and steroid-induced gastric ulcers

  3. Contraindication: pregnancy (can induce labor and uterine rupture)

C. Colloidal bismuth compounds

  • Example: bismuth subsalicylate

  1. Mechanism of action: selective binding to ulcer coating, thereby protecting the ulcer from gastric acid

  2. Uses

    a. Control of nonspecific diarrhea

    b. Prophylaxis of traveler's diarrhea, dyspepsia, and heartburn

    c. Control of *H. pylori* (in combination therapy)

IV. Drugs Used in the Treatment of *H. pylori* Infection

  • *H. pylori* organisms can be identified in antral samples from most patients with duodenal and gastric ulcers.

A. Eradication requires multiple drug therapy to enhance the rate of ulcer healing, when compared with treatment with only H$_2$-receptor antagonists.

B. The therapeutic regimen usually includes a proton pump inhibitor in combination with two or more of the following drugs: amoxicillin, bismuth, clarithromycin, metronidazole, or tetracycline.

Triple drug therapy with metronidazole; a bismuth compound; and an antibiotic such as tetracycline, amoxicillin, or clarithromycin is recommended in some patients to overcome drug resistance.

V. Antidiarrheal Drugs (Box 21-3)

A. Inhibitors of acetylcholine (ACh) release

  • Examples: diphenoxylate, difenoxin, loperamide

  • These drugs are also known as opioid antidiarrheals (see Chapter 19).

> **BOX 21-3**
>
> ## ANTIDIARRHEAL DRUGS
>
> ### Locally Acting Drugs
> Bismuth subsalicylate
> Kaolin-pectin
> Polycarbophil
>
> ### Opioids
> Difenoxin with atropine
> Diphenoxylate with atropine
> Loperamide

1. Mechanism of action
   a. These drugs inhibit ACh release through presynaptic opioid receptors in the enteric nervous system, disrupting peristalsis, decreasing intestinal motility, and increasing intestinal transit time.
   b. Loperamide does *not* cross the blood-brain barrier.
2. Uses
   a. Control and relief of acute, nonspecific diarrhea
   b. Treatment of chronic diarrhea associated with inflammatory bowel disease
3. Contraindication: ulcerative colitis (can induce toxic megacolon)

B. Locally acting agents
1. Mechanism of action
   a. Inhibit intestinal secretions
   b. Adsorb water and other substances
2. Uses
   a. Bismuth: management of infectious diarrhea, especially traveler's diarrhea
   b. Adsorbents (kaolin-pectin)
      • Can also bind potentially toxic substances

VI. Prokinetic Drugs
   • Example: metoclopramide
A. Mechanism of action
1. Enhance gastric motility without stimulating gastric secretions
2. Augment cholinergic release of ACh from postganglionic nerve endings, sensitizing muscarinic receptors on smooth muscle cells
3. Block dopamine D_2 and 5-HT$_3$ receptors (antiemetic action)
B. Uses and clinical effects
1. GERD: reduced reflux and increased gastric emptying due to the decrease of the resting tone of the lower esophageal sphincter

Loperamide produces less sedation and less abuse potential than diphenoxylate; atropine is added to diphenoxylate to act as a deterrent of abuse.

> **BOX 21-4**
>
> **ANTIEMETICS**
>
> **Anticholinergic Drugs**
> Scopolamine
>
> **Antihistamines**
> Diphenhydramine
> Meclizine
>
> **Dopamine D$_2$-Receptor Antagonists**
> Metoclopramide
> Phenothiazines
> Prochlorperazine
> Promethazine
>
> **Serotonin 5-HT$_3$ Receptor Antagonists**
> Alosetron
> Dolasetron
> Granisetron
> Ondansetron
> Palonosetron

2. Nausea and vomiting: antiemetic effect produced by blockade of dopamine D$_2$ receptors in the chemoreceptor trigger zone
3. Gastroparesis: promotion of motility
C. Adverse effects: extrapyramidal or dystonic reactions

VII. Antiemetic Drugs (Box 21-4)
  A. Physiology of emesis (incompletely understood process)
    1. Coordination of stimuli takes place in the vomiting center, located in the reticular formation of the medulla.
    2. Input arises from the chemoreceptor trigger zone, vestibular apparatus, and afferent nerves.
  B. Antiemetic drugs
    1. Serotonin 5-HT$_3$ receptor antagonists
      • Examples: ondansetron, granisetron
      a. Safe and effective antiemetics
      b. Uses
        • The -setrons are used for chemotherapy-induced emesis and postsurgery nausea and vomiting.
        • Alosetron is used for the treatment of women who exhibit severe diarrhea-predominant irritable bowel syndrome (IBS) and have failed conventional therapy.

Note common ending -setron in 5-HT$_3$ receptor antagonists: ondansetron, granisetron

2. Marijuana derivatives
   - Example: dronabinol
   - Use: nausea and vomiting in patients with acquired immunodeficiency syndrome (AIDS) or cancer
3. Metoclopramide: dopamine D_2 receptor antagonist
4. Antihistamines
   - Examples: diphenhydramine, hydroxyzine
   - Use: nausea and vomiting associated with motion sickness
5. Phenothiazines
   - Examples: prochlorperazine, promethazine
   - Dopamine D_2 receptor antagonists

VIII. Drugs Used to Treat Irritable Bowel Syndrome (IBS)
   A. Tricyclic antidepressants: Low doses of amitriptyline or desipramine are used for treatment of chronic abdominal pain associated with IBS.
   B. Antispasmodics: Anticholinergics, such as dicyclomine or hyoscyamine, are sometimes used to treat IBS.
   C. Selective serotonin ($5-HT_4$) partial agonist: Tegaserod is approved for the short-term treatment of IBS in women who exhibit constipation as their primary symptom.
      - See Table 21-1 for 5-HT receptor subtypes and their important pharmacology.
   D. Serotonin $5-HT_3$ receptor antagonist: Alosetron is used for the treatment of women who exhibit severe diarrhea-predominant IBS and have failed conventional therapy.

TABLE 21-1: 5-Hydroxytrypamine (5-HT) Receptor Subtypes and Important Pharmacology

Receptor Subtype	Distribution	Second Messenger	Agonists	Antagonists	Uses
$5-HT_{1A}$	Raphe nuclei, hippocampus	Multiple, G_i dominates	Buspirone (partial)		Anxiolytic
$5-HT_{1D}$	Brain	G_i, ↓ cAMP	Sumatriptan and other triptans, ergots		Migraine
$5-HT_{2A}$	Platelets, smooth and striated muscle, cerebral cortex	G_q, ↑ IP_3		Clozapine, olanzapine, risperidone	Psychosis
$5-HT_3$	Area postrema, sensory and enteric nerves	Na^+-K^+ ion channel		Ondansetron, granisetron	Emesis
$5-HT_4$	CNS and myenteric neurons, smooth muscle	G_s, ↑ cAMP	Metoclopramide, cisapride, tegaserod partial		Prokinetic and irritable bowel syndrome

cAMP, cyclic adenosine monophosphate; CNS, central nervous system; IP_3, inositol-triphosphate.

IX. Drugs Used in the Treatment of Inflammatory Bowel Disease
  • Crohn's disease and ulcerative colitis are often considered together as inflammatory bowel disease.
  A. Salicylates (see Chapter 18)
    1. 5-Aminosalicylic acid (5-ASA, mesalamine): active anti-inflammatory agent
      a. Mechanism of action: inhibitor of cyclooxygenase (COX) pathway
      b. Uses: ulcerative colitis, Crohn's disease (sometimes)
      c. Adverse effects: abdominal pain, nausea, vomiting, headache
    2. Sulfasalazine
      • Combination of sulfapyridine and mesalamine
      a. Mechanism of action: production of beneficial effects due to antibacterial action of sulfapyridine and anti-inflammatory (most important) properties of mesalamine
      b. Uses: ulcerative colitis, Crohn's disease (maintain remission), rheumatoid arthritis
      c. Adverse effects
        (1) Malaise
        (2) Nausea, abdominal discomfort
        (3) Headache
        (4) Typical sulfonamide adverse effects (e.g., blood dyscrasias, skin reactions)
    3. Olsalazine
      • Two 5-ASA molecules linked by a diazo bond (RN = NR'), cleaved by bacteria in colon
      • Used in the treatment of ulcerative colitis
  B. Immunosuppressive agents (see Chapter 17)
    1. Hydrocortisone and other glucocorticoids can induce remission of ulcerative colitis and Crohn's disease.
    2. Infliximab, a monoclonal antibody to tumor necrosis factor-α, is used to treat moderate to severe Crohn's disease.

X. Laxatives (Table 21-2)
  A. General considerations
    • Laxative abuse occurs frequently.
    • Contraindications to these drugs include unexplained abdominal pain and intestinal obstruction.
  B. Types of laxatives (Box 21-5)
    1. Bulk-forming laxatives: psyllium, methylcellulose
      • Natural and semisynthetic polysaccharides and cellulose derivatives (similar to dietary fiber)
    2. Osmotic laxatives
      • The osmotic effect of these laxatives increases water in the colon.
      a. Saline cathartics: magnesium salts, sodium phosphate
        • Used when prompt, complete evacuation is necessary
      b. Other osmotic drugs: lactulose, sorbitol

TABLE 21-2:
Effects of Common Laxatives

Type	Site of Action	Mechanism	Uses	Adverse Effects
Bulk-Forming				
Psyllium	Small and large intestines	Increase bulk and moisture content in stool, stimulating peristalsis	Prevent straining during defecation	Esophageal or bowel obstruction if taken with insufficient liquid Flatulence
Osmotic				
Lactulose	Colon	Retain ammonia in colon, producing osmotic effect that stimulates bowel evacuation	Prevent and treat portal systemic encephalopathy Treat constipation	Abdominal discomfort Flatulence
Saline cathartics, magnesium citrate	Small intestine	Induce cholecystokinin release from duodenum, producing osmotic effect that produces distention, promoting peristalsis	Evacuate colon before diagnostic examination or surgery Accelerate excretion of parasites or poisons from GI tract	Electrolyte disturbance
Stimulant				
Senna	Colon	Act directly on intestinal smooth muscle to increase peristalsis	Facilitate defecation in diminished colonic motor response Evacuate colon before diagnostic examination or surgery	Urine discoloration Abdominal cramping Fluid and electrolyte depletion
Stool Softener				
Docusate	Small and large intestine	Lower surface tension Facilitate penetration of fat and water into stool	Short-term treatment of constipation Evacuate colon before diagnostic examination or surgery Prevent straining during defecation Modify fluid from ileostomy, colostomy	GI cramping

GI, gastrointestinal.

BOX 21-5

LAXATIVES

Bulk-Forming Laxatives

Methylcellulose
Psyllium

Osmotic Laxatives

Lactulose
Saline cathartics (magnesium citrate, magnesium hydroxide, sulfate phosphate, sodium phosphate)
Sorbitol

Balanced Polyethanol Glycol (PEG)

PEG and isotonic salt solution

Stimulants

Bisacodyl
Cascara sagrada
Castor oil
Senna

Stool Softeners

Docusate
Glycerin
Mineral oil

3. Balanced polyethylene glycol: polyethylene glycol (PEG) plus isotonic salt solution
4. Stimulant laxatives: castor oil, cascara, senna, bisacodyl
   • Castor oil, a primary irritant, increases intestinal motility.
5. Stool softeners: surfactants (e.g., docusate) and lubricants (e.g., mineral oil, glycerin)

Drugs Used in the Treatment of Rheumatic Disorders and Gout

TARGET TOPICS

- NSAIDs and COX-2 inhibitors in the treatment of arthritic disease
- Disease-modifying antirheumatic drugs (DMARDs)

- Drugs used in the treatment of gout

I. Antiarthritic Drugs (Box 22-1)
- The drugs used to treat rheumatoid arthritis act at various sites (Fig. 22-1).
A. Nonsteroidal anti-inflammatory drugs (NSAIDs) and cyclooxygenase-2 (COX-2) inhibitors (see Chapter 18)
  - NSAIDs and COX-2 inhibitors primarily provide symptomatic relief in the initial therapy of rheumatoid arthritis, rheumatic fever, and other inflammatory joint conditions, as well as treatment of acute pain syndromes.
  - Celecoxib, approved in 1998 for the treatment of rheumatoid arthritis and osteoarthritis, along with rofecoxib and valdecoxib, became widely used to treat inflammatory diseases.
  - After 2004, reports suggesting increased cardiovascular risk compared to placebo from long-term use of selective COX-2 inhibitors including rofecoxib, celecoxib, and valdecoxib, as well as the nonselective NSAID naproxen have resulted in the removal of rofecoxib and valdecoxib from the market and much stronger warnings on the long-term use of all NSAIDs except aspirin.

> COX-2 inhibitors decrease the formation of the prostaglandin PGI_2, producing adverse effects on vasculature and kidney.

B. Corticosteroids
  - Examples: prednisone, methylprednisolone
  1. Mechanism of action
    a. Decrease phospholipase A_2 and COX-2 activity (see Chapter 23)
    b. Decrease immune component
  2. Use: acute episodes of rheumatoid arthritis
    - Steroids result in dramatic improvement but do not arrest the disease process.

BOX 22-1

ANTIARTHRITIC DRUGS

Nonsteroidal Anti-inflammatory Drugs (NSAIDs)
Diclofenac
Diflunisal
Indomethacin
Oxaprozin
Piroxicam
Sulindac
Tolmetin

Cyclooxygenase-2 (COX-2) Inhibitors
Celecoxib

Corticosteroids
Prednisone
Methylprednisolone

Disease-Modifying Antirheumatic Drugs (DMARDs)

Antimetabolites
Methotrexate

Immunologic Drugs
Adalimumab
Anakinra
Etanercept
Infliximab
Leflunomide
Mycophenolate

Antimalarial Drugs
Hydroxychloroquine

Gold Salts
Auranofin
Aurothioglucose

Chelators
Penicillamine

Miscellaneous
Sulfasalazine

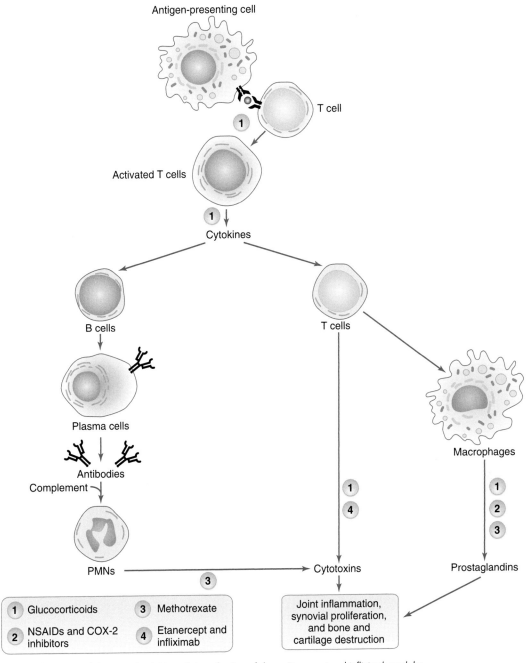

22-1: *Pathogenesis of rheumatoid arthritis and sites of action of drugs. Etanercept and infliximab work by inactivating tumor necrosis factor. COX-2, cyclooxygenase-2; NSAID, nonsteroidal anti-inflammatory drug; PMN, polymorphonuclear neutrophil.*

C. Disease-modifying antirheumatic drugs (DMARDs)
- Examples: methotrexate, immunosuppressive drugs, antimalarial drugs, gold salts, penicillamine, infliximab, anakinra, mycophenolate
1. General characteristics
   a. Suppress proliferation and activity of lymphocytes and polymorphonuclear neutrophils (PMNs)
   b. Counteract joint inflammation and destruction
   c. Slow progression of joint erosion in rheumatoid arthritis and systemic lupus erythematosus (SLE)
2. Methotrexate
   a. Mechanism of action: inhibition of human folate reductase, lymphocyte proliferation, and production of cytokines and rheumatoid factor
   b. Uses: rheumatoid arthritis, immunosuppression, cancer chemotherapy (see Chapter 29)
      - More effective when used in combination with other drugs, such as etanercept or infliximab
   c. Adverse effects
      (1) Macrocytic anemia (caused by folate deficiency)
      (2) Bone marrow suppression
      (3) Pulmonary fibrosis
      (4) Teratogenic activity
3. Immunosuppressive drugs
   a. Mechanism of action
      (1) Leflunomide suppresses mononuclear and T-cell proliferation; its active metabolite inhibits dihydroorotate dehydrogenase (DHODH), an important enzyme in *de novo* pyrimidine synthesis.
      (2) Etanercept, infliximab, and adalimumab inhibit tumor necrosis factor-α.
      (3) Anakinra targets interleukin 1 receptor (IL-1Ra).
      (4) Mycophenolate is converted to mycophenolic acid, which inhibits lymphocyte purine synthesis; it is used to treat rheumatoid arthritis, but even more widely used to prevent allograft rejection.
   b. Uses: Crohn's disease (severe), rheumatoid arthritis
   c. Adverse effects: headache, nausea and vomiting, serum sickness–like reaction
4. Antimalarial drugs (see Chapter 28)
   - Example: hydroxychloroquine
   a. Mechanism of action (unclear): may inhibit lymphocyte function and chemotaxis of PMNs
   b. Use (other than malaria prophylaxis and treatment): adjunct to NSAIDs in the treatment of rheumatoid arthritis, juvenile chronic arthritis, Sjögren's syndrome, and SLE
   c. Adverse effects: retinal degeneration, dermatitis
5. Gold compounds
   - Examples: aurothioglucose, auranofin
   a. Mechanism of action: alter morphology and function of macrophages, which may be a major mode of action

Methotrexate widely used to treat rheumatoid arthritis

Leflunomide inhibits pyrimidine synthesis.

Mycophenolate inhibits purine synthesis.

   b. Use: early stages of adult and juvenile rheumatoid arthritis
   c. Adverse effects
    (1) Cutaneous reactions such as erythema and exfoliative dermatitis
    (2) Blood dyscrasias
    (3) Renal toxicity
  6. Penicillamine: oral chelating agent
   a. Mechanism of action: chelates heavy metals
    • Penicillamine should not be used in combination with gold
     compounds to treat rheumatoid arthritis.
   b. Uses
    (1) Wilson's disease
    (2) Cystinuria
    (3) Resistant cases of rheumatoid arthritis
   c. Adverse effects: aplastic anemia, renal disease (membranous
    glomerulonephritis)
  7. Sulfasalazine
   • Uses: rheumatoid arthritis, ankylosing spondylitis, ulcerative colitis (see
   Chapter 21)

> Don't use penicillamine with gold salts.

II. Drugs Used in the Treatment of Gout (Box 22-2)
 A. Types of gout
  • Gout is a disorder of uric acid metabolism that results in deposition of
  monosodium urate in joints and cartilage (Fig. 22-2).
  1. Primary gout is caused by overproduction (from increase in *de novo*
   synthesis) or underexcretion (e.g., diabetes, starvation states) of uric acid.
  2. Secondary gout is caused by accumulation of uric acid due to one of the
   following factors:
   a. Disease, such as leukemia
   b. Drugs that interfere with uric acid disposition, such as diuretics (e.g.,
    thiazides, furosemide, ethacrynic acid)

BOX 22-2

DRUGS USED IN THE TREATMENT OF GOUT

Acute Therapy
Colchicine
Indomethacin and other NSAIDs

Prevention
Allopurinol
Probenecid
Rasburicase
Sulfinpyrazone

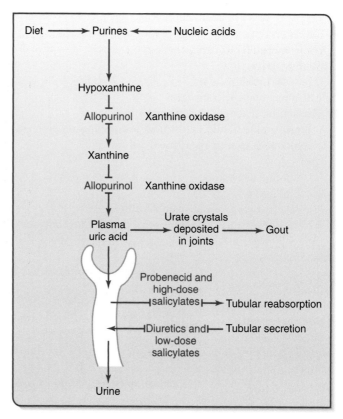

22-2: *Sites of action of drugs that affect uric acid metabolism and excretion.*

  B. Treatment of acute attacks
     1. Colchicine
       a. Mechanism of action: binds to microtubule and inhibits leukocyte migration and phagocytosis, thereby blocking the ability to inflame the joint
         • Colchicine is *not* an analgesic.
       b. Use: reduction of pain and inflammation of acute attacks of gouty arthritis
       c. Adverse effects: diarrhea, nausea and vomiting
     2. Indomethacin and other NSAIDs
       a. All these drugs are effective in the relief of pain and inflammation due to acute gouty arthritis (see Chapter 18).
       b. Additional uses for indomethacin
         (1) Ankylosing spondylitis and osteoarthritis of the hip
         (2) Patent ductus arteriosus
  C. Prevention of acute attacks
     • The goal is to prevent gouty attacks by decreasing the serum concentration of uric acid (see Fig. 22-2).

1. Uricosuric drugs
   - These drugs block active reabsorption of uric acid in the proximal tubule, increasing urinary excretion of uric acid.
   a. Sulfinpyrazone
      (1) Mechanism of action: uricosurgic; also inhibits platelet aggregation
      (2) Use: chronic gouty arthritis
   b. Probenecid: oral uricosuric agent
      (1) Mechanism of action: uricosurgic; also inhibits the renal excretion of penicillins
      (2) Uses
          (a) Hyperuricemia associated with chronic gout or drug-induced hyperuricemia
          (b) Chronic gouty arthritis with frequent attacks (in combination with colchicine)
              - Probenecid is *not* effective in the treatment of acute attacks of gout.
2. Allopurinol
   a. Mechanism of action: inhibits xanthine oxidase and thus inhibits synthesis of uric acid
   b. Use: prevention of primary and secondary gout
   c. Adverse effects: maculopapular rash, toxic epidermal necrolysis, vasculitis
3. Rasburicase
   - Recombinant form of nonhuman urate oxidase
   a. Mechanism of action: converting uric acid to allantoin, which is effectively excreted by the kidneys
   b. Uses: patients with hematologic malignancies (children) or solid tumors who are at particular risk for tumor lysis syndrome (TLS).
   c. Adverse reactions: severe hypersensitivity reactions including anaphylactic shock and anaphylactoid reactions

Probenecid can aggravate inflammation from gout if administered during the initial stages of an acute attack.

Allopurinol potentiates the effects of 6-mercaptopurine and azathioprine.

Allopurinol should *not* be used in acute attacks of gout; it exacerbates symptoms.

23 **CHAPTER**

Drugs Used in the Treatment of Hypothalamic, Pituitary, Thyroid, and Adrenal Disorders

TARGET TOPICS

- Drugs used in the diagnosis and treatment of hypothalamic and pituitary disorders
- Drugs used in the treatment of thyroid disorders
- Glucocorticoids and mineralocorticoids
- Drugs used to treat disorders of adrenal function

I. General Considerations
- A hormone is a substance secreted by one tissue or gland that is transported via the circulation to a site where it exerts its effects on different tissues.
  A. Uses for hormones and synthetic analogues
    1. Diagnostic tools in endocrine disorders
    2. Replacement therapy in endocrine disorders
    3. Treatment of nonendocrine disorders
  B. Interactions among the hypothalamic, pituitary, and peripheral glands (Table 23-1 and Fig. 23-1)

II. Hypothalamic Hormones and Related Drugs (Box 23-1)
  A. Sermorelin (growth hormone–releasing hormone)
    1. Mechanism of action: causes rapid elevation of growth hormone in the blood
    2. Use: assessment of responsiveness and treatment of growth hormone deficiency

TABLE 23-1:
Relationships Among Hypothalamic, Pituitary, and Target Gland Hormones

Hypothalamic	Pituitary	Target Organ	Target Organ Hormones
GHRH (+), SRIH (−), CRH (+)	GH (+) ACTH (+)	Liver Adrenal cortex	Somatomedins Glucocorticoids Mineralocorticoids Androgens
TRH (+) GnRH or LHRH (+)	TSH (+) FSH (+) LH (+)	Thyroid Gonads	T_4, T_3 Estrogen Progesterone Testosterone
Dopamine (−), PRH (+)	Prolactin (+)	Breast	—

+, stimulant; −, inhibitor; ACTH, adrenocorticotropic hormone; CRH, corticotropin-releasing hormone; FSH, follicle-stimulating hormone; GH, growth hormone; GHRH, growth hormone–releasing hormone; GnRH or LHRH, gonadotropin-releasing hormone; LH, luteinizing hormone; PRH, prolactin-releasing hormone; SRIH, somatotropin-releasing inhibiting hormone; TRH, thyrotropin-releasing hormone; TSH, thyroid-stimulating hormone.

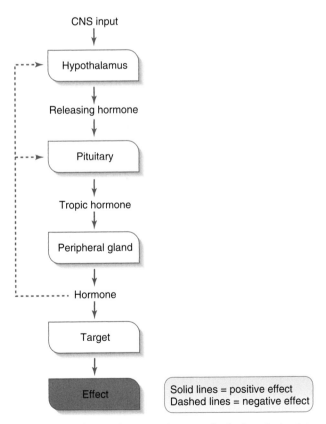

23-1: *Regulation of hormone synthesis and secretion. A negative feedback mechanism is an example of a negative effect. CNS, central nervous system.*

BOX 23-1

HYPOTHALAMIC HORMONES AND RELATED DRUGS

Corticorelin
Gonadorelin
Leuprolide
Nafarelin
Octreotide
Protirelin
Sermorelin
Somatostatin
GnRH antagonists
   Ganirelix
   Cetrorelix

B. Somatostatin (growth hormone–inhibiting hormone)
- Octreotide (synthetic analogue)
1. Mechanism of action: inhibits release of pituitary and gastrointestinal hormones
2. Uses
   a. Symptomatic treatment of hormone-secreting tumors, including pituitary tumors, carcinoid tumors, insulinomas, vasoactive intestinal peptide tumors (VIPomas)
   b. Esophageal varices (octreotide)
3. Adverse effects: abdominal pain, diarrhea, nausea, and vomiting

C. Protirelin (thyrotropin-releasing hormone; TRH)
1. Mechanism of action: stimulates synthesis and release of thyrotropin and prolactin from the anterior pituitary
2. Use: assessment of thyroid function in patients with pituitary or hypothalamic dysfunction

D. Corticotropin-releasing hormone (CRH; corticorelin)
1. Mechanism of action: stimulates release of corticotropin and β-endorphin from the anterior pituitary
2. Use: differentiation between hypothalamic and pituitary causes of corticotropin deficiency or excess

E. Gonadotropin-releasing hormone (GnRH)–related preparations
- Examples: leuprolide, nafarelin, gonadorelin
1. Mechanism of action
   a. Stimulate secretion of follicle-stimulating hormone (FSH) and luteinizing hormone (LH): pulsatile intravenous administration every 1 to 4 hours
   b. Inhibit gonadotropin release: continuous administration of longer-lasting synthetic analogues

The ending -relin indicates a hypothalamic-related hormone.

Pulsatile administration of GnRH increases but continuous administration inhibits gonadotropin release from pituitary.

2. Uses
   a. Shorter-acting preparations: treatment of delayed puberty, induction of ovulation in women with hypothalamic amenorrhea, stimulation of spermatogenesis in men with hypogonadotropic hypogonadism (infertility)
   b. Long-acting GnRH analogues: suppression of FSH and LH in polycystic ovary syndrome, endometriosis, precocious puberty, prostate cancer
3. Adverse effects: menopausal symptoms, amenorrhea, testicular atrophy
4. GnRH antagonist: ganirelix, cetrorelix
   - Used to prevent premature surges of LH during controlled ovarian hyperstimulation.
   - May be effective in endometriosis, uterine fibrinoids in women, and prostate cancer in men.

III. Anterior Pituitary Hormones and Related Drugs (Box 23-2)
   A. Growth hormone–related preparations
      - Somatropin, somatrem, recombinant human growth hormone (rhGH)
      - Growth hormone is required for stimulating normal growth in children and adolescents as well as for controlling metabolism in adults.
      - Disorders characterized by an excess of growth hormone include gigantism (*before* puberty) and acromegaly (*after* fusion of epiphyseal plates of the long bones).
      - Disorders characterized by a deficiency of growth hormone include dwarfism.
      1. Mechanism of action
         a. Increase production of somatomedins in the liver and other tissues
         b. Oppose the actions of insulin
      2. Uses: hypopituitary dwarfism, cachexia, Turner's syndrome (single X chromosome)

Excess growth hormone production results in gigantism and acromegaly; deficiency results in dwarfism.

BOX 23-2

ANTERIOR PITUITARY HORMONES AND RELATED DRUGS

$ACTH_{1-24}$
Corticotropin
Cosyntropin
Human chorionic gonadotropin
Menotropins
Prolactin
Somatrem
Somatropin (recombinant human growth hormone)
Thyrotropin
Urofollitropin

3. Adverse effects
   a. Impaired glucose tolerance may develop over long periods.
   b. Only synthetic growth hormone is used today (Creutzfeldt-Jakob disease resulted from the use of cadaveric growth hormone).

B. Thyrotropin (thyroid-stimulating hormone; TSH)
   1. Mechanism of action
      a. Stimulates growth of thyroid gland
      b. Stimulates the synthesis and release of thyroid hormones
   2. Use: diagnosis of hypothyroidism

C. Adrenocorticotropin (ACTH; corticotropin)–related preparations
   • Examples: corticotropin, $ACTH_{1-24}$, cosyntropin
   1. Regulation of secretion
      a. Corticotropin levels undergo daily cyclic changes (circadian rhythms).
         • Peak plasma levels occur about 6:00 AM, and the lowest levels occur about midnight.
      b. Stress increases the release of corticotropin.
   2. Mechanism of action
      a. Stimulate growth of the adrenal gland
      b. Stimulate the production and release of glucocorticoids, mineralocorticoids, and androgens from the adrenal cortex
   3. Use: differentiation between primary (adrenal malfunction) and secondary (pituitary malfunction) adrenocortical insufficiency
   4. Adverse effects (corticotropin or glucocorticoids): Cushing's syndrome
      a. General: weight gain, cushingoid appearance ("moon face"), sodium retention, edema
      b. Musculoskeletal: osteoporosis, myopathy, growth retardation (children)
      c. Ophthalmic: cataracts, glaucoma
      d. Other: diabetes mellitus, peptic ulcer disease, psychosis, decreased resistance to infection

D. Urofollitropin (follicle-stimulating hormone; FSH)
   1. Mechanism of action: stimulates ovarian follicle growth (females) and spermatogenesis (males)
   2. Uses: infertility, polycystic ovary syndrome
   3. Adverse effects: multiple births, ovarian enlargement

E. Prolactin and related preparations
   1. Prolactin
      a. Regulation of secretion
         (1) Stress, suckling, phenothiazines (dopamine antagonists), and TRH stimulate the release of prolactin.
         (2) Dopamine and dopamine agonists in the central nervous system (CNS), such as bromocriptine, tonically inhibit the release of prolactin.
      b. Mechanism of action: stimulates milk production
      c. Use: not available for clinical use

Stress markedly affects multiple hormonal systems.

ACTH and glucocorticoids cause iatrogenic Cushing's syndrome.

> **BOX 23-3**
>
> **POSTERIOR PITUITARY HORMONES AND RELATED DRUGS**
>
> Desmopressin
> Oxytocin

   2. Inhibitors of prolactin release (bromocriptine, pergolide)
      • Uses: prevention of breast tenderness and engorgement in women who are not breastfeeding; inhibition of lactation; treatment of amenorrhea and galactorrhea associated with hyperprolactinemia due to pituitary adenomas

IV. Posterior Pituitary Hormones and Related Drugs
   • These hormones are produced in the hypothalamus and are transported to the posterior pituitary (neurohypophysis), where they are stored and released into the circulation (Box 23-3).
   A. Vasopressin (antidiuretic hormone; ADH)
      1. General considerations
         • The synthetic analogue is desmopressin.
         a. Disorders characterized by an absence of ADH include diabetes insipidus (severe polyuria, hypernatremia).
         b. Disorders characterized by an excess of ADH include syndrome of inappropriate antidiuretic hormone (SIADH), water retention, hyponatremia, and possible pulmonary disease.
      2. Regulation of secretion
         a. Increases in plasma osmolality (e.g., dehydration) result in increased secretion of ADH.
         b. Decreases in blood pressure (e.g., due to hemorrhage) increase ADH secretion.
      3. Mechanism of action
         a. Modulates renal tubular reabsorption of water, increasing permeability of the distal tubule and collecting ducts to water
            • This effect is mediated by an increase in cAMP associated with stimulation of the V_2 receptor.
         b. At high concentrations, causes vasoconstriction (helps maintain blood pressure during hemorrhage)
            • This effect occurs via the stimulation of the V_1 receptor coupled to the polyphosphoinositide pathway.
      4. Uses
         a. Central (neurogenic) diabetes insipidus
            • Thiazide diuretics are used to treat nephrogenic (peripheral) diabetes insipidus because they paradoxically cause a reduction in the polyuria of patients with diabetes insipidus.

Excess ADH results in SIADH, water retention, hyponatremia, and possible pulmonary disease; absence of ADH results in diabetes insipidus.

V_2 = cAMP pathway

V_1 = polyphosphoinositide pathway

      b. Esophageal variceal bleeding and colonic diverticular bleeding (some cases)

      c. Ventricular fibrillation or pulseless ventricular tachycardia

   5. Adverse effects: overhydration, hypertension

   6. Drugs that affect the secretion or action of ADH

      a. Diuretics, carbamazepine, morphine, tricyclic antidepressants increase ADH release.

      b. Ethanol decreases ADH release.

        • Lithium and demeclocycline, which reduce the action of ADH at the collection ducts of the nephron, are used to treat SIADH.

  B. Oxytocin

     • This substance, which is secreted by the supraoptic and paraventricular nuclei on the hypothalamus, is used to induce labor and stimulate uterine contractions (see Chapter 26).

V. Thyroid Hormones and Related Drugs (Box 23-4)

     • Thyroid hormones are required for normal growth and development.

     • These substances play a role in metabolism (calorigenic activity).

  A. Thyroxine (T_4)- and triiodothyronine (T_3)-related preparations

     • T_3 is less tightly bound than T_4 to the transport protein, thyroxine-binding globulin (TBG).

     • T_3 is approximately four times more potent than T_4.

   1. Regulation of thyroid function

      a. Thyrotropin (TSH) from the anterior pituitary stimulates the synthesis and secretion of T_4 and T_3.

      b. Iodine deficiency results in decreased thyroid hormone synthesis, leading to increased TSH release and goiter.

   2. Drugs that affect thyroid function (Table 23-2)

   3. Levothyroxine (T_4)

      a. Pharmacokinetics

        (1) Slow-acting: 1 to 3 weeks required for full therapeutic effect

        (2) Half-life ($t_{1/2}$): 9 to 10 days in hyporthyroid patients

> Thyroid hormone may cause hyperthyroid symptoms and allergic skin reactions.

BOX 23-4

THYROID HORMONES AND RELATED DRUGS

β-Adrenergic receptor antagonists
Iodide (radioactive iodine)
Iodinated contrast media
Levothyroxine
Liothyronine
Methimazole
Propylthiouracil

TABLE 23-2:
Drugs That Affect
Thyroid Function

Drugs	Effect on Thyroid Gland
Amiodarone	Altered thyroid synthesis, causing hypo- or hyperthyroidism
Androgens	Decreased TBG, causing decrease in T_4
Carbamazepine	Induced cytochrome P-450 system, causing hypothyroidism
Estrogens	Increased TBG, causing increase in T_4
Glucocorticoids	Decreased TBG, causing decrease in T_4
Iodides	Altered thyroid synthesis, causing hyperthyroidism
Levodopa	Altered thyroid synthesis, causing hypothyroidism
Lithium	Altered thyroid synthesis, causing hypothyroidism
Phenobarbital	Induced cytochrome P-450 system, causing hypothyroidism
Phenytoin	Induced cytochrome P-450 system, causing hypothyroidism
Rifampin	Induced cytochrome P450 system, causing hypothyroidism
Salicylates	Displaced from TBG, causing hyperthyroidism
Tamoxifen	Increased TBG, causing increase in T_4

T_4, thyroxine; TBG, thyroxine-binding globulin.

     b. Uses: thyroid replacement and suppression therapy
     c. Adverse effects: cardiotoxicity, excessive thermogenesis, increased sympathetic activity, insomnia, anxiety, tension
   4. Triiodothyronine (T_3), liothyronine (synthetic T_3)
     • Faster acting than T_4, but not usually used because T_4 is converted to T_3 in the body

> T_4 is converted to T_3 in peripheral tissues.

B. Antithyroid agents
   1. Thioamides
     • Examples: propylthiouracil, methimazole
     a. Mechanism of action: inhibit synthesis of T_3 and T_4
       (1) Prevent oxidation of iodide to iodine
       (2) Inhibit coupling of two iodotyrosyl residues (iodinated tyrosine molecules) to form T_3 or T_4

> Thioamides inhibit organification of iodide.

     b. Uses: hyperthyroidism, thyrotoxicosis
     c. Adverse effects: hypothyroidism, hepatotoxicity, leukopenia, agranulocytosis; should be used in caution during pregnancy and nursing

> Propylthiouracil also inhibits conversion of peripheral T_4 to T_3.

   2. Iodide (sodium or potassium iodide, intravenous or oral; iodinated contrast media, ipodate or diatrizoate)
     a. Mechanism of action: rapidly inhibits release of T_3 and T_4 in pharmacologic doses by inhibition of proteolysis of thyroglobulin; effects are transient because the thyroid gland "escapes" the block after a few weeks.

> Propylthiouracil is less likely to cross the placenta than methimazole.

     b. Uses
       (1) Preparation for surgical thyroidectomy (decreases size and vascularity of gland)
       (2) Treatment of thyrotoxicosis
     c. Adverse effects: blocked uptake of radioactive iodine, induction of hyperthyroidism
     • Iodide should be avoided if therapy with radioactive iodine is necessary.

3. Radioactive iodine (^{131}I)
- ^{131}I, the radioactive isotope of iodine, is administered orally as sodium iodide^{131}.
   a. Mechanism of action: trapped by the thyroid gland and incorporated into thyroglobulin
      - Emission of beta radiation destroys the cells of the thyroid gland.
   b. Use: hyperthyroidism
   c. Adverse effects: bone marrow suppression, angina, radiation sickness
4. β-Adrenergic receptor antagonists (see Chapter 5)
- Use: reduction of symptoms of thyrotoxicosis, such as tremor, palpitations, anxiety, heat intolerance, tachycardia, and arrhythmias

VI. Adrenocorticosteroids (Box 23-5)
   A. Glucocorticoids
   - Examples: cortisone, hydrocortisone, dexamethasone
   1. Synthesis and secretion
      a. Synthesized from cholesterol
         - Adrenocorticosteroids are not stored by the adrenal gland but are released as soon as they are produced.
      b. Regulated by ACTH and exhibits a similar circadian rhythm
   2. Mechanism of action: suppression of the release of arachidonic acid from phospholipids by inhibiting phospholipase A_2 (lipocortin) and expressing COX-2, resulting in an anti-inflammatory action (see Chapter 2 for signaling mechanism)

BOX 23-5

ADRENAL HORMONES AND RELATED DRUGS

Glucocorticoids

Short- to Medium-Acting
Cortisone
Hydrocortisone (cortisol)
Prednisolone
Prednisone

Intermediate-Acting
Fluprednisolone
Triamcinolone

Long-Acting
Betamethasone
Dexamethasone

Mineralocorticoids
Desoxycorticosterone
Fludrocortisone

Glucocorticoid Antagonists and Synthesis Inhibitors
Aminoglutethimide
Ketoconazole
Metyrapone
Mifepristone
Mitotane

Mineralocorticoid Antagonists
Spironolactone
Eplerenone

3. Uses
   a. Substitution therapy in adrenocortical insufficiency
   b. Nonendocrine disorders (Tables 23-3 and 23-4)
   c. Diagnostic functions
      • Adrenocorticosteroids suppress ACTH production to identify the source of a particular hormone or establish whether production of a hormone is influenced by secretion of ACTH.

TABLE 23-3: Nonadrenal Disorders Treated with Corticosteroids

Nature of the Condition	Disorder
Allergic reactions	Angioedema, anaphylaxis
Bone and joint disorders	Rheumatoid arthritis, systemic lupus erythematosus
Collagen vascular disorders	Systemic lupus erythematosus
Eye diseases	Iritis, keratitis, chorioretinitis
Gastrointestinal disorders	Crohn's disease, ulcerative colitis
Hematologic disorders	Idiopathic cytopenic purpura
Neurologic disorders	Acute spinal cord injury, multiple sclerosis flare, increased intracranial pressure
Organ transplants	Kidney transplant
Pulmonary diseases	Chronic obstructive pulmonary disease or asthma flares
Renal disease	Glomerulonephropathies (Goodpasture's syndrome)
Skin disorders	Psoriasis, dermatitis, eczema
Thyroid diseases	Malignant exophthalmos, subacute thyroiditis

TABLE 23-4: The Relative Potencies of Various Steroids Compared to Cortisol (Arbitrary Value = 1.0)

Drugs	RGP	RMP	Duration of Action (hr)
Short-Acting			
Cortisol (hydrocortisone)	1.0	1.0	2.0
Cortisone	0.8	0.8	2
Intermediate-Acting			
Prednisone	4.0	0.3	12–36
Prednisolone	5.0	0.3	12–36
Methylprednisolone	5.0	0	12–36
Triamcinolone	5	0	24–36
Long-Acting			
Betamethasone	25–40	0	>48
Dexamethasone	30	0	>48
Mineralocorticoids			
Fludrocortisone	10	125	
Deoxycortisone	0	20	
Aldosterone	0.3	3000	

RGP, relative glucocorticoid potency (liver glycogen deposition, or anti-inflammatory activity); RMP, relative mineralocorticoid potency (sodium retention).

- Urine levels of steroid metabolites are of diagnostic value.
4. Adverse effects
  a. Adrenal suppression due to negative feedback mechanisms
     (1) The degree of suppression is a function of the dose and length of therapy.
     (2) When therapy is discontinued, the dose must be tapered.
  b. Iatrogenic Cushing's syndrome
  c. Metabolic effects
     (1) Hypokalemic alkalosis due to the mineralocorticoid effects of the glucocorticoid
     (2) Glycosuria due to the effect on glucose metabolism
  d. Edema due to Na^+ and fluid retention
  e. Increased susceptibility to infection
  f. Peptic ulcer disease
  g. Musculoskeletal effects
     (1) Myopathy: skeletal muscle weakness
     (2) Osteoporosis
  h. Behavioral disturbances: psychosis, euphoria, insomnia, restlessness
  i. Ophthalmic effects: permanent visual impairment, exophthalmos, retinopathy, cataracts

B. Mineralocorticoids
   - Aldosterone: naturally occurring hormone
   - Fludrocortisone: oral synthetic adrenocorticosteroid with both mineralocorticoid and glucocorticoid activity (only mineralocorticoid effects at usual doses)
   1. Synthesis and secretion
      - Angiotensin II is the primary stimulus for aldosterone secretion.
   2. Mechanism of action
      a. Increase the retention of Na^+ and water
      b. Increase the excretion of K^+ and H^+
   3. Use: adrenocortical insufficiency (administered with glucocorticoids)

C. Antagonists of adrenocortical agents
   1. Glucocorticoid antagonists and synthesis inhibitors
      a. Metyrapone
         (1) Mechanism of action: inhibits 11β-hydroxylase, thus inhibiting production of cortisol
         (2) Uses
             (a) Diagnostic test for the production of ACTH
             (b) Treatment of Cushing's syndrome; available only for compassionate use
      b. Aminoglutethimide
         (1) Mechanism of action: inhibits enzymatic conversion of cholesterol to pregnenolone, leading to reduced synthesis of all adrenocortical hormones
         (2) Use: Cushing's syndrome
      c. Ketoconazole
         - Antifungal agent

Glucocorticoids: taper doses on discontinuation

Long-term use of glucocorticoids causes osteoporosis and cataracts.

      (1) Mechanism of action: inhibits mammalian synthesis of glucocorticoids and steroid hormones by inhibiting the cytochrome P-450 system and 11β-hydroxylase

      (2) Use: Cushing's syndrome

   d. Mifepristone (RU 486)

     • Glucocorticoid receptor antagonist and progesterone antagonist (see Chapter 26)

   e. Mitotane: adrenocortical cytotoxic antineoplastic agent

     • Use: adrenocortical carcinoma

2. Mineralocorticoid antagonists

   • Examples: spironolactone, eplerenone (see Chapter 15)

   a. Mechanism of action: competitive inhibitor of aldosterone

   b. Uses

      (1) Hypertension (in combination with thiazide diuretics as a potassium-sparing diuretic)

      (2) Primary hyperaldosteronism (treatment and diagnosis)

      (3) Hirsutism (women)

      (4) Ascites associated with cirrhosis

      (5) Severe congestive heart failure

Drugs Used in the Treatment of Diabetes Mellitus and Errors of Glucose Metabolism

---

TARGET TOPICS

- Insulins
- Oral hypoglycemic agents
- Metformin
- Thiazolidinediones ("insulin sensitizers")
- Glucagon

I. General Considerations (Table 24-1)
   A. Types of diabetes mellitus
      1. Type 1: an autoimmune disease characterized by a loss of pancreatic β cells
      2. Type 2: a disease characterized by β cells that are desensitized to a glucose challenge and peripheral tissues that are resistant to insulin
   B. Complications
      - Chronic hyperglycemia results in neuropathy, retinopathy, nephropathy, peripheral vascular disease, and coronary artery disease.
   C. Drugs that impair glucose tolerance include corticosteroids, thiazide diuretics, and combination oral contraceptives.

II. Hypoglycemic Agents (Box 24-1)
   A. Insulin
      1. Synthesis and secretion
         - Insulin, a polypeptide hormone, is composed of two chains joined together by disulfide linkages.
         a. Synthesis: by β cells of the pancreas and by proteolytic enzymes into insulin and C peptide
         b. Release: regulated by blood glucose levels
      2. Physiologic action
         a. Promotion of glucose uptake by the liver, muscle cells, and adipocytes, resulting in decreased serum glucose levels
         b. Translocation of the glucose transporter to the cell surface

Use C peptide levels to differentiate between exogenous insulin (overdose) and endogenous insulin (overproduction/insulinoma).

TABLE 24-1:
Characteristics of Type 1 and Type 2 Diabetes Mellitus

Characteristic	Type 1	Type 2
Age of onset	Usually <25 yr	Usually >40 yr
Acuteness of onset	Usually sudden	Usually gradual
Presenting features	Polyuria, polydipsia, polyphagia, acidosis	Often asymptomatic
Body habitus	Often thin	Usually overweight
Control of diabetes	Difficult	Easy
Ketoacidosis	Frequent	Seldom, unless under stress
Insulin requirement	Always	Often unnecessary
Control by oral agents	Never	Frequent
Control by diet alone	Never	Frequent
Complications	Frequent	Frequent

BOX 24-1

DRUGS USED IN THE TREATMENT OF DIABETES MELLITUS

Insulins

Lente
Lispro and aspart
NPH
Regular
Ultralente
Glargine

Sulfonylureas

Chlorpropamide
Glimepiride
Glipizide
Glyburide
Tolbutamide

Biguanide

Metformin

α-Glucosidase Inhibitors

Acarbose
Miglitol

Thiazolidinediones

Pioglitazone
Rosiglitazone

Meglitinides

Repaglinide

NPH, neutral protamine Hagedorn.

---

3. Insulin preparations
   - Different insulin preparations have different effects on plasma glucose use (Fig. 24-1 and Table 24-2).
   - Beef insulin is no longer used in the United States.
   a. Human insulin is produced using recombinant DNA technology.
   b. Pork insulin is more immunogenic than human insulin.
4. Uses: diabetes mellitus, hyperkalemia
5. Adverse effects: hypoglycemia, lipodystrophy (change in the subcutaneous fat at the site of injection)

24-1: *Effects of various insulin preparations on plasma glucose levels in a fasting individual.*

TABLE 24-2:
Therapeutic Time Course of Insulin Preparations

Preparation	Onset of Action	Duration of Action	Peak Effect
Rapid-Acting Insulin			
Insulin lispro and aspart	0–15 min	<5 hr	30–90 min
Short-Acting Insulin			
Insulin injection (regular insulin)	30–45 min	5–7 hr	2–4 hr
Intermediate-Acting Insulin			
Insulin zinc suspension (lente insulin) or isophane insulin suspension (neutral protamine Hagedorn insulin; NPH)	1–4 hr	18–24 hr	6–14 hr
Long-Acting Insulin			
Extended insulin zinc suspension (ultralente insulin)	4–6 hr	≥30 hr	18–26 hr
Insulin glargine	1.5 hr	>24 hr	No peak

B. Oral hypoglycemic agents
1. Sulfonylureas
- First-generation drugs: chlorpropamide, tolbutamide
- Second-generation drugs: glipizide, glyburide, glimepiride

    a. Mechanism of action
- (1) Stimulate the release of insulin from the functional β cells of the pancreas
- (2) Bind to ATP-sensitive potassium-channel receptors on the β cells, depolarizing the membrane

    b. Use: type 2 diabetes mellitus

    c. Adverse effects
- (1) Hypoglycemia
- (2) Disulfiram-like reaction after ingestion of ethanol (most prominent with chlorpropamide)
  - Ethanol also inhibits gluconeogenesis; thus, hypoglycemia can occur more readily in patients receiving oral hypoglycemic drugs.

> Sulfonamide hypersensitivity: cross-hypersensitivity with sulfonamides, thiazides, furosemide

2. Meglitinides
   - Example: repaglinide

   a. Mechanism of action: binds to a site on the β cells in the pancreas and closes ATP-dependent potassium channels; similar to the sulfonylureas

   b. Uses: adjunct to diet and exercise in the treatment of type 2 diabetes mellitus; unique in that it has a rapid onset and short duration, thereby when taken just prior to meals, replicates physiologic insulin profiles

> Repaglinide can be used in patients with sulfonanide hypersensitivity.

3. Biguanides
   - Example: metformin

   a. Mechanism of action
   - (1) Do *not* stimulate insulin release
   - (2) Improve glucose tolerance
     - (a) Increase peripheral utilization of glucose
     - (b) Decrease hepatic gluconeogenesis
   - (3) Do *not* induce weight gain
   - (4) Reduce macrovascular complications of type 2 diabetes mellitus

   b. Use: type 2 diabetes mellitus

   c. Adverse effects: lactic acidosis, especially in patients who have cardiac, renal, or hepatic disease

> Metformin may cause lactic acidosis.

4. Thiazolidinediones ("insulin sensitizers")
   - Examples: rosiglitazone, pioglitazone (troglitazone removed from the market)

   a. Mechanism of action
   - (1) Decrease hepatic gluconeogenesis
   - (2) Enhance uptake of glucose by skeletal muscle cells
   - (3) Act via the peroxisome proliferator-activated receptor-γ, a nuclear receptor that alters gene transcription

   b. Use: type 2 diabetes mellitus, especially in patients with insulin resistance

   c. Adverse effects: elevated hepatic enzymes, hepatic failure

5. α-Glucosidase inhibitors
   - Examples: acarbose, miglitol

   a. Mechanism of action: inhibitor of α-glucosidases in enterocytes of the small intestine, resulting in delayed carbohydrate digestion and reduced absorption

b. Use: type 2 diabetes mellitus
  - α-Glucosidase inhibitors effectively lower postprandial serum glucose but have minimal effects on fasting glucose.

c. Adverse effects: abdominal pain, diarrhea, flatulence

III. Hyperglycemic Agent: Glucagon

A. Regulation of secretion
  - Glucagon is synthesized by the α cells of the pancreas.
  1. Stimulators: α-adrenergic agents, amino acids
  2. Inhibitors: glucose, secretin, somatostatin, free fatty acids

B. Physiologic actions
  - Glucagon increases blood glucose by stimulating glycogenolysis and gluconeogenesis in the liver.
  - Many of the actions of glucagon oppose those of insulin (e.g., hyperglycemia, increased gluconeogenesis).

C. Uses
  1. Severe hypoglycemia in unconscious patients (emergency use)
  2. Diagnostic uses
    a. Radiologic and contrast procedures (reduction of gastrointestinal spasms)
    b. Glycogen storage disease
    c. Pheochromocytoma and insulinoma
    d. Growth hormone dysfunction
  3. Treat overdoses of beta blockers.

Endogenous hormones that counterregulate insulin: glucagon, cortisol, epinephrine

Treat hypoglycemia with intravenous glucose or glucagon.

Beta blocker overdose treated with glucagon

Drugs Used in the Treatment of Bone and Calcium Disorders

TARGET TOPICS

- Parathyroid hormone
- Vitamin D and calcitonin
- Bisphosphonates
- Estrogens and raloxifene

I. General Considerations
- Parathyroid hormone (PTH) and vitamin D play a role in the regulation of calcium and phosphorus (Fig. 25-1 and Table 25-1).
  A. Parathyroid hormone
  1. Regulation of secretion: stimulated by hypocalcemia
  2. Use: no therapeutic use at present
     - PTH analogues (teriparatide) may be used in the treatment of osteoporosis.
  B. Disorders of parathyroid function
  1. Hypoparathyroidism
     - Often occurs after accidental damage to or removal of the parathyroid gland during thyroid surgery
     - Leads to a decrease in serum calcium and an increase in serum phosphate
  2. Hyperparathyroidism
     - May be seen with adenomas or carcinomas of the parathyroid gland or occur as a result of a compensatory mechanism when chronic hypocalcemia (malabsorption, vitamin D deficiency) is present

Regulators of calcium and phosphorus: PTH, vitamin D, calcitonin

II. Drugs That Affect Calcium Levels (Box 25-1)
  A. Calcitonin
   - This peptide is produced by the parafollicular cells of the thyroid gland.
   1. Regulation of secretion: stimulation of release by hypercalcemia
   2. Mechanism of action: inhibits bone resorption and increases kidney excretion of calcium and phosphate, thereby lowering serum calcium and phosphate levels
   3. Uses
      a. Administered parenterally to treat hypercalcemia

25-1: The effects of vitamin D, parathyroid hormone (PTH), and calcitonin on serum calcium (Ca^{2+}) and phosphate (PO_4^{3-}) on bone mineral homeostasis.

TABLE 25-1:
Actions of Parathyroid Hormone and Vitamin D on Intestine, Kidney, and Bone

Area of Action	Parathyroid Hormone	Vitamin D
Intestine	↑ Calcium and phosphate absorption by ↑1,25-(OH)$_2$D production	↑ Calcium and phosphate absorption by 1,25-(OH)$_2$D
Kidney	↓ Calcium excretion ↑ Phosphate excretion	Calcium and phosphate excretion may be ↓ by 25-(OH)D and 1,25-(OH)$_2$D
Bone	↑ Calcium and phosphate resorption in high doses Low doses may ↑ bone formation	↑ Calcium and phosphate resorption by 1,25-(OH)$_2$D Bone formation may be ↑ by 24,25-(OH)$_2$D
Net effect on serum levels	↑ Serum calcium ↓ Serum phosphate	↑ Serum calcium ↑ Serum phosphate

---

BOX 25-1

DRUGS THAT AFFECT CALCIUM LEVELS

Drugs That Increase Calcium Levels
Calcium
Parathyroid hormone
Vitamin D (calciferol, dihydrotachysterol, calcitriol)

Drugs That Decrease Calcium Levels
Bisphosphonates (etidronate, pamidronate, alendronate, risedronate, clodronate, ibandronate, tiludronate)
Calcitonin
Estrogens and raloxifene
Phosphate
Plicamycin (cytotoxic antibiotic)

      b. Paget's disease

      c. Postmenopausal osteoporosis (intranasal)

B. Vitamin D

- Vitamin D deficiency causes rickets in children and osteomalacia in adults.

  1. Sources and formation

    a. Sterols are converted by sunlight to ergocalciferol (vitamin D_2) and cholecalciferol (vitamin D_3) in the skin.

      - Dihydrotachysterol: ergocalciferol analogue

    b. Sterols are metabolized by the liver and kidney to active forms of vitamin D (see Table 25-1).

      (1) Calcitriol: $1,25\text{-}(OH)_2D_3$

      (2) Secalcifediol: $24,25\text{-}(OH)_2D_3$

  2. Uses

    a. Rickets: prevention; given with calcium to supplement the diet of infants

    b. Hypoparathyroidism: given with calcium supplements

    c. Osteoporosis: prevention and treatment

    d. Chronic renal disease

  3. Hypervitaminosis D

    a. Hypercalcemia

    b. Fatigue

    c. Nephrocalcinosis, calcification of soft tissues

C. Calcium

  1. Pharmacokinetics: limited gastrointestinal absorption (<30%)

  2. Uses

    a. Bone and normal growth

    b. Osteoporosis: prevention and treatment

    c. Hypocalcemia

    d. Chronic renal disease

  3. Adverse effects: constipation

D. Phosphate

- Quickly lowers serum calcium levels when given intravenously

E. Bisphosphonates

- Examples: etidronate, pamidronate, alendronate, risedronate, clodronate, ibandronate, tiludronate

  1. Mechanism of action: bind to hydroxyapatite in bone, inhibiting osteoclast activity

  2. Uses

    a. Postmenopausal bone loss

    b. Hypercalcemia due to malignancy

    c. Osteoporosis and compression fractures

    d. Paget's disease

  3. Adverse effects: reflux esophagitis (gastroesophageal reflux disease; GERD)

    - To avoid this condition, patients should:

    a. Take these drugs on an empty stomach, with at least 8 oz water, immediately upon awakening

---

Vitamin D deficiency: rickets (children) and osteomalacia (adults)

Calcitriol is the preferred drug for management of hypocalcemia in dialysis-dependent renal failure patients.

Hypervitaminosis D: hypercalcemia, fatigue, nephrocalcinosis, calcification of soft tissues

Note common ending -dronate for all bisphosphonates.

Alendronate is given once a week to prevent osteoporosis.

Bisphosphonates irritate the stomach and esophagus.

Ibandronate is given once a month to prevent osteoporosis.

No evidence that "natural" estrogens are more or less efficacious or safe than "synthetic" estrogens when given at equiestrogenic doses

When prescribing solely for the prevention of osteoporosis, use only for women at significant risk of osteoporosis; nonestrogen drugs should always be considered as alternatives.

Drugs used in the prevention and treatment of postmenopausal osteoporosis: estrogens with or without progestins, bisphosphonates, raloxifene, calcium, fluoride

      b. Remain in an upright position for at least 30 minutes after taking drug

      c. Do *not* drink or eat anything for 30 minutes after taking drug

F. Estrogens and raloxifene (selective estrogen receptor modulator; SERM)

  1. Mechanism of action: reduces bone resorption

  2. Uses: postmenopausal osteoporosis (reduces bone loss)

    • *Cannot* restore bone

  3. Adverse effects

    • Similar to oral contraceptives but to a lesser extent because of lower estrogen content

    • The Women's Health Initiative (WHI) Trial reported an increase in the incidence of strokes in both the estrogen-alone and the estrogen-progestin subgroups as compared to placebo groups.

G. Plicamycin (cytotoxic antibiotic)

  1. Mechanism of action: inhibits osteoclast activity

  2. Use: hypercalcemia (intravenous), especially associated with cancer (e.g., breast cancer)

26 CHAPTER

Drugs Used in Reproductive Endocrinology

TARGET TOPICS

- Oxytocin and prostaglandins
- Estrogens and progestins
- Oral contraceptives
- Androgens and antiandrogens

I. Drugs That Act on the Uterus (Box 26-1)
  A. Oxytocin
  - This peptide hormone is synthesized in the hypothalamus and stored in the posterior pituitary until it is needed.
  - It plays a facilitatory role in parturition and is an essential element in the milk-ejection reflex; suckling → oxytocin release → milk "let-down."
  - It is associated with mating, parental, and social behaviors.
  - There is speculation that it facilitates the emotional bond between mother and child.
  - Oxytocin may have a protective role against stress-related diseases.
  1. Mechanism of action
     a. Stimulates contraction of uterine muscle
     b. Stimulates smooth muscles of mammary glands
  2. Uses
     a. Induction of labor (administered intravenously)
     b. Control of postpartum hemorrhage (administered intravenously)
     c. Promotion of milk ejection (administered intranasally)
  3. Adverse effects: uterine rupture, water intoxication, hypertension, fetal death
  4. Contraindications
     a. Fetal distress
     b. Prematurity
     c. Abnormal fetal presentation
     d. Cephalopelvic disproportion

  B. Prostaglandins
  - Examples: dinoprostone (PGE_2), carboprost ($PGF_{2\alpha}$), misoprostol (PGE_1 analogue)

Oxytocin is used to induce labor and to manage postpartum bleeding.

BOX 26-1

DRUGS THAT ACT ON THE UTERUS

Drugs That Cause Contraction

Ergot alkaloids: ergonovine, methylergonovine
Oxytocin
Prostaglandins: dinoprostone (PGE_2), carboprost ($PGF_{2\alpha}$), misoprostol (PGE_1 analogue)

Drugs That Cause Relaxation

β_2-Adrenoceptor agonist: terbutaline, ritodrine
Magnesium sulfate
Nonsteroidal anti-inflammatory drugs (NSAIDs)

---

  1. Mechanism of action: potent stimulation of uterine tissue
  2. Uses
     a. Induction of abortion
     b. Softening of the cervix (cervical ripening) before induction of labor (administered intravaginally)
     c. Facilitation of labor
  3. Adverse effects
     a. Prolonged vaginal bleeding
     b. Severe uterine cramps
  C. Ergot alkaloids and related compounds
     • Examples: ergonovine, methylergonovine
  1. Mechanism of action: increase the motor activity of the uterus, resulting in forceful, prolonged contractions
  2. Use: prevention of postpartum bleeding
  3. Adverse effects: nausea, vomiting, abdominal pain, prolactin suppression
  D. Other drugs that affect the uterus
  1. Nonsteroidal anti-inflammatory drugs (NSAIDs)
     a. Mechanism of action: inhibit prostaglandin synthesis
     b. Use: relief of cramps associated with menstruation (dysmenorrhea)
        • The therapeutic effect is attributed to blocking of the increased endometrial synthesis of prostaglandins during menstruation.
  2. β_2-Adrenoceptor agonist (terbutaline, ritodrine)
     a. Mechanism of action: mediate relaxation of uterine smooth muscle
     b. Use: prevention of premature labor (tocolytic agent)
  3. Magnesium sulfate
     a. Mechanism of action: relax uterine muscle
     b. Uses: prevention of premature labor (tocolytic agent); treatment of preeclampsia and eclampsia

Ergot alkaloids should only be used post partum.

BOX 26-2

GONADAL HORMONES AND INHIBITORS

Estrogens

Conjugated estrogens
Estradiol
Ethinyl estradiol

Selective Estrogen Receptor Modulators (SERMs)

Clomiphene
Raloxifene
Tamoxifen
Toremifene

Progestins

Norethindrone
Norgestimate
Norgestrel
Progesterone

Antiprogestins

Danazol
Mifepristone

Androgens

Methyltestosterone
Testosterone

Antiandrogens

Bicalutamide
Finasteride
Flutamide
GnRH analogues
Ketoconazole
Nilutamide

II. Estrogens and Related Drugs (Box 26-2)
   A. Estrogens
      1. Synthesis and secretion
         a. Formation in ovarian follicles: controlled by follicle-stimulating hormone (FSH)
         b. Major secretory product of the ovary: estradiol
      2. Physiologic actions
         a. Necessary for the normal maturation of females
         b. Important for the proliferation of endometrial tissue and normal menstrual cycling
      3. Pharmacokinetics
         a. Metabolized by the liver; high "first-pass" metabolism
         b. Transdermal and intravaginal preparations may avoid negative effects caused by increased protein synthesis (clotting factors, lipoproteins, etc.) that occur in the liver with oral preparations.
      4. Uses
         a. Oral contraception
         b. Estrogen replacement therapy (ERT) in individuals with primary hypogonadism and in postmenopausal women
         c. Osteoporosis: prevention and treatment; consider alternative treatments
         d. Suppression of ovulation in women with intractable dysmenorrhea or excessive ovarian androgen secretion
         e. Androgen-dependent cancers (e.g., carcinoma of the prostate gland)

The Women's Health Initiative (WHI) Trial reported an increase in the incidence of strokes in both the estrogen-alone and the estrogen-progestin subgroups as compared to placebo groups.

5. Adverse effects
   a. Postmenopausal bleeding during ERT
   b. Nausea
   c. Breast tenderness
   d. Increased incidence of migraine headaches, cholestasis, hypertension, gallbladder disease, thrombophlebitis, thromboembolism, increased platelet aggregation, and accelerated blood clotting

6. Contraindications
   a. Estrogen-dependent neoplasms (e.g., endometrial carcinoma)
   b. Known or suspected carcinoma of the breast
   c. Liver disease
   d. History of thromboembolic disorders
   e. Smoking

B. Selective estrogen receptor modulators (SERMs)
   • Agonists in some tissues and antagonists in other tissues
   • Sometimes called partial agonists
   1. Clomiphene
      a. Mechanism of action: blocks estrogen negative feedback, causing an increase in FSH and luteinizing hormone (LH)
      b. Use: to stimulate ovulation in the treatment of infertility
      c. Adverse effects: multiple pregnancies (incidence 5–10%), hot flashes
   2. Tamoxifen and toremifene
      a. Mechanism of action: acts as an estrogen receptor antagonist in the breast
      b. Uses: breast cancer (receptor positive) prophylaxis and treatment
      c. Adverse effects: hot flashes, nausea and vomiting (incidence 25%)
   3. Raloxifene (see Chapter 25)
      • Partial agonist in bone but does not stimulate the endometrium or breast

C. Progestins
   • Progesterone is the most important progestin in humans.
   • The newer third-generation progestins (norgestimate, desogestrel) have less androgenic effects.
   1. Synthesis and secretion
      a. Synthesis: ovary, testes, adrenal cortex, placenta
      b. Synthesis and secretion: corpus luteum stimulated by LH
   2. Physiologic actions
      a. Contributes to the development of a secretory endometrium
      b. Suppresses uterine contractility, especially during pregnancy
   3. Uses
      a. Hormonal contraception
      b. Dysmenorrhea, endometriosis, uterine bleeding disorders
      c. Hirsutism
      d. Hormonal replacement therapy (estrogens and progestins)
      e. Acne vulgaris (norgestimate and ethinyl estradiol)

D. Antiprogestins
   1. Mifepristone (RU 486): postcoital contraceptive agent

Women who smoke should not use estrogens.

Tamoxifen is an estrogen antagonist in the breast but an agonist in the uterus and bone.

    2. Danazol
- Weak progestational, androgenic, and glucocorticoid drug

    a. Mechanism of action: decreases secretion of FSH and LH

    b. Uses

      (1) Endometriosis

      (2) Fibrocystic disease of the breast

      (3) Hereditary angioedema

    c. Adverse effects: androgenic effects, weight gain, seborrhea, hirsutism, edema, alopecia

III. Contraceptives

  A. Types

    1. Oral estrogen-progestin combination contraceptives
- Estrogen (ethinyl estradiol or mestranol) and progestin (norethindrone, norgestrel, or norgestimate)

    a. Monophasic combination tablets: same combination of estrogen and progestin given for 20 to 21 days and stopped for 7 to 8 days each month

    b. Biphasic combination: same estrogen dose for 21 days, with a higher progestin dose in the last 10 days of each month

    c. Triphasic combination: generally the same estrogen dose for 21 days, with a varying progestin dose over the 3 weeks of administration

    2. Continuous progestins

    a. Daily progestin tablets: for patients for whom estrogen administration is undesirable

    b. Implantable progestin preparation
- The Norplant system, a subcutaneous implant of levonorgestrel, allows secretion of progestin in the blood for up to 5 years.
- Capsules are implanted under the skin and can be removed at any time.
- Implants are not used much anymore because of complications.

    3. Topical preparations

    a. Ethinyl estradiol plus etonogestrel vaginal ring; insert for 3 weeks of the cycle

    b. Ethinyl estradiol plus norelgestromin transdermal patch system for once-a-week dosing.

  B. Mechanism of action

    1. Combination contraceptives: selectively inhibit pituitary function (LH and FSH release), thus blocking ovulation

    2. Progestin-only contraceptives: affect ovarian function and cervical mucus

  C. Uses: contraception, morning-after contraception, endometriosis; norgestimate-containing oral contraceptives for the treatment of acne vulgaris

  D. Adverse effects

    1. Venous thrombotic disease, myocardial infarction, cerebrovascular disease, and cholestatic jaundice

    2. Norgestimate, a third-generation progestin, has high progestational, slight estrogenic, and low androgenic activity; it has little effect on serum lipoproteins and has very little negative effect on carbohydrate metabolism.

IV. Androgens and Inhibitors (see Box 26-2)
- Testosterone is the most important androgen in humans.

A. Androgens
1. Synthesis and secretion
   - Stimulated by LH
   a. Produced primarily by testes (Leydig cells) in males and by ovaries and adrenal cortex in females
   b. Converted to 5α-dihydrotestosterone (DHT) by the enzyme 5α-reductase in some tissues (e.g., prostate, skin)
2. Physiologic actions
   a. Stimulates libido (increased sex drive) in both males and females
   b. Accounts for the major changes that occur in males at puberty
   c. Has anabolic activity
3. Uses
   a. Replacement therapy in hypogonadism or hypopituitarism
   b. Acceleration of growth in childhood
   c. Anabolic agent (especially in debilitating diseases such as AIDS-associated wasting syndrome and breast cancer and in geriatric patients)
4. Adverse effects
   a. Masculinization (in women)
   b. Azoospermia, decrease in testicular size
5. Abuse potential
   - Because androgens stimulate muscle growth, some athletes misuse these agents in attempts to improve athletic performance.

B. Androgen suppression and antiandrogens
1. Androgen suppression
   - Gonadotropin-releasing hormone (GnRH) analogues such as leuprolide and goserelin produce gonadal suppression when blood levels are continuous rather than pulsatile.
2. Finasteride
   a. Mechanism of action: inhibits the androgen-metabolizing enzyme 5α-reductase, thus inhibiting formation of DHT and androgen necessary for prostate growth and function
   b. Uses: benign prostatic hyperplasia (BPH), male pattern baldness
   c. Adverse effects
      (1) Teratogenic properties: pregnant women are cautioned about working with finasteride because breathing the dust could result in teratogenesis.
      (2) Impotence, decreased libido
3. Receptor antagonists
   a. Flutamide, bicalutamide, nilutamide
      - Uses: carcinoma of the prostate
   b. Cyproterone
      - Uses: hirsutism (women), excessive libido (men)
4. Ketoconazole
   a. Mechanism of action: decreases testosterone synthesis (males)
   b. Use: carcinoma of the prostate (experimental)

Finasteride is extremely teratogenic.

Note common ending -lutamide for androgen receptor blockers.

CHAPTER

27

Antimicrobial Drugs

I. General Considerations
- Antibacterial drugs exhibit selective toxicity by destroying pathogenic microorganisms yet causing minimal side effects in the host.
- It is important to reach and maintain adequate blood levels to destroy microorganisms and prevent development of microbial resistance.
  A. Mechanism of action
  - Antibacterial drugs act at a number of different sites (Fig. 27-1).
  B. Mechanisms of microbial resistance
  - Resistance often correlates with the frequency of antimicrobial use, the total quantity of drug dispensed, the location of the patient when receiving the medication, and the immune status of the patient.
    1. Pathogens or cells fail to absorb the drug, or they inactivate or remove it (i.e., pump it out).
    2. The target receptors are modified or the production of target molecules is increased.
    3. Altered metabolic pathways bypass the drug target.
    4. Multidrug resistance is often transmitted by plasmids.
  C. Functions
    1. Antibacterial selection (Table 27-1)
       a. Bactericidal: kill disease-causing microorganisms
       b. Bacteriostatic: prevent bacterial growth and multiplication
    2. Prophylaxis (Table 27-2)
  D. Adverse effects
    1. Organ-directed toxicity
       a. Ototoxicity: aminoglycosides, vancomycin, minocycline
       b. Hematopoietic toxicity: chloramphenicol, sulfonamides
       c. Hepatotoxicity: tetracyclines, isoniazid, erythromycin, clindamycin, sulfonamides, amphotericin B
       d. Renal toxicity: cephalosporins, vancomycin, aminoglycosides, sulfonamides, amphotericin B

Drugs that cause hepatotoxicity: tetracyclines, isoniazid, erythromycin, clindamycin, sulfonamides, amphotericin B

Drugs that cause renal toxicity: cephalosporins, vancomycin, aminoglycosides, sulfonamides, amphotericin B

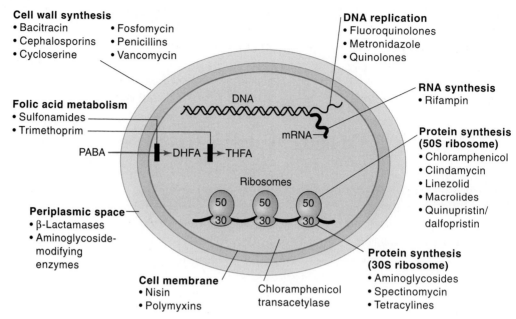

Cell wall synthesis
- Bacitracin
- Cephalosporins
- Cycloserine
- Fosfomycin
- Penicillins
- Vancomycin

DNA replication
- Fluoroquinolones
- Metronidazole
- Quinolones

RNA synthesis
- Rifampin

Folic acid metabolism
- Sulfonamides
- Trimethoprim

Protein synthesis (50S ribosome)
- Chloramphenicol
- Clindamycin
- Linezolid
- Macrolides
- Quinupristin/ dalfopristin

PABA → DHFA → THFA

DNA

mRNA

Ribosomes

Periplasmic space
- β-Lactamases
- Aminoglycoside-modifying enzymes

Protein synthesis (30S ribosome)
- Aminoglycosides
- Spectinomycin
- Tetracylines

Cell membrane
- Nisin
- Polymyxins

Chloramphenicol transacetylase

27-1: *Sites of action of antimicrobial drugs and enzymes that inactivate these drugs. DHFA, dihydrofolic acid; PABA, p-aminobenzoic acid; THFA, tetrahydrofolic acid.*

2. Idiosyncrasies (unexpected individual reactions)
   a. Hemolytic anemias (in G6PD-deficient people): sulfonamides, nitrofurantoin
   b. Photosensitivity: tetracyclines, fluoroquinolones
3. Hypersensitivity reactions
   - These reactions are most notable with penicillins and sulfonamides but can occur with most antimicrobial drugs.
4. Superinfections
   a. Candidiasis
      - Treatment: oral nystatin (local effects), miconazole (local vaginal effects), fluconazole (oral medication for vaginal candidiasis)
   b. Pseudomembranous colitis caused by *Clostridium difficile*
      - Treatment: oral metronidazole or vancomycin
   c. Staphylococcal enterocolitis
      - Treatment: oral vancomycin
E. Drug-drug interactions
   1. Synergism: aminoglycosides + penicillins, sulfamethoxazole + trimethoprim
   2. Potentiation: imipenem + cilastatin; ampicillin + clavulanic acid
   3. Antagonism: penicillin + chloramphenicol

II. Cell Wall Synthesis Inhibitors (Box 27-1)
   - These drugs inhibit various intracellular or extracellular steps in the synthesis of the cell wall (see Fig. 27-1).

TABLE 27-1:
Antibiotics of
Choice for Various
Infections

Drug	Organism (Disease)
Amoxicillin, clarithromycin (omeprazole*)	*Helicobacter pylori* (peptic ulcer)
Ampicillin	*Listeria* (meningitis)
Ceftriaxone, cefexime	*Neisseria gonorrhoeae* (gonorrhea)
Cephalosporins (third generation)	*Haemophilus influenzae* (pneumonia, meningitis) *Klebsiella* (meningitis)
Doxycycline	*Borrelia burgdorferi* (Lyme disease) *Rickettsiae* (Rocky Mountain spotted fever)
Erythromycin	*Legionella* (legionnaires' disease)
Fluconazole, miconazole, nystatin	*Candida* (candidiasis)
Isoniazid, rifampin, ethambutol, pyrazinamide	*Mycobacterium tuberculosis* (tuberculosis)
Macrolides	*Mycoplasma pneumoniae* (atypical pneumonia) *Legionella* (legionnaires' disease) *Corynebacterium diphtheriae* *Chlamydia*
Metronidazole	*Trichomonas* (trichomoniasis) anaerobes
Penicillin G	*Neisseria meningitidis* (meningitis) *Treponema pallidum* (syphilis) Infections caused by streptococci, pneumococci, other meningococci, *Bacillus anthracis*, *Clostridium*, *Bacteroides* (except *B. fragilis*)
Fluoroquinolones	*Campylobacter* (diarrhea) *Shigella*
Tetracycline	*Vibrio cholerae* (cholera)
Other tetracyclines	*Chlamydia* (pneumonia, lymphogranuloma venereum)
Trimethoprim-sulfamethoxazole	*Salmonella*, *Shigella* (diarrhea)
Metronidazole or vancomycin (oral)	*Clostridium difficile* (diarrhea)

*Omeprazole is not an antibiotic but is used in combination with antibiotics for treatment of *H. pylori*.

TABLE 27-2:
Prophylactic Use of
Anti-infective Drugs

Drug	Use
Cefazolin	Surgical procedures
Cefoxitin, cefotetan	Surgical procedures in which anaerobic infections are common
Ampicillin or penicillin	Group B streptococcal infections
Trimethoprim-sulfamethoxazole	*Pneumocystis carinii* pneumonia UTIs
Rifampin	*Haemophilus influenzae* type B Meningococcal infection
Chloroquine	Malaria
Isoniazid	Tuberculosis
Azithromycin	*Mycobacterium avium* complex in patients with AIDS
Ciprofloxacin	*Bacillus anthracis* (anthrax)
Ampicillin or azithromycin	Dental procedures in patients with valve abnormalities

AIDS, acquired immunodeficiency syndrome; UTI, urinary tract infection.

BOX 27-1

β-LACTAM DRUGS AND OTHER CELL WALL SYNTHESIS INHIBITORS

Penicillins

Amoxicillin
Ampicillin
Mezlocillin
Nafcillin
Oxacillin
Penicillin G
Penicillin V
Piperacillin
Ticarcillin

Cephalosporins

First-Generation Drugs
Cefazolin
Cephalexin
Cephalothin (prototype; no longer
  available in the United States)
Cephradine
Second-Generation Drugs
Cefaclor
Cefamandole
Cefotetan

Cefoxitin
Cefuroxime
Third-Generation Drugs
Cefixime
Cefoperazone
Ceftazidime
Ceftizoxime
Ceftriaxone
Fourth-Generation Drugs
Cefepime

Other β-Lactam Drugs

Aztreonam
Ertapenem
Imipenem-cilastatin
Meropenem

Other Cell Wall Synthesis Inhibitors

Bacitracin
Fosfomycin
Vancomycin

- β-Lactam antibiotics are most often used.
- A. Penicillins
  - Key characteristics: β-lactam ring, penicillinase sensitivity, acid labile, tubular secretion, inhibition of cell wall synthesis, hypersensitivity
  1. Pharmacokinetics
     a. Absorption
        - May be destroyed by gastric acid
        - Acid-resistant: penicillin V; oral administration
     b. Distribution: poor movement across the noninflamed blood-brain barrier
     c. Excretion: unchanged in urine by tubular secretion, which is inhibited by probenecid
  2. Pharmacodynamics
     a. Mechanism of action

Exceptions: Nafcillin and, to a lesser extent, oxacillin depend on biliary secretion.

       (1) Bind to specific penicillin-binding proteins (PBPs) located inside the bacterial cell wall, thus inhibiting the cross-linking in bacterial cell wall synthesis

       (2) Inhibit transpeptidase enzymes

  b. Causes of resistance

       (1) Inactivation by β-lactamases (most common)

       (2) Alteration in target PBPs (methicillin-resistant species, e.g., methicillin-resistant *Staphylococcus aureus,* or MRSA)

       (3) Permeability barrier, preventing drug penetration

         • Contributes to the resistance of many gram-negative bacteria

3. Uses

  a. Penicillin G

       (1) Pharyngitis (hemolytic streptococcus)

       (2) Syphilis *(Treponema pallidum)*

       (3) Pneumonia (pneumococcus, streptococcus)

       (4) Meningitis (meningococcus, pneumococcus)

  b. Benzathine penicillin G

     • Intramuscular injection: low blood levels for up to 3 weeks

     • Useful in situations in which organisms are very sensitive (e.g., *T. pallidum* in syphilis)

  c. Ampicillin and amoxicillin (extended spectrum penicillins)

     • Ampicillin is usually given by injection; amoxicillin is given orally

       (1) Urinary tract infections (UTIs) *(Escherichia coli)*

       (2) Infectious diarrhea *(Salmonella)*

       (3) Otitis media or sinusitis *(Haemophilus)*

       (4) Meningitis *(Listeria)*

       (5) Endocarditis (prevention)

  d. Ticarcillin (antipseudomonal penicillin) potent against nosocomial *(Pseudomonas)* infections

     • Usually combined with an aminoglycoside

  e. Piperacillin (antipseudomonal penicillin)

     • More active against *Pseudomonas* than ticarcillin

  f. Penicillinase-resistant β-lactam antibiotics (nafcillin, oxacillin)

     • Used against penicillinase-producing microorganisms

       (1) Endocarditis

       (2) Osteomyelitis (staphylococci)

4. Adverse effects: allergic reactions (most serious)

B. Cephalosporins

  • Key characteristics: β-lactam ring, increased resistance to penicillinases, inhibition of cell wall synthesis, acid resistance (some agents), nephrotoxicity, tubular secretion

1. Mechanism of action: similar to penicillins but penicillinase-resistant

2. Uses

  a. First-generation (cefazolin [parenteral]; cephalexin [oral])

  • Cephalothin, the prototype first-generation cephalosporin, *is no longer available in the United States.*

Alterations in PBPs: responsible for methicillin resistance in staphylococci and penicillin resistance in pneumococci

Primary use of penicillin G: infections with gram-positive (+) bacteria

Antipseudomonal penicillins and cephalosporins are combined with aminoglycosides to prevent resistance.

Antistaphylococcal penicillins (e.g., nafcillin): ineffective against infections with MRSA

Ampicillin rash: nonallergic rash; high incidence in patients with Epstein-Barr virus infection (mononucleosis)

Exceptions:
Cefoperazone and
ceftriaxone are mostly
eliminated by biliary
secretion.

- Cefazolin has good activity against gram-positive bacteria and modest activity against gram-negative bacteria.
  - (1) Cellulitis (staphylococcus, streptococcus)
  - (2) Surgical prophylaxis
  b. Second-generation (cefaclor, cefoxitin, cefotetan, cefuroxime, cefamandole)
  - Increased activity against gram-negative bacteria *(E. coli, Klebsiella, Proteus, Haemophilus influenzae, Moraxella catarrhalis)*
    - (1) Pelvic inflammatory disease, diverticulitis, surgical prophylaxis
    - (2) Pneumonia, bronchitis *(H. influenzae)*
  c. Third-generation (ceftriaxone, cefotaxime, ceftazidime, cefoperazone, ceftizoxime, cefexime)
  - Decreased activity against gram-positive bacteria but increased activity against gram-negative bacteria *(Enterobacter, Serratia)*
  - Activity against *Pseudomonas aeruginosa* in a subset of drugs (ceftazidime, cefoperazone)
    - (1) Meningitis *(Neisseria gonorrhoeae)*
    - (2) Community-acquired pneumonia, Lyme disease, meningitis, osteomyelitis (ceftazidime)
    - (3) Gonorrhea: ceftriaxone (parenteral) or cefixime (oral) are drugs of choice

Many third-generation
cephalosporins that
penetrate into the CNS
are useful in treatment of
meningitis.

  d. Fourth-generation (cefepime)
  - Extensive gram-positive and gram-negative activity and increased resistance to β-lactamases
  - Use: neutropenic fever (parenteral)
3. Adverse effects
- Disulfiram-like effect with alcohol (some second- and third-generation cephalosporins)
- Dose-dependent nephrotoxicity, especially when used with other nephrotoxic drugs (e.g., aminoglycosides, amphotericin B)

Cross-sensitivity to
cephalosporins: less than
5% of patients with
penicillin allergy

C. Other β-lactam drugs
  1. Aztreonam
  - This monobactam, which is given intravenously, has no activity against gram-positive or anaerobic bacteria.
    a. Use: infections with gram-negative rods, including *Serratia, Klebsiella,* and *Pseudomonas*
    b. Adverse effects: pseudomembranous colitis, candidiasis

Aztreonam has no cross-
allergenicity with other
β-lactams.

Note the common ending
-penem for all
carbapenems.

  2. Carbapenems
  - Examples: imipenem, meropenem, ertapenem
    a. Meropenem and ertapenem: not inactivated by dehydropeptidases
    b. Imipenem
      (1) Rapidly inactivated by renal tubule dehydropeptidases
      (2) Must be given with cilastatin, a dehydropeptidase inhibitor

Imipenem must be given
with cilastatin to prevent
inactivation by renal
tubule
dehydropeptidases.

    c. Ertapenem: highly stable against β-lactamases; good activity against many gram-positive, gram-negative, and anaerobic microorganisms, particularly the *Enterobacteriaceae*
    d. Uses: broad-spectrum activity, including anaerobes

   e. Adverse effects: nausea, vomiting, pseudomembranous colitis, confusion, myoclonia, seizures (not with meropenem)

  3. Clavulanic acid: β-lactamase inhibitor

   • Other β-lactamase inhibitors: sulbactam and tazobactam

   a. Given in combination with β-lactamase–sensitive penicillins, such as ampicillin, amoxicillin, ticarcillin, and piperacillin

   b. Not active against methicillin-resistant *Staphylococcus aureus* (MRSA)

 D. Other cell wall synthesis inhibitors

  1. Vancomycin

   a. Mechanism of action

    • Prevents chain elongation and cross-linking by binding to the D-ala-D-ala terminus of the peptidoglycan peptide, thus inhibiting cell wall synthesis

   b. Uses

    • Active against only gram-positive bacteria

    (1) Infections caused by penicillin-resistant *S. aureus* and MRSA, enterococci, and other gram-positive bacteria in penicillin-allergic patients

    (2) *C. difficile*—caused diarrhea

     • Oral administration results in poor gastrointestinal (GI) absorption.

   c. Adverse effects

    (1) Ototoxicity

    (2) Nephrotoxicity

    (3) "Red man syndrome" (flushing from histamine release when given too quickly)

  2. Fosfomycin

   a. Mechanism of action: inhibits cell wall synthesis by inhibiting the first step of peptidoglycan formation

   b. Uses

    (1) Uncomplicated lower UTIs in women

    (2) Infections caused by gram-positive (enterococci) and gram-negative bacteria

   c. Adverse effects: asthenia, diarrhea, dizziness

  3. Bacitracin (see Box 27-1)

   • Given in combination with polymyxin or neomycin ointments for prophylaxis of superficial infections

   a. Mechanism of action: inhibits the transmembrane transport of peptidoglycan units

   b. Uses: skin and ocular infections (gram-positive cocci) (topical applications)

III. Drugs That Affect the Cell Membrane (Box 27-2)

 A. Polymyxin B

  1. Mechanism of action: bactericidal

   • Interacts with specific lipopolysaccharide component of the outer cell membrane, increasing permeability to polar molecules

---

BOX 27-2

DRUGS THAT AFFECT THE CELL MEMBRANE

Nisin
Polymyxin

BOX 27-3

PROTEIN SYNTHESIS INHIBITORS

Inhibitors of the 30S Ribosomal Subunit

Aminoglycosides
Amikacin
Gentamicin
Streptomycin
Tobramycin

Tetracyclines
Demeclocycline
Doxycycline
Minocycline
Tetracycline

Inhibitors of the 50S Ribosomal Subunit

Macrolides
Azithromycin
Clarithromycin
Erythromycin

Other Antibiotics

Chloramphenicol
Clindamycin
Linezolid
Mupirocin
Quinupristin-dalfopristin
Telithromycin

---

2. Use: infections with gram-negative bacteria (topical)
B. Nisin (under study)
- 34-Amino acid peptide produced by *Lactococcus*
1. Mechanism of action
- Interacts with and perturbs the cell membrane by forming ion channels
2. Uses: vancomycin-resistant enterococcus (VRE), *C. difficile*

IV. Protein Synthesis Inhibitors (Box 27-3)
- These drugs reversibly or irreversibly bind to the 30S or 50S ribosomal subunit (see Fig. 27-1).
A. Aminoglycosides
- Examples: amikacin, gentamicin, streptomycin, tobramycin
- Key characteristics: irreversible binding to the 30S ribosomal subunit; bactericidal action; several mechanisms of resistance; adverse effects: nephrotoxicity, ototoxicity, and neuromuscular junction blockade

Aminoglycosides: irreversible inhibitors of protein synthesis

1. Pharmacokinetics
   a. Usually given by intramuscular or intravenous injection (poorly absorbed from the GI tract)
   b. Dosage monitoring using plasma levels
   c. Often used for once-a-day dosing
   d. Eliminated by glomerular filtration
2. Pharmacodynamics
   a. Mechanism of action: irreversible bactericidal inhibitor of protein synthesis
      (1) Undergo active transport across cell membrane via an oxygen-dependent process after crossing the outer membrane via a porin channel
      (2) Once bound to specific 30S ribosome proteins, inhibit protein synthesis
         (a) Interfere with the "initiation complex" of peptide formation
         (b) Misread mRNA, causing the incorporation of incorrect amino acids into the peptide
         (c) Synergy with β-lactam antibiotics
   b. Causes of resistance
      (1) Adenylation, acetylation, or phosphorylation (occurs via plasmids) as the result of the production of an enzyme by the inactivating microorganism
      (2) Alteration in porin channels or proteins involved in the oxygen-dependent transport of aminoglycosides
      (3) Deletion or alteration of the receptor on the 30S ribosomal subunit that binds the aminoglycosides
3. Uses
   • Infections with aerobic gram-negative bacteria *(E. coli, Proteus, Klebsiella, Serratia, Enterobacter)*
   • Infection with *P. aeruginosa* (in combination with antipseudomonal penicillins, such as piperacillin or third-generation cephalosporins)
   a. Streptomycin: tuberculosis
   b. Amikacin, gentamicin, tobramycin: gram-negative coverage often in combination with penicillin or cephalosporin
   c. Neomycin: skin and eye infections (topical), preparation for colon surgery (oral)
4. Adverse effects
   a. Ototoxicity
   b. Nephrotoxicity (acute tubular necrosis)
   c. Neuromuscular junction blockade (high doses; see Chapter 6)

B. Tetracyclines
   • Examples: minocycline, doxycycline
   • Key characteristics: chelation; bacteriostatic action; inhibition of protein synthesis; broad spectrum of action; multiple drug resistance
   • Adverse effects: GI toxicity, bone growth retardation, tooth discoloration, and photosensitivity

Aminoglycosides: treatment of gram-negative infections

1. Pharmacokinetics
   a. Absorption: decreased by chelation with divalent and trivalent cations (e.g., metals, especially calcium)
   b. Distribution: high concentration in the bones, teeth, kidneys, and liver
   c. Excretion
      (1) Tetracycline: cleared by the kidney
      (2) Minocycline, doxycycline: cleared more by the liver
2. Pharmacodynamics
   a. Mechanism of action: bacteriostatic inhibitor of protein synthesis
      • Tetracyclines bind reversibly to the 30S subunit of the ribosome, blocking binding of aminoacyl-tRNA to the acceptor site (A site) on the mRNA-ribosome complex, thus inhibiting protein synthesis.
   b. Causes of resistance
      (1) Decreased intracellular accumulation caused by impaired influx or increased efflux via an active transport protein pump (encoded on a plasmid)
      (2) Ribosomal protection by synthesis of proteins that interfere with the binding of tetracyclines to the ribosome
      (3) Enzymatic inactivation of tetracyclines
3. Uses
   • Infections with gram-positive and gram-negative bacteria, including *Mycoplasma pneumoniae, Chlamydia,* and *Vibrio cholerae*
   a. Rocky Mountain spotted fever *(Rickettsia)*
   b. Lyme disease (doxycycline)
   c. Syndrome of inappropriate antidiuretic hormone (SIADH) (demeclocycline)
   d. Syphilis and gonorrhea (alternative treatment)
   e. Plague *(Yersinia pestis)* (doxycycline)
4. Adverse effects
   a. Nausea, diarrhea *(C. difficile)*
   b. Inhibition of bone growth (fetuses, infants, and children)
   c. Discoloration of teeth
   d. Superinfections (e.g., candidiasis)
   e. Photosensitivity

C. Macrolides
   • Examples: erythromycin, clarithromycin, azithromycin
   • Key characteristics: bacteriostatic or bactericidal inhibitors of protein synthesis, elimination by biliary secretion
1. Mechanism of action
   a. Bind reversibly to the 50S ribosomal unit
   b. Block peptidyl transferase and prevent translocation from the aminoacyl site to the peptidyl site
2. Causes of resistance
   a. Plasma-encoded reduced permeability
   b. Intracellular metabolism of the drug
   c. Modification of the ribosomal binding site

Tetracyclines: antibiotic of choice for chlamydial infection, brucellosis, mycoplasma pneumonia, rickettsial infections, some spirochetes (Lyme disease)

Note common ending of -thromycin for all macrolides.

3. Uses
- Secondary drugs for infections caused by gram-positive bacteria in penicillin-sensitive patients
    a. Erythromycin: legionnaires' disease, *Mycoplasma* pneumonia, neonatal genital or ocular infections, chlamydial infections
    b. Azithromycin: *Mycobacterium avium* complex prophylaxis in patients with advanced HIV; sinusitis and otitis media *(H. influenzae, M. catarrhalis);* chlamydial infections
    c. Clarithromycin: infection caused by *Helicobacter pylori* in addition to the uses for azithromycin
4. Adverse effects
- Erythromycin, a potent inhibitor of the cytochrome P-450 system, increases the effects of carbamazepine, clozapine, cyclosporine, digoxin, midazolam, quinidine, and the protease inhibitors.
    a. GI effects: anorexia, nausea, vomiting, diarrhea
    b. Hepatotoxicity: cholestatic hepatitis
    c. Pseudomembranous colitis

D. Other protein synthesis inhibitors
1. Chloramphenicol
    a. Mechanism of action
    - Inhibits protein synthesis at the 50S ribosome; bacteriostatic
    - Inhibits peptidyl transferase
    b. Uses
       (1) *Salmonella* infections (typhoid)
       (2) Ampicillin-resistant *H. influenzae* meningitis
    c. Adverse effects
       (1) Aplastic anemia and bone marrow toxicity
       (2) Gray baby syndrome (deficiency of glucuronyl transferase)
2. Clindamycin
    a. Mechanism of action: inhibits protein synthesis at the 50S ribosome; bacteriostatic
    b. Uses: severe gram-positive anaerobic infections (*Bacteroides* and others; aspiration pneumonia)
    c. Adverse effects: severe diarrhea, pseudomembranous colitis *(C. difficile)*
3. Linezolid
    a. Mechanism of action: binds to the 50S ribosome, interfering with protein synthesis
    b. Uses: infections caused by MRSA or VRE; given orally
    c. Adverse effects: diarrhea, nausea, vomiting, headache
    - Patients should avoid consuming tyramine-containing foods (e.g., aged cheese, red wine), because linezolid inhibits monoamine oxidase (MAO).
4. Quinupristin-dalfopristin
    a. Mechanism of action: interferes with protein synthesis; bactericidal
    b. Uses: infections caused by MRSA, enterococcus; given by injection
       (1) Severe bacteremia
       (2) Pneumonia

Erythromycin inhibits cytochrome P-450.

Azithromycin does not inhibit cytochrome P-450.

Chloramphenicol: inhibitor of microsomal oxidation that increases blood levels of phenytoin, tolbutamide, and warfarin

Chloramphenicol: potential to cause lethal aplastic anemia

Clindamycin is effective against anaerobes.

Linezolid inhibits MAO.

Quinupristin-dalfopristin inhibits drug metabolism.

      c. Adverse effects: nausea, vomiting, diarrhea

      d. Drug interactions: potent inhibitors of CYP3A4; increase plasma levels of cyclosporine, diazepam, nucleoside reverse transcriptase inhibitors, warfarin

  5. Telithromycin

    • Broad-spectrum antibiotic, binds to the 50S ribosomal subunit, similar to macrolides

    • Used for upper and lower respiratory tract infections

  6. Mupirocin

      a. Mechanism of action: interferes with protein synthesis

      b. Uses: impetigo, nasal colonization by MRSA (eradication)

      c. Adverse effects: nasal irritation, pharyngitis

V. Antimetabolites Used for Microorganisms (Box 27-4)

  • These antimicrobials interfere with the metabolism of folic acid (see Fig. 27-1).

  A. Sulfonamides

    • Key characteristics: competitive inhibition of *p*-aminobenzoic acid (PABA); synergistic action with trimethoprim; primary use is for UTIs

    • Adverse effects: acute hemolytic anemia, crystalluria

    1. Pharmacodynamics

      a. Mechanism of action: bacteriostatic

      • Competitively inhibit dihydropteroate synthase (Fig. 27-2)

      • Have a synergistic action when given with trimethoprim, causing a sequential blockade of the formation of tetrahydrofolate

      b. Causes of resistance

      • Mutations cause excess production of PABA.

    2. Uses

    • Usually given in combination with other drugs such as trimethoprim

    • Infections with *Nocardia, Chlamydia trachomatis,* and some protozoa

---

BOX 27-4

ANTIMETABOLITES

Sulfonamides

Sulfamethoxazole
Sulfasalazine
Sulfisoxazole

Dihydrofolate Reductase Inhibitors

Co-trimoxazole (trimethoprim-sulfamethoxazole)
Trimethoprim

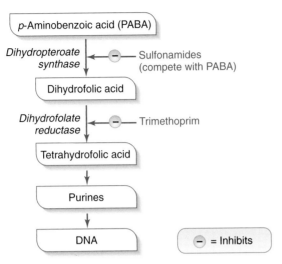

27-2: *Sequential inhibition of tetrahydrofolic acid synthesis. Dihydropteroate is inhibited by sulfonamides and sulfones (dapsone). Dihydrofolate reductase is inhibited by trimethoprim (bacteria, protozoa); pyrimethamine (protozoa); and methotrexate (mammals). Trimethoprim is used in the treatment of certain infections; pyrimethamine is used in the treatment of malaria; and methotrexate is used as an anticancer and immunosuppressive agent.*

- Infections caused by many gram-positive and gram-negative bacteria, especially enteric bacteria such as *E. coli, Salmonella, Shigella,* and *Enterobacter*
  a. UTIs (trimethoprim-sulfamethoxazole)
  b. Respiratory infections
  c. Ulcerative colitis (sulfasalazine)
  d. Burn therapy (silver sulfadiazine; good for *P. aeruginosa*)

Primary use for sulfonamides: UTIs

3. Adverse effects
   a. Blood dyscrasias: agranulocytosis, leukemia, aplastic anemia (rare)
   b. Crystalluria and hematuria
   c. Hypersensitivity reactions: Stevens-Johnson syndrome
4. Contraindications
   a. Relative contraindications: preexisting bone marrow suppression, blood dyscrasias, megaloblastic anemia secondary to folate deficiency
   b. Absolute contraindications: glucose-6-phosphate dehydrogenase (G6PD) deficiency, megaloblastic anemia, porphyria, neonatal period
   c. Sulfonamide hypersensitivity

B. Trimethoprim
1. Mechanism of action: inhibits dihydrofolate reductase; bacteriostatic
2. Uses
   a. Prostatitis
   b. Vaginitis
   c. Otitis media and bronchitis (in combination with sulfonamide)
3. Adverse effects: similar to those of sulfonamides

BOX 27-5

DNA GYRASE INHIBITORS: FLUOROQUINOLONES

Ciprofloxacin
Gatifloxacin
Levofloxacin
Lomefloxacin
Moxifloxacin
Norfloxacin
Ofloxacin
Sparfloxacin
Trovafloxacin

C. Combination product (co-trimoxazole; trimethoprim-sulfamethoxazole)
   • Agent of choice for *P. carinii* pneumonia (PCP), symptomatic *Shigella* enteritis, symptomatic *Salmonella* infections resistant to ampicillin and chloramphenicol, UTIs, upper respiratory infections

VI. Inhibitors of DNA Gyrase: Fluoroquinolones (Box 27-5)
   • Fluoroquinolones interfere with bacteria DNA synthesis (see Fig. 27-1).
   • These drugs are classified by "generation" based on activity.
   • Example of first-generation: norfloxacin; activity against common pathogens that cause urinary tract infections; similar to nalidixic acid
   • Examples of second-generation: ciprofloxacin, ofloxacin; excellent activity against gram-negative bacteria, including gonococcus, many gram-positive cocci, mycobacteria, and *Mycoplasma pneumoniae*
   • Examples of third-generation: levofloxacin, gatifloxacin, sparfloxacin; less activity against gram-negative bacteria but greater activity against some gram-positive cocci, such as *S. pneumoniae,* enterococci, and MRSA

Note the common ending of -floxacin for most fluoroquinolones.

   • Examples of fourth-generation: moxifloxacin, trovafloxacin; broadest spectrum fluoroquinolones with good activity against anaerobes
   A. Pharmacokinetics
      • Good oral bioavailability; absorption is affected by antacids containing divalent and trivalent cations
      • Excretion of most fluoroquinolones is by tubular secretion; blocked by probenecid
   B. Mechanism of action: bactericidal by inhibition of DNA gyrase, the enzyme responsible for counteracting the excessive supercoiling of DNA during replication or transcription
   C. Resistance: due to a change in the gyrase enzyme or decreased permeability

D. Uses
  • Infections with aerobic gram-negative rods, including Enterobacteriaceae, *Pseudomonas,* and *Neisseria*
  • Infections caused by *Campylobacter jejuni, Salmonella, Shigella,* and *Mycobacterium avium* complex
  1. Sinusitis, bronchitis, pneumonia
  2. UTIs
  3. Neutropenic fever (ciprofloxacin)
  4. Anthrax prophylaxis (ciprofloxacin)
E. Adverse effects
  1. Nausea
  2. Interactions with other drugs
    • Patients taking fluoroquinolones should avoid calcium, theophylline, and caffeine.
  3. Interference with collagen synthesis
    a. Causes tendon rupture
    b. Should be avoided during pregnancy
  4. Sparfloxacin prolongs QT interval; potential to cause arrhythmias
  5. Trovafloxacin has hepatotoxic potential

Ciprofloxacin may cause rupture of the Achilles tendon.

Trovafloxacin use is limited to life- and limb-threatening infections.

28 CHAPTER

Other Anti-infective Drugs

TARGET TOPICS

- Treatment of tuberculosis
- Treatment of viral infections
- Treatment of parasitic infections
- Treatment of fungal infections

I. Antimycobacterial Drugs (Box 28-1)
- The management of tuberculosis is summarized in Table 28-1.
  A. Isoniazid (INH)
   1. Pharmacokinetics
      - Metabolism occurs by acetylation (*N*-acetyltransferase; NAT), which is under genetic control.
      - Individuals are either "fast" or "slow" acetylators.
   2. Mechanism of action: bactericidal
      - Inhibits synthesis of mycolic acids, thus inhibiting mycobacterial cell wall synthesis
   3. Use: tuberculosis *(Mycobacterium tuberculosis)*
      a. Prophylaxis in tuberculin converters (positive skin test)
      b. Treatment with rifampin, ethambutol, pyrazinamide, or streptomycin (see Table 28-1)
   4. Adverse effects
      a. Hepatic damage (especially in individuals >35 years of age)
      b. Peripheral neuritis (reversed by pyridoxine; more prominent in "slow" acetylators)
  B. Rifampin
   1. Mechanism of action
      - Binds to the β-subunit of bacterial DNA-dependent RNA polymerase, inhibiting binding of the enzyme to DNA and blocking RNA transcription
   2. Uses
      a. Tuberculosis *(Mycobacterium tuberculosis)*
         (1) Prophylaxis in cases of INH resistance or in individuals who are older than 35 years of age
         (2) Treatment in combination with other drugs (see Table 28-1)

Use rifampin for prophylactic treatment in those older than 35 years of age.

BOX 28-1

ANTIMYCOBACTERIAL DRUGS

Dapsone (leprosy)
Ethambutol
Isoniazid
Pyrazinamide
Rifabutin
Rifampin
Streptomycin

Alternative Drugs Used in Treatment of Tuberculosis

Amikacin
Ciprofloxacin
Ofloxacin
Ethionamide
para-Aminosalicylic acid (PAS)
Capreomycin
Cycloserine

TABLE 28-1:
Management of Tuberculosis

Therapeutic Goal and Drug-Related Patient Features	Initial Drug Treatment	Subsequent Drug Treatment
Prevention of Tuberculosis		
Not resistant to isoniazid	Isoniazid (6 mo)	None
HIV-negative; resistant to isoniazid; >35 years of age	Rifampin (6 mo)	None
HIV-positive	Rifampin* or rifabutin (12 mo)	None
Treatment of Tuberculosis		
Not resistant to isoniazid	Combination of isoniazid, rifampin, ethambutol, and pyrazinamide for 2 months	Combination of isoniazid and rifampin (4 more months if HIV-negative or 7 more months if HIV-positive)
Possibly resistant to isoniazid	Combination of isoniazid, rifampin, pyrazinamide, and either ethambutol or streptomycin (6 mo)	Individualized therapy based on microbial susceptibility testing
Resistant to multiple drugs[†]	Combination of at least four drugs believed to be active in patient population (6 mo)	Individualized therapy based on microbial susceptibility testing

*In HIV-infected patients, substitution of rifabutin for rifampin minimizes drug interactions with protease inhibitors and nucleoside reverse transcriptase inhibitors.
[†]Patients suspected of having multidrug resistance include those from certain demographic populations, those who have failed to respond to previous treatment, and those who have experienced a relapse of tuberculosis. HIV, human immunodeficiency virus.

b. Prophylaxis in contacts of *Neisseria meningitidis* and *Haemophilus influenzae* type B

c. Legionnaires' disease (in combination with azithromycin)

d. Leprosy *(Mycobacterium leprae)* (combination therapy)

3. Adverse effects

a. Red-orange discoloration of urine, tears, saliva

b. Hepatotoxicity

c. Drug interactions

- Rifampin, a potent inducer of the cytochrome P-450 hepatic enzyme systems, can reduce the plasma concentrations of many drugs, including anticonvulsants, contraceptive steroids, cyclosporine, warfarin, terbinafine, ketoconazole, methadone.
- Rifabutin is a less potent inducer of the cytochrome P-450 hepatic enzyme system; thus, it causes less robust drug-drug interactions.

C. Ethambutol

1. Mechanism of action: unknown; possibly inhibits RNA synthesis

2. Use: tuberculosis (combination therapy; see Table 28-1)

3. Adverse effects: optic neuritis, reduction in red-green visual acuity
- Annual eye examination is necessary.

D. Pyrazinamide

1. Mechanism of action: unknown; requires metabolic conversion to pyrazinoic acid

2. Use: tuberculosis (combination therapy; see Table 28-1)

3. Adverse effects: hyperuricemia, hepatotoxicity, photosensitivity

E. Rifabutin

- Rifabutin is a less potent inducer of cytochrome P-450 hepatic enzymes than is rifampin.

1. Mechanism of action: inhibition of mycobacterial RNA polymerase

2. Uses

a. Substitute for rifampin in the treatment of tuberculosis in HIV-infected patients

b. Prevention and treatment of *Mycobacterium avium* complex

F. Streptomycin: This aminoglycoside is used more frequently because of increased incidence of drug-resistant *M. tuberculosis* strains; other uses include tularemia *(Francisella tularensis),* plague *(Yersinia pestis),* and, until recently, in combination with a penicillin for the treatment of endocarditis.

G. Alternative drugs used in treatment of tuberculosis: amikacin, ciprofloxacin, ofloxacin, ethionamide, para-aminosalicylic acid (PAS), capreomycin, cycloserine

H. Dapsone

1. Mechanism of action: bacteriostatic inhibitor of folic acid synthesis

2. Use: leprosy *(M. leprae)*

3. Adverse effects

a. Optic neuritis, neuropathy

b. Glucose-6-phosphate dehydrogenase (G6PD) deficiency, which leads to hemolytic anemia

Treatment with rifampin often results in permanent discoloration of soft contact lenses.

Rifampin: potent inducer of cytochrome P-450 hepatic enzymes

Ethambutol use requires eye examinations.

BOX 28-2

ANTIVIRAL DRUGS

Drugs Used in the Treatment and Prophylaxis of Influenza

Amantadine
Oseltamivir
Rimantadine
Zanamivir

Antiherpes Drugs

Acyclovir
  Acyclovir congeners: famciclovir, penciclovir, valacyclovir
Cidofovir
Foscarnet
Ganciclovir

Interferons

Interferon alfa
Interferon beta

Antiretroviral Drugs

Nucleoside Reverse Transcriptase Inhibitors
Abacavir
Didanosine (ddI)
Emtricitabine

Lamivudine (3TC)
Stavudine (d4T)
Zalcitabine (ddC)
Zidovudine (AZT)

Nonnucleoside Reverse Transcriptase Inhibitors
Delavirdine
Efavirenz
Nevirapine
Tenofovir

Protease Inhibitors
Amprenavir
Indinavir
Lopinavir
Nelfinavir
Ritonavir
Saquinavir

Fusion Inhibitor
Enfuvirtide

Other Antiviral Drugs

Ribavirin

II. Antiviral Drugs (Box 28-2)
  • The mechanism of viral replication and the effects of antiviral drugs are shown in Figure 28-1.
  A. Drugs used in the prevention and treatment of influenza
    1. Amantadine and rimantadine
      a. Mechanism of action
        • Blocks the uncoating of the virus particle and the subsequent release of viral nucleic acid into the host cell
        • May also interfere with penetration of the cell wall by absorbed virus
      b. Uses
        (1) Influenza A (prophylaxis)
        (2) Parkinson's disease (see Chapter 11)
      c. Adverse effects: dizziness, anxiety, impaired coordination
    2. Oseltamivir and zanamivir
      a. Mechanism of action: inhibit viral neuraminidase

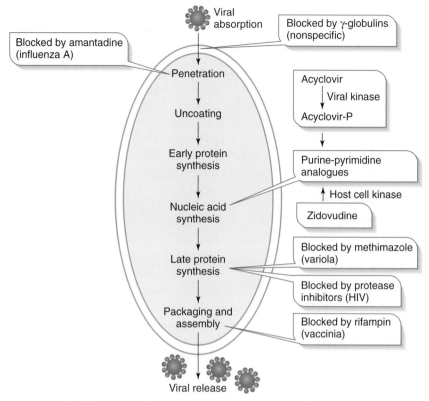

28-1: *Mechanism of viral replication and the site of action of antiviral drugs.*

    b. Use: influenza (prevention and treatment of symptoms)

    c. Adverse effects: nausea, vomiting, bronchitis

B. Interferons

    1. Mechanism of action: inhibit viral penetration and uncoating along with peptide elongation

    2. Uses

        a. Interferon alfa (systemic): hairy-cell leukemia, AIDS-related Kaposi's sarcoma, condyloma acuminatum, chronic hepatitis B and hepatitis C

        b. Interferon beta: multiple sclerosis

    3. Adverse effects: neutropenia, anemia, influenza symptoms

C. Ribavirin

    • The antiviral action of this synthetic nucleoside requires intracellular phosphorylation.

    1. Mechanism of action: selectively inhibits viral DNA and RNA synthesis

    2. Use

        a. Inhalation therapy in respiratory syncytial virus (RSV) infections and influenza

        b. Hepatitis C

    3. Adverse effects: respiratory depression, hemolytic anemia

D. Antiherpes drugs
1. Acyclovir and ganciclovir
a. Mechanism of action
- These drugs are phosphorylated by viral thymidine kinases; the phosphorylated metabolites inhibit viral DNA polymerase.
b. Resistance: involves loss of thymidine kinase activity
c. Uses: herpes simplex, herpes genitalis, herpes zoster, varicella zoster, cytomegalovirus (ganciclovir)
- Acyclovir congeners: famciclovir, penciclovir, valacyclovir
d. Adverse effects: nephrotoxicity, confusion, coma, encephalopathy
2. Foscarnet
a. Mechanism of action
- No dependence on thymidine kinase, with no phosphorylation necessary.
- Selective inhibition of the viral-specific DNA polymerases
b. Uses: cytomegalovirus, herpes simplex virus, varicella zoster virus
c. Adverse effects: renal impairment, headache, seizures
3. Cidofovir
- This acyclic phosphonate nucleotide analogue is used for the treatment of cytomegalovirus (CMV) retinitis or herpesvirus infections.
- It is not dependent upon intracellular activation for its antiviral activity.
- Hepatotoxicity is a major dose-limiting toxicity.
E. Antiretroviral drugs
- These drugs may have serious side effects (Table 28-2).

Drug	Adverse Effect(s)
Nucleoside Reverse Transcriptase Inhibitors	
Didanosine (ddI)	Peripheral neuropathy, pancreatitis (dose-dependent)
Lamivudine (3TC)	Headache, elevated hepatic enzymes, hyperbilirubinemia (dosereduction is necessary in renal disease)
Stavudine (d4T)	Peripheral sensory neuropathy
Zalcitabine (ddC)	Peripheral sensory neuropathy, esophageal ulcers
Zidovudine (AZT)	Bone marrow suppression, anemia
Nonnucleoside Reverse Transcriptase Inhibitors	
Delavirdine	Rash, pruritus
Nevirapine	Rash, elevated hepatic enzymes
Protease Inhibitors	
Indinavir	Hyperbilirubinemia, nephrolithiasis
Nelfinavir	Diarrhea, anaphylactoid reactions, inhibition of metabolism of many drugs
Ritonavir	Multiple drug interactions
Saquinavir	Gastrointestinal disturbance, rhinitis

TABLE 28-2:
Adverse Effects of Antiretroviral Agents

1. Nucleoside reverse transcriptase inhibitors
   - Zidovudine (AZT), didanosine (ddI), lamivudine (3TC), stavudine (d4T), zalcitabine (ddC), abacavir, emtricitabine
   a. Mechanism of action: inhibit viral RNA–directed DNA polymerase (reverse transcriptase) following phosphorylation
   b. Use: HIV infection (treatment and prevention)
2. Nonnucleoside reverse transcriptase inhibitors (NNRTI)
   - Delavirdine, nevirapine, efavirenz, tenofovir
   a. Mechanism of action
     - Directly inhibit reverse transcriptase, with no activation required
     - Not incorporated into viral DNA
   b. Use: HIV infection
3. Protease inhibitors (PI)
   - Indinavir, nelfinavir, ritonavir, saquinavir, amprenavir, lopinavir
   a. Mechanism of action: competitively inhibit HIV protease
     (1) Indinavir and ritonavir: inhibit the cytochrome P-450 system
     (2) Saquinavir: metabolized by the cytochrome P-450 system but does not inhibit the enzyme
   b. Use: HIV infection
   c. Adverse effects: effects on carbohydrate and lipid metabolism including hyperglycemia and insulin resistance, hyperlipidemia, and altered body fat distribution (buffalo hump, gynecomastia, and truncal obesity)
4. Fusion inhibitor: enfuvirtide
   - It interferes with the entry of HIV-1 into host cells by inhibiting the fusion of the virus and cell membranes
   - Reserved for individuals who have advanced disease or show resistance to current HIV treatments

III. Antiparasitic Drugs (Box 28-3)
   A. Antimalaria drugs
     1. Chloroquine
        a. Pharmacokinetics
          (1) Extensive tissue binding, with a very large volume of distribution (13,000 L)
          (2) Slow release from the tissues
          (3) Liver metabolism, renal excretion
        b. Mechanism of resistance: membrane P-glycoprotein pump that expels chloroquine from the parasite
        c. Uses: clinical cure and prophylaxis (all species of *Plasmodium*)
          - Treatment of infections caused by *Plasmodium vivax* and *Plasmodium ovale* requires use of chloroquine in combination with primaquine.
        d. Adverse effects: visual impairment, hearing loss, tinnitus, aplastic anemia
     2. Mefloquine
        - Use: chloroquine-resistant and multidrug-resistant falciparum malaria (prophylaxis and treatment)

Note common ending -navir for protease inhibitors, whereas many antivirals have the ending: -vir.

The preferred NNRTI-based regimen combines efavirenz with lamivudine or emtricitabine and zidovudine or tenofovir; the preferred PI-based regimen combines lopinavir, ritonavir with zidovudine, and lamivudine or emtricitabine (available on the World Wide Web at www.aidsinfo.nih.gov).

Adverse effects of protease inhibitors are very similar to the cushingoid syndrome.

Chloroquine should be avoided or used cautiously in patients with ocular, hematologic, neurologic, or hepatic diseases.

> ### BOX 28-3
>
> ### ANTIPARASITIC DRUGS
>
> **Antimalarial Drugs**
> Chloroquine
> Mefloquine
> Primaquine
>
> **Antihelmintic Drugs**
> Ivermectin
> Mebendazole
> Praziquantel
> Pyrantel pamoate
> Thiabendazole
>
> **Other Antiprotozoal Drugs**
> Metronidazole
> Pentamidine

3. Primaquine
   a. Mechanism of action: active against late hepatic stages (hypnozoites and schizonts) of *P. vivax* and *P. ovale*
   b. Uses
      (1) Malaria (in combination with chloroquine)
      (2) *Pneumocystis carinii* pneumonia (PCP) (alternative therapy; in combination with clindamycin)
   c. Adverse effects: anorexia, weakness, hemolytic anemia, leukopenia
B. Other antiprotozoal drugs
   1. Metronidazole
      a. Uses
         (1) Urogenital trichomoniasis *(Trichomonas vaginalis),* giardiasis *(Giardia),* amebiasis *(Entamoeba histolytica)*
         (2) Aspiration pneumonia
         (3) Anaerobic infections (including *Clostridium difficile, Bacteroides fragilis*)
      b. Adverse effects: metallic taste, disulfiram-like effect
   2. Pentamidine
      • Uses: PCP in HIV-infected individuals, *Trypanosoma gambiense*
C. Antihelmintic drugs
   1. Praziquantel
      a. Mechanism of action
         • Increases calcium permeability, depolarizing cells
         • Results in contraction followed by paralysis of worm musculature

Individuals with G6PD deficiency who take primaquine are susceptible to hemolytic anemia.

Metronidazole: Patients who are taking this drug should not consume alcohol.

Praziquantel is useful for flukes and tapeworms.

   b. Uses
      (1) Schistosomiasis
      (2) Infections with flukes (trematodes) and tapeworms (cestodes)
   c. Adverse effects
      (1) Headaches, dizziness, drowsiness
      (2) Gastrointestinal (GI) disturbances
2. Thiabendazole and mebendazole
   a. Mechanism of action: block microtubule formation
   b. Uses
      (1) Thiabendazole: strongyloidiasis, cutaneous larva migrans
          (alternative drug)
      (2) Mebendazole: ascariasis, trichuriasis, hookworm, pinworm
          (Enterobius vermicularis), cysticercosis *(Taenia solium), Echinococcus*
          infestations
   c. Adverse effects: abdominal pain, diarrhea
3. Pyrantel pamoate
   a. Mechanism of action
      • Acts as a depolarizing neuromuscular blocking agent on the nicotinic
        receptor
      • Increases the effects of acetylcholine and inhibits cholinesterase in the
        worm
   b. Uses: ascariasis, pinworm *(E. vermicularis),* hookworm, whipworm
      (Trichuris trichiura), Trichostrongylus
   c. Adverse effects: nausea, vomiting, diarrhea, anorexia
4. Ivermectin
   a. Mechanism of action: increases chloride permeability, thus polarizing
      cells, which leads to paralysis
   b. Uses: strongyloidiasis, onchocerciasis

IV. Antifungal Drugs (Box 28-4)
   • Antifungal agents are commonly used in debilitated and immunosuppressed
     patients with conditions such as leukemia, lymphoma, immunodeficiencies,
     and diabetes.
   • The mechanisms of action of some antifungal agents are shown in Figure 28-2.
   A. Amphotericin B (polyene antibiotic)
      1. Pharmacokinetics
         • The drug is given intravenously or intrathecally; it is *not* absorbed orally.
         • Placement of the active drug in a lipid delivery system (liposomal
           amphotericin B) results in increased efficacy and decreased toxicity.
      2. Mechanism of action
         • Binds to ergosterol in fungal cell membranes, causing an increase in
           membrane permeability
      3. Use: severe systemic fungal infection (drug of choice)
      4. Adverse effects
         a. Nephrotoxicity
         b. Pancytopenia, anemia
         c. Hepatotoxicity

*Increased fungal
infections in
immunosuppressed
patients*

BOX 28-4

ANTIFUNGAL DRUGS

Azole Derivatives

Fluconazole
Itraconazole
Ketoconazole
Voriconazole

Other Drugs

Amphotericin B
Liposomal amphotericin B
Caspofungin
Flucytosine
Griseofulvin
Nystatin
Terbinafine

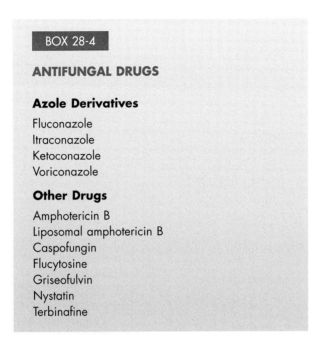

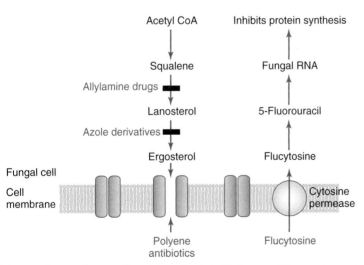

28-2: *Mechanism of action of some antifungal drugs. Amphotericin B and nystatin are polyenes; terbinafine is an allylamine; and ketoconazole, fluconazole, and itraconazole are azoles. CoA, coenzyme A.*

B. Flucytosine
   1. Mechanism of action: conversion to fluorouracil (an antimetabolite) only in fungal cells
      • Competes with uracil by interfering with pyrimidine metabolism and disrupting both RNA and protein synthesis

Resistance develops to flucytosine rapidly when it is used alone.

2. Uses: systemic fungal infections due to *Candida* species, including *C. glabrata,* and *Cryptococcus neoformans* (in combination with amphotericin B)
3. Adverse effects: nausea, vomiting, diarrhea, bone marrow suppression

C. Azole drugs
   - Examples: ketoconazole, itraconazole, fluconazole, voriconazole
   1. Pharmacokinetics
      - The four drugs listed as examples are absorbed orally.
      - Fluconazole has good central nervous system (CNS) penetration.
   2. Mechanism of action
      - Azoles inhibit ergosterol synthesis by preventing conversion of lanosterol to ergosterol (essential component of the fungal cell membrane) (see Fig. 28-2).
   3. Uses
      a. Mucocutaneous candidiasis and nonmeningeal coccidioidomycosis
      b. Cryptococcal meningitis (fluconazole)
      c. *Aspergillus* (itraconazole)
   4. Adverse effects
      a. Elevation of serum transaminase levels
      b. Gynecomastia (blocks adrenal steroid synthesis)
      c. Inhibition of cytochrome P-450 enzymes (especially ketoconazole)

Azole derivatives: inhibition of cytochrome P-450 enzymes

D. Caspofungin
   1. An intravenous drug that inhibits the synthesis of glucan, a major fungal cell wall component.
   2. Use: invasive aspergillosis in patients who failed amphotericin B therapy

E. Griseofulvin
   1. Mechanism of action
      - Decreases microtubule function, disrupting the mitotic spindle structure of the fungal cell and causing an arrest of the M phase of the cell cycle
      - Concentrates in keratinized tissue, so selectively localizes in the skin, with an affinity for diseased skin
   2. Uses: dermatophytic infections such as ringworm and athlete's foot *(Microsporum, Trichophyton)*

F. Terbinafine
   1. Mechanism of action
      a. Inhibits the fungal enzyme squalene epoxidase
      b. Interferes with ergosterol biosynthesis (like azoles)
      c. Concentrates in keratinized tissue (like griseofulvin)
   2. Use
      a. Dermatophytosis (topical),
      b. Onychomycosis (oral, replaces griseofulvin)
   3. Adverse effects (rare): headache, GI upset

G. Nystatin
   1. Polyene antifungal with mechanism similar to amphotericin B
   2. Use
      a. Orally (not absorbed from the GI tract) for intestinal candidiasis
      b. Topically for candidiasis of the oral and vaginal cavity

Nystatin swish is often used for the treatment of oral thrush.

29 CHAPTER

Chemotherapeutic Drugs

TARGET TOPICS

- Alkylating agents
- Antimetabolites
- Antibiotics
- Plant alkaloids
- Hormones
- Monoclonal antibodies
- Signal transduction inhibitors

I. General Considerations (Box 29-1)
  - Cancer is a disease in which the cellular control mechanisms that govern proliferation and differentiation are changed.
  A. Drugs used in cancer chemotherapy target important biosynthetic processes in proliferating cells (Fig. 29-1).
  B. The goal of cancer chemotherapy is to destroy cancer cells selectively with as few effects on normal cells as possible.
  C. Adverse effects of chemotherapeutic drugs (Table 29-1)
    - Individual drugs have "signature" adverse effects in addition to the number of adverse effects that are characteristic to the group that are listed below:
    1. Bone marrow suppression
    2. Toxicity to mucosal cells of the gastrointestinal tract, which leads to nausea, ulcers, and diarrhea
    3. Toxicity to skin and hair follicles, which results in hair loss
    4. Teratogenic effects
    5. Sterility
    6. Immunosuppression

II. Drugs That Alter DNA
  A. Alkylating drugs
    1. Cyclophosphamide
      - Prodrug that requires activation by the cytochrome P-450 system
      a. Mechanism of action: cell cycle–nonspecific (CCNS)
        - Cross-links DNA strands, stopping DNA processing
      b. Uses
        (1) Chronic lymphocytic leukemia (CLL), acute lymphocytic leukemia (ALL), non-Hodgkin's lymphoma, multiple myeloma

Ondansetron and other -setron drugs are used to treat the nausea and vomiting associated with anticancer drugs.

BOX 29-1

CHEMOTHERAPEUTIC DRUGS

Drugs That Alter DNA

Alkylating Drugs
Busulfan
Carboplatin
Carmustine
Cisplatin
Cyclophosphamide
Dacarbazine
Lomustine
Mechlorethamine
Melphalan
Promethazine

Antibiotics
Bleomycin
Dactinomycin
Daunorubicin
Doxorubicin
Epirubicin
Idarubicin
Mitoxantrone

Antimetabolites

Folic Acid Antagonist
Methotrexate

Purine Antagonists
Cladribine
Fludarabine
6-Mercaptopurine
6-Thioguanine

Pyrimidine Antagonists
Capecitabine
Cytarabine
5-Fluorouracil
Gemcitabine

Mitotic Inhibitors
Docetaxel
Paclitaxel
Vinblastine
Vincristine

Podophyllotoxins
Etoposide
Teniposide

Camptothecans
Irinotecan
Topotecan

Hormones and Hormone Regulators

Hormones
Prednisone

Modulators of Hormone Release and Action
Anastrozole
Aminoglutethimide
Bicalutamide
Exemestane
Flutamide
Goserelin
Letrozole
Leuprolide
Nafarelin
Nilutamide
Tamoxifen
Toremifene

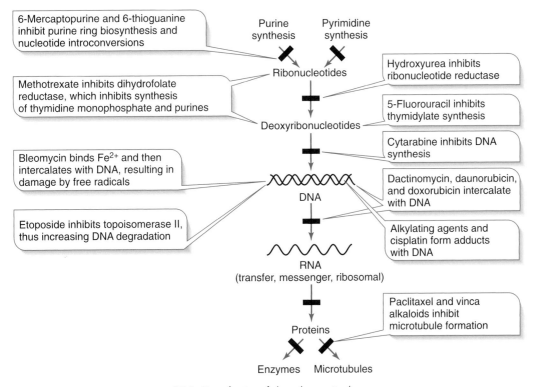

29-1: *Sites of action of chemotherapeutic drugs.*

(2) Breast, ovarian, and lung cancers
(3) Immunologic disorders such as lupus nephritis, nephrotic syndrome, Wegener's granulomatosis, rheumatoid arthritis, and graft-versus-host disease or graft rejection

2. Busulfan
   a. Mechanism of action: cell cycle–nonspecific (CCNS), bifunctional alkylating agent
   b. Use: chronic granulocytic leukemia (drug of choice)
3. Mechlorethamine (nitrogen mustard): a CCNS drug used to treat Hodgkin's disease, non-Hodgkin's lymphoma, and mycosis fungoides
4. Carmustine and lomustine: nitrosourea drugs
   a. Mechanism of action: cell cycle–nonspecific (CCNS)
   b. Use: primary and metastatic brain tumors
5. Cisplatin and carboplatin
   a. Mechanism of action
      • Cross-links to any nucleic acid or protein structure that forms irreversible covalent bonds, thereby inhibiting DNA replication, RNA transcription, and protein synthesis

"Signature" adverse effect of cyclophosphamide: hemorrhagic cystitis

"Signature" adverse effect of busulfan: pulmonary fibrosis

The nitrosoureas are unique anticancer agents because they cross the blood-brain barrier.

TABLE 29-1:
Therapeutic Uses and Adverse Effects of Drugs Used in Cancer Chemotherapy

Drug	Use: Type(s) of Cancer*	Important Adverse Effect(s)
Aminoglutethimide	Breast, prostate	Adrenal suppression, dizziness, rash
Anastrozole	Breast	Hot flashes
Bleomycin	Testicular, ovarian, cervical, thyroid	Pulmonary fibrosis; very little bone marrow toxicity
Busulfan	CML, polycythemia vera	Interstitial pulmonary fibrosis
Carmustine/lomustine	Brain	Leukopenia, thrombocytopenia, hepatotoxicity
Cisplatin	Head and neck, lung, testicular, cervical, thyroid, ovarian	Ototoxicity, severe nephrotoxicity, mild bone marrow suppression
Cyclophosphamide	Leukemias/lymphomas	Hemorrhagic cystitis, alopecia
Cytarabine	Leukemias	Bone marrow suppression, CNS toxicity, immunosuppression
Dactinomycin	Wilms' tumor	Hepatotoxicity
Daunorubicin/doxorubicin	Acute leukemia, Hodgkin's disease, breast and lung	Cardiomyopathy (daunorubicin)
Etoposide	Lung, testicular	Bone marrow suppression
5-Fluorouracil	Colon, stomach, prostate, breast	Bone marrow suppression, GI toxicity
Imatinib	CML, gastrointestinal stromal tumors	Fluid retention
Irinotecan	Colon	Bone marrow suppression
Leuprolide	Prostate, breast	Hot flashes
Melphalan	Multiple myeloma	Bone marrow suppression
6-Mercaptopurine	Leukemias	Bone marrow suppression
Methotrexate	Wilms' tumor, choriocarcinoma, leukemias	Bone marrow suppression, oral and GI tract ulceration, diarrhea, hepatotoxicity†
Paclitaxel (Taxol)	Breast, ovarian	Bone marrow suppression
Procarbazine	Hodgkin's disease	Secondary malignancies, teratogenic
Tamoxifen	Breast	Hot flashes
Trastuzumab	Breast	Fever and chills
Vinblastine	Lymphomas	Bone marrow suppression
Vincristine	Acute lymphocytic leukemia	Neurotoxicity/peripheral neuropathy, low bone marrow suppression

*Not a complete list; for most cancers, drug combinations are used.
†Adverse effects, especially toxicity, may be reversed with folic acid ("leucovorin rescue").
CML, chronic myelogenous leukemia; CNS, central nervous system; GI, gastrointestinal.

      b. Uses
        (1) Genitourinary cancers: testicular (in combination with vinblastine and bleomycin), ovarian, urinary bladder
        (2) Non–small cell lung cancer

  6. Melphalan
    • Uses: breast and ovarian cancers, multiple myeloma

  7. Drugs related to alkylating agents: procarbazine, dacarbazine
    • Procarbazine is used in the treatment of Hodgkin's disease; highly teratogenic and a known carcinogen that can cause secondary malignancy
    • Dacarbazine is used in the treatment of metastatic malignant melanoma, osteogenic sarcoma, soft-tissue sarcoma, and Hodgkin's disease.

B. Intercalating agents: antibiotics
  1. Dactinomycin (actinomycin D)
    a. Mechanism of action: cell cycle–nonspecific (CCNS)
      • Intercalates between base pairs of DNA, preventing DNA and RNA synthesis
    b. Uses
      (1) Trophoblastic tumors
      (2) Wilms' tumor in combination with surgery and vincristine
      (3) Ewing's sarcoma

  2. Daunorubicin and doxorubicin
    • Liposomal preparation of daunorubicin and doxorubicin decrease the incidence of severe toxicity seen with the conventional formulations while taking advantage of the unique delivery properties of liposomes and the cytotoxic effects of the anthracyclines
    • Newer congeners: epirubicin and idarubicin; less cardiotoxicity
    a. Mechanism of action: cell cycle–nonspecific (CCNS)
      (1) Intercalate between base pairs of DNA
      (2) Inhibit topoisomerase II, causing faulty DNA repairs
    b. Uses
      (1) Daunorubicin: acute granulocytic leukemia (AGL), acute lymphocytic leukemia (ALL)
      (2) Doxorubicin: breast, endometrial, ovarian, testicular, thyroid, and lung cancers; sarcomas
    c. Adverse effects: Dexrazoxane is a chemoprotectant agent for the prevention of anthracycline-associated cardiomyopathy; it is an intracellular iron chelator that decreases the ability of iron to react with superoxide anions and H_2O_2 to produce highly toxic superhydroxide radicals leading to cardiotoxicity.

  3. Mitoxantrone: similar to the anthracyclines; sometimes substituted for doxorubicin or daunorubicin because it has considerably less cardiotoxicity

  4. Bleomycin
    • Concentrates in skin and lungs
    a. Mechanism of action: cell cycle–specific (CCS); most active during the G_2 and M phases

---

"Signature" adverse effects of cisplatin: nephrotoxicity, ototoxicity

Procarbazine is highly carcinogenic.

Note the common ending of -rubicin for anthracycline anticancer drugs.

"Signature" adverse effect of daunorubicin and doxorubicin: cardiotoxicity (cardiomyopathy)

"Signature" adverse effect of bleomycin: pulmonary fibrosis

- • Causes formation of free radicals, which affects DNA
    b. Uses
        (1) Squamous cell carcinoma of the head, neck, and skin
        (2) Lymphomas
        (3) Testicular cancer

III. Antimetabolites

Methotrexate is also a potent immunosuppressant drug.

A. Folic acid antagonists: methotrexate (MTX)
    1. Mechanism of action: cell cycle–specific (CCS)
        • Inhibits conversion of folic acid to tetrahydrofolic acid (dihydrofolate reductase inhibitor)

Leucovorin rescue (folinic acid) can be used to overcome the effects of high blood levels of methotrexate.

    2. Uses
        a. Choriocarcinoma (women)
        b. ALL, non-Hodgkin's lymphoma
        c. Tumors of the breast, testis, bladder, and lung
        d. Systemic lupus erythematosus, rheumatic arthritis, Crohn's disease

"Signature" adverse effect of methotrexate: acute and chronic hepatotoxicity

B. Purine antagonist: 6-mercaptopurine (6-MP), thioguanine
    1. Mechanism of action: cell cycle–specific (CCS)
        • Inhibits purine synthesis
    2. Use: ALL induction

Effects of purine antagonists are potentiated by allopurinol.

    3. Newer purine antagonist congeners: fludarabine, cladribine

C. Pyrimidine antagonists
    1. 5-Fluorouracil (5-FU)
        a. Mechanism of action: cell cycle–specific (CCS); most active during the S phase
            • Active metabolite inhibits thymidylate synthase and interferes with DNA and RNA synthesis

Leucovorin (folinic acid) potentiates the effects of 5-FU.

            • Leucovorin (folinic acid) enhances its binding to thymidylate synthase
        b. Uses: gastric, breast, colorectal, and skin neoplasms
    2. Cytarabine (Ara-C)
        a. Mechanism of action: cell cycle–specific (CCS); active during the S phase
            • Active metabolite inhibits DNA polymerase, thus interfering with DNA synthesis.
        b. Uses: AGL, non-Hodgkin's lymphoma
    3. Newer pyrimidine antagonist congeners: capecitabine, gemcitabine

IV. Mitotic Inhibitors
    A. Vinca alkaloids
        1. Vinblastine
            a. Mechanism of action: cell cycle–specific (CCS); active during the M phase; metaphase
                • Binds to tubulin (microtubular protein) and prevents polymerization

Vinblastine: BLASTs the bone marrow

            b. Uses
                (1) Hodgkin's and non-Hodgkin's lymphomas

(2) Testicular carcinoma (in combination with cisplatin and bleomycin)
2. Vincristine
    a. Mechanism of action: similar to vinblastine
    b. Uses: same as for vinblastine, plus ALL and Wilms' tumor
B. Paclitaxel (taxol) and docetaxel
    1. Mechanism of action: cell cycle–specific (CCS); active during the G_2 and M phases
      • Binds to tubulin and prevents depolymerization
    2. Uses
      a. Refractory ovarian and breast cancers
      b. Non–small cell lung cancer

> "Signature" adverse effect of vincristine (dose-limiting): neurotoxicity, such as peripheral neuropathy
>
> Taxanes stabilize and vinca alkaloids inhibit formation of microtubular structure.

V. Podophyllotoxin: Etoposide (VP-16), Teniposide
  A. Mechanism of action: cell cycle–specific (CCS); active during the G_2 phase
    • Inhibits topoisomerase II
  B. Uses
    1. Non-Hodgkin's lymphoma
    2. Testicular cancer
    3. Small cell lung cancer

VI. Camptothecin: Irinotecan, Topotecan
  • Cytotoxic plant alkaloids that are topoisomerase I inhibitors.
  • Topotecan is used as a second-line treatment for ovarian cancers.
  • Irinotecan is used in the first-line treatment of metastatic colorectal cancer in combination with 5-fluorouracil (5-FU) and leucovorin.

VII. Hormones and Hormone Regulators
  A. Hormones
    1. Corticosteroids (prednisone; see Chapter 23)
      a. Mechanism of action: inhibits cytokine production and T-cell production
      b. Uses: often used in combination with other antineoplastic agents
        (1) ALL in children
        (2) CLL
        (3) Multiple myeloma
        (4) Hodgkin's and non-Hodgkin's lymphomas
  B. Modulation of hormone release and action
    1. Aminoglutethimide
      a. Mechanism of action: blocks first step in adrenal steroid synthesis and inhibits estrogen synthesis (aromatase inhibitor)
      b. Use: metastatic breast cancer (equivalent to tamoxifen but with more adverse effects); also used for the suppression of adrenal function in Cushing's syndrome
    2. Aromatase inhibitors: anastrozole, exemestane, letrozole
      a. Mechanism of action: inhibits aromatase, the enzyme that catalyzes the final step in estrogen synthesis
      b. Uses: treatment of advanced breast cancer

> Aminoglutethimide treatment must always be given in combination with hydrocortisone to prevent adrenal insufficiency.

Patients often complain of hot flashes.

Note the common ending -lutamide for the androgen antagonists.

3. Estrogen antagonists: tamoxifen, toremifene
   a. Mechanism of action
      (1) Blocks estrogen receptors in cancer cells that require estrogen for growth and development
      (2) Acts as a weak agonist at estrogen receptors in other tissues
   b. Uses
      (1) Breast and endometrial cancers
      (2) Metastatic melanoma (some effect)
4. Androgen antagonists: flutamide, bicalutamide, nilutamide
   a. Mechanism of action: inhibits the uptake and binding of testosterone and dihydrotestosterone by prostatic tissue
   b. Use: treatment of metastatic prostatic carcinoma in combination with luteinizing hormone–releasing hormone (LHRH) agonists such as leuprolide
5. Gonadotropin-releasing hormone (GnRH) analogues: leuprolide, goserelin, nafarelin (see Chapter 26)
   a. Pharmacokinetics
      • Synthetic analogue of a naturally occurring GnRH
      • Administered as an injection
   b. Uses
      (1) Advanced prostate or breast cancers (hormonal antagonist)
      (2) Endometriosis

VIII. Monoclonal Antibodies
   A. Alemtuzumab
      • Binds to CD52 antigen on normal and malignant β-lymphocytes
      • CD52 antigen also found on T lymphocytes, natural killer cells, macrophages, and platelets
      • Approved for chronic lymphocytic leukemia (CLL)
   B. Gemtuzumab ozogamicin
      • Directed toward the CD33 antigen that is expressed on leukemic cells and myelomonocytic cells
      • Coupled to calicheamicin, a cytotoxic molecule
      • Used for the treatment of acute myelogenous leukemia (AML) in adults over 60 years of age in first relapse and have a CD33-positive tumor
   C. Rituximab
      • Binds to CD20 antigen on B cells
      • Used in B-cell non-Hodgkin's lymphoma
   D. Tositumomab
      • Targets the CD20 antigen found on pre-B- and mature B-lymphocytes
      • Used for treatment of CD20-positive follicular non-Hodgkin's lymphoma (NHL) whose disease is refractory to rituximab and has relapsed following chemotherapy
   E. Trastuzumab
      • Binds to the HER2 protein on the surface of tumor cells
      • Used for metastatic breast tumors that over express HER2 protein

IX. Signal Transduction Inhibitors
  A. Imatinib
   • Inhibits the Bcr-Abl tyrosine protein kinase found in chronic myelogenous leukemia (CML)
   • Used for the treatment of CML in patients who have failed alpha interferon therapy and for the treatment of metastatic and unresectable malignant gastrointestinal stromal tumors (GIST)

Alfa is the name of one of the alpha interferons.

CHAPTER

30

Toxicology and Drugs of Abuse

TARGET TOPICS

- Symptoms of poisoning
- Treatment of poisoning
- Teratogenic substances
- Substances of abuse

I. General Principles of Toxicology
- Toxicology is the study of the hazardous effects of chemicals, including drugs, on biologic systems.
- Toxicity is a reflection of how much, how fast, and how long an individual is exposed to a poison.
  A. Primary determinants of toxicity
  1. Dose and dose rate
  2. Duration of exposure
  3. Route of exposure
  B. Factors that affect toxicity
  1. Biotransformation
     - Methanol is converted to formaldehyde and formic acid (toxic metabolites).
  2. Genetic factors
     - Individuals are "fast" or "slow" acetylators of isoniazid.
  3. Immune status: hypersensitivity reactions such as penicillin or sulfonamide hypersensitivity
  4. Photosensitivity: skin photosensitivity due to demeclocycline
  5. Species differences
     - Malathion is rapidly metabolized by humans but not by insects.
  6. Age
     - Both toxicodynamic and toxicokinetic parameters vary with age.
  7. Gender
     - Hormonal status affects both toxicodynamic and toxicokinetic parameters.
  8. Environmental factors
  9. Nutritional status/protein binding
  10. Drug interactions

- Interactions between drugs and between drugs and environmental chemicals may occur by both toxicokinetic and toxicodynamic mechanisms.

II. Symptoms and Treatment of Acute Poisoning (Tables 30-1 and 30-2)
   A. Obtain important historical information and determine the severity of exposure.
   B. Check vital signs.
   C. Remove stomach contents if indicated.
      1. Gastric lavage
         - Not recommended after 4 hours after poisoning
         a. Contraindications
            (1) After 30 minutes of ingestion of corrosive material
            (2) Ingestion of hydrocarbon solvents (aspiration pneumonia)
            (3) Coma, stupor, delirium, or seizures (present or imminent)
         b. Substance used to reduce absorption of poison
            - Activated charcoal adsorbs many toxins if given immediately before or after lavage.
      2. Induced emesis
         a. Same contraindications as for gastric lavage
         b. Makes use of syrup of ipecac (slow-acting oral emetic)
   D. History and physical examination provide clues to potential exposure.
      - Oral statements may be unreliable.
      - Always treat symptoms.
      - Physical examination should focus on clues of intoxication.
      - Vital signs are checked.
         1. Hypertension with tachycardia: amphetamines, cocaine, antimuscarinics
         2. Hypotension and bradycardia: beta blockers, calcium channel blockers, clonidine, sedative-hypnotics
         3. Hypotension with tachycardia: tricyclic antidepressants, phenothiazines, theophylline (acute), β-agonists
         4. Rapid respiration: salicylates, carbon monoxide, chemicals producing metabolic acidosis or cellular asphyxia (cyanide)
         5. Hyperthermia: sympathomimetics, anticholinergics, salicylates, uncouplers of oxidative phosphorylation (dinitrophenol), chemicals producing seizures or muscular rigidity
         6. Hypothermia: phenothiazines, ethanol, and other sedatives
         7. Eyes
            - Pupil constriction (miosis): opioids, phenothiazines (α-blockade), cholinesterase inhibitors, alpha blockers
            - Pupil dilation (mydriasis): amphetamines, cocaine, lysergic acid diethylamide (LSD), anticholinergics, phencyclidine (PCP)
         8. Skin
            - Flushed, hot, and dry: atropine, antimuscarinics
            - Excessive sweating: cholinesterase inhibitors, sympathomimetics, nicotine
         9. Cyanosis: hypoxemia, methemoglobinemia (nitrites)

Rapid review of adverse effects of chemicals is high yield for board examinations.

TABLE 30-1:
Symptoms and Treatment of Poisoning

Agent	Clinical Features	Treatment	Comments
Alkalies (hydroxides in soaps, cleansers, drain cleaners)	GI irritation	Supportive care H$_2$O	No emesis or lavage More potent than strong acids
Bleach (sodium hypochlorite)	Irritation, delirium	Supportive care; milk, ice cream, or beaten eggs; antacids	No emesis
Carbon monoxide	Headaches, dizziness, metabolic acidosis, retinal hemorrhage	Supportive care, oxygen	Cherry-red blood
Corrosives	GI irritation, seizures, weakness	Milk, antacids, calcium gluconate (antidote for oxalates); milk of magnesia (antidote for mineral acids)	No emesis or lavage
Cyanide	Seizures, ECG changes	Amyl nitrite or sodium nitrite plus sodium thiosulfate	Rapid treatment necessary
Ethylene glycol	Renal failure; metabolic acidosis with anion gap	Ethanol IV or fomepizole (antidotes), sodium bicarbonate for acidosis, supportive care	Culprit: toxic metabolite (oxalic acid)
Heavy metals			
Arsenic	Vomiting, diarrhea, seizures, neuropathy, nephropathy	Chelation (dimercaprol or penicillamine); succimer for chronic exposure	Delayed reaction: white lines on fingernails (Mees' lines)
Iron	GI irritation, blood loss, acidosis	Deferoxamine	Keep away from children
Lead	Abdominal pain, lead lines on gums, basophilic stippling, weakness, behavioral changes, peripheral neuropathy, encephalopathy	Chelation (dimercaprol, EDTA, succimer, or penicillamine)	In old paints and glazes
Mercury	Renal failure, GI irritation, behavioral changes	Chelation (dimercaprol); milk or eggs; succimer for chronic exposure	Delayed reaction: "mad as a hatter"
Hydrocarbons	Pulmonary infiltrates, CNS depression, seizures, tinnitus	Supportive care	No emesis or lavage Delayed reaction: chemical pneumonitis
Methanol	Visual disturbance, metabolic acidosis, respiratory failure	Ethanol IV or fomepizole (antidotes), sodium bicarbonate for acidosis, supportive care	Culprit: toxic metabolite (formic acid)
Salicylates	Respiratory alkalosis, metabolic acidosis, increased temperature, tinnitus, respiratory failure, seizures	Supportive care, alkalinize urine, dialysis, cool down	Uncouple oxidative phosphorylation
Strychnine	Seizures, respiratory failure, rigidity	Supportive care, activated charcoal	Glycine antagonist in spinal cord, blocking nerve impulses

CNS, central nervous system; ECG, electrocardiogram; EDTA, ethylenediamine-tetraacetate; GI, gastrointestinal.

TABLE 30-2:
Specific Antidotes for Selected Drugs and Toxins

Antidote	Poison
Drugs That Chelate Metals	
Calcium disodium edetate (EDTA)	Lead
Deferoxamine	Iron
Dimercaprol	Arsenic, gold, mercury, lead
Penicillamine	Lead, copper, arsenic, gold
Succimer	Lead; also used for chronic exposure to arsenic and mercury
Substances That Act Against Specific Drugs or Toxins	
Acetylcysteine	Acetaminophen
Amyl nitrite	Cyanide
Atropine	Cholinesterase inhibitor
Digoxin-specific Fab antibodies	Cardiac glycosides (e.g., digitalis)
Esmolol	Theophylline, caffeine, metaproterenol
Ethanol	Methanol or ethylene glycol
Flumazenil	Benzodiazepine
Fomepizole	Ethylene glycol, methanol
Glucagon	Beta blockers
Naloxone	Opioids
Oxygen	Carbon monoxide
Physostigmine	Anticholinergics
Pralidoxime (2-PAM)	Organophosphates; contraindicated for carbamates
Pyridoxine	Isoniazid
Sodium bicarbonate	Cardiac depressants (tricyclic antidepressants, quinidine)

Fab, fragment antigen binding.

10. Jaundice (liver toxicity): acetaminophen, erythromycin estolate (cholestatic), carbon tetrachloride, troglitazone, valproic acid
11. Abdomen
    - Ileus: typical of antimuscarinics, opioids, and sedatives
    - Hyperactive bowel sounds, cramping, and diarrhea: common with organophosphates, iron, arsenic, theophylline, and mushrooms
12. Nervous system
    - Twitching and muscular hyperactivity: anticholinergics, sympathomimetics, cocaine
    - Muscular rigidity: antipsychotics (especially haloperidol), strychnine, fentanyl
    - Seizures (treat with intravenous diazepam or lorazepam): theophylline, isoniazid, cocaine, amphetamines, tricyclics, diphenhydramine, lidocaine, meperidine
    - Flaccid coma: opioids, sedative/hypnotics, central nervous system depressants
E. Provide symptomatic and supportive treatment.
F. Use specific antidotes when appropriate (see Table 30-2).
G. Increase the rate of excretion when appropriate.
    - Use cathartics (e.g., magnesium sulfate, sorbitol); alter urine pH (e.g., ammonium chloride to acidify urine, sodium bicarbonate to alkalinize

The smaller the volume of distribution (V_d), the more effective the hemodialysis.

urine); osmotic diuretics (e.g., mannitol); hemodialysis; peritoneal dialysis; and hemoperfusion

1. Acidification of urine: increased excretion of weak organic bases (e.g., phencyclidine, amphetamine)
2. Alkalinization of urine: increased excretion of weak organic acids (e.g., salicylates, phenobarbital)

III. Teratogenic Effects of Specific Drugs (Table 30-3)

TABLE 30-3:
Teratogenic Effects
of Selected Drugs

Drug	Adverse Effects
Alkylating agents and antimetabolites (anticancer drugs)	Cardiac defects; cleft palate; growth retardation; malformation of ears, eyes, fingers, nose, or skull; other anomalies
Carbamazepine	Abnormal facial features; neural tube defects, such as spina bifida; reduced head size; other anomalies
Diethylstilbestrol (DES)	Effects in female offspring: clear cell vaginal or cervical adenocarcinoma; irregular menses and reproductive abnormalities, including decreased rate of pregnancy and increased rate of preterm deliveries Effects in male offspring: cryptorchism, epididymal cysts, hypogonadism
Ethanol	Fetal alcohol syndrome (growth retardation; hyperactivity; mental retardation; microcephaly and facial abnormalities; poor coordination; other anomalies)
Phenytoin	Fetal hydantoin syndrome (cardiac defects; malformation of ears, lips, palate, mouth, and nasal bridge; mental retardation; microcephaly, ptosis, strabismus; other anomalies)
Retinoids (systemic)	Spontaneous abortions; hydrocephaly; malformation of ears, face, heart, limbs, and liver; microcephaly; other anomalies
Tetracycline	Hypoplasia of tooth enamel, staining of teeth
Thalidomide	Deafness; heart defects; limb abnormalities (amelia or phocomelia); renal abnormalities; other anomalies
Valproate	Cardiac defects; central nervous system defects; lumbosacral spina bifida; microcephaly
Warfarin anticoagulants	Fetal warfarin syndrome (chondrodysplasia punctata; malformation of ears and eyes; mental retardation; nasal hypoplasia; optic atrophy; skeletal deformities; other anomalies)

Other substances known to be teratogenic: arsenic, cadmium, lead, lithium, methyl mercury, penicillamine, polychlorinated biphenyls, and trimethadione. Other drugs that should be avoided during the second and third trimesters of pregnancy: angiotensin-converting enzyme inhibitors, angiotensin receptor blockers, chloramphenicol, indomethacin, prostaglandins, sulfonamides, and sulfonylureas. Other drugs that should be used with great caution during pregnancy: antithyroid drugs, aspirin, barbiturates, benzodiazepines, corticosteroids, fluoroquinolones, heparin, opioids, and phenothiazines.

IV. Dependence and Drugs of Abuse
- Repeated drug use may lead to dependence (Table 30-4).
  A. Physical dependence
     - Examples: ethanol (Table 30-5), barbiturates, opioids
     - Repeated administration produces an altered or adaptive physiologic state in which signs and symptoms of withdrawal (abstinence syndrome) occur if the drug is not present.

Disulfiram discourages ethanol use.

TABLE 30-4:
Drugs of Abuse

Drug	Effect	Withdrawal	Treatment
Alcohol	Slurred speech, unsteady gait, nystagmus, lack of coordination, mood changes	Tremor, tachycardia, insomnia, seizures, delusions, hypertension	Clonidine, lorazepam, chlordiazepoxide, disulfiram
Amphetamines	Psychomotor agitation, pupil dilation, tachycardia, euphoria, hypertension, paranoia, seizures	Dysphoria, fatigue	Supportive care
Barbiturates	Same as alcohol	Anxiety, seizures, hypertension, irritability	Same as alcohol
Benzodiazepines	CNS depression, respiratory depression	Anxiety, hypertension, irritability	Supportive care, flumazenil
Caffeine	CNS stimulation, hypertension	Lethargy, headache, irritability	Supportive care
Cocaine	CNS stimulation, arrhythmias, psychomotor agitation, pupil dilation, tachycardia, euphoria, paranoia (similar to amphetamines)	Dysphoria, fatigue (same as amphetamines)	Supportive care
Lysergic acid diethylamide (LSD)	Anxiety, paranoia, pupil dilation, tremors, tachycardia, hallucinations. Severe agitation may respond to diazepam	None	No specific treatment
Marijuana	Euphoria, dry mouth, increased appetite, conjunctival injection	Irritability, nausea	No specific treatment
Methylenedioxy-methamphetamine (MDMA, ecstasy)	Amphetamine-like hyperthermia, hypertension, jaw-clenching	Dysphoria, fatigue, brain damage	Reduce body temperature
Nicotine	CNS stimulation, increased GI motility	Anxiety, dysphoria, increased appetite	Bupropion, clonidine
Opioids	Pinpoint pupils, respiratory depression, hypotension	Dysphoria, nausea, diarrhea	Supportive care, naloxone, methadone, clonidine
Phencyclidine hydrochloride (PCP)	Aggressive behavior, horizontal-vertical nystagmus, ataxia, seizures, hallucinations	None	Life support, diazepam, haloperidol

CNS, central nervous system; GI, gastrointestinal.

TABLE 30-5:
Stages of Ethanol
Poisoning*

Degree of Poisoning	Blood Alcohol Level (mg/dL)	Symptoms
Acute, mild	50–150	Decreased inhibitions, visual impairment, lack of muscular coordination, slowing of reaction time
Moderate	150–300	Major visual impairment, more pronounced symptoms of mild intoxication, slurred speech
Severe	300–500	Approaching stupor, severe hypoglycemia, seizures, death
Coma	>500	Unconsciousness, slowed respiration, complete loss of sensations, death (frequent)

*Disulfiram inhibits acetaldehyde dehydrogenase, which causes acetaldehyde to accumulate in the blood, resulting in nausea and vomiting if alcohol is consumed.

B. Psychological dependence
  • Examples: amphetamines, cocaine, LSD
  • Affected individuals use a drug repeatedly for personal satisfaction and engage in compulsive drug-seeking behavior.
C. Substance dependence (addiction)
  • Chronic use of a drug results in a cluster of symptoms (e.g., craving, withdrawal symptoms, drug-seeking behavior) indicating that the individual continues to use the substance despite substance-related problems (e.g., medical, financial, social).

Common Laboratory Values

Test	Conventional Units	SI Units
Blood, Plasma, Serum		
Alanine aminotransferase (ALT, GPT at 30°C)	8–20 U/L	8–20 U/L
Amylase, serum	25–125 U/L	25–125 U/L
Aspartate aminotransferase (AST, GOT at 30°C)	8–20 U/L	8–20 U/L
Bilirubin, serum (adult): total; direct	0.1–1.0 mg/dL; 0.0–0.3 mg/dL	2–17 μmol/L; 0–5 μmol/L
Calcium, serum (Ca^{2+})	8.4–10.2 mg/dL	2.1–2.8 mmol/L
Cholesterol, serum	Rec: <200 mg/dL	<5.2 mmol/L
Cortisol, serum	8:00 AM: 6–23 μg/dL; 4:00 PM: 3–15 μg/dL 8:00 PM: ≤50% of 8:00 AM	170–630 nmol/L; 80–410 nmol/L Fraction of 8:00 AM: ≤0.50
Creatine kinase, serum	Male: 25–90 U/L Female: 10–70 U/L	25–90 U/L 10–70 U/L
Creatinine, serum	0.6–1.2 mg/dL	53–106 μmol/L
Electrolytes, serum		
Sodium (Na^+)	136–145 mEq/L	135–145 mmol/L
Chloride (Cl^-)	95–105 mEq/L	95–105 mmol/L
Potassium (K^+)	3.5–5.0 mEq/L	3.5–5.0 mmol/L
Bicarbonate (HCO_3^-)	22–28 mEq/L	22–28 mmol/L
Magnesium (Mg^{2+})	1.5–2.0 mEq/L	1.5–2.0 mmol/L
Estriol, total, serum (in pregnancy)		
24–28 wk; 32–36 wk	30–170 ng/mL; 60–280 ng/mL	104–590 nmol/L; 208–970 nmol/L
28–32 wk; 36–40 wk	40–220 ng/mL; 80–350 ng/mL	140–760 nmol/L; 280–1210 nmol/L
Ferritin, serum	Male: 15–200 ng/mL Female: 12–150 ng/mL	15–200 μg/L 12–150 μg/L
Follicle-stimulating hormone, serum/plasma (FSH)	Male: 4–25 mIU/mL Female: Premenopause, 4–30 mIU/mL Midcycle peak, 10–90 mIU/mL Postmenopause, 40–250 mIU/mL	4–25 U/L 4–30 U/L 10–90 U/L 40–250 U/L
Gases, arterial blood (room air)		
pH	7.35–7.45	[H^+] 36–44 nmol/L
P_{CO_2}	33–45 mmHg	4.4–5.9 kPa
P_{O_2}	75–105 mmHg	10.0–14.0 kPa
Glucose, serum	Fasting: 70–110 mg/dL 2 hr postprandial: <120 mg/dL	3.8–6.1 mmol/L <6.6 mmol/L
Growth hormone–arginine stimulation	Fasting: <5 ng/mL Provocative stimuli: >7 ng/mL	<5 μg/L >7 μg/L

continued

Test	Conventional Units	SI Units
Blood, Plasma, Serum—cont'd		
Immunoglobulins, serum		
IgA	76–390 mg/dL	0.76–3.90 g/L
IgE	0–380 IU/mL	0–380 kIU/L
IgG	650–1500 mg/dL	6.5–15 g/L
IgM	40–345 mg/dL	0.4–3.45 g/L
Iron	50–170 µg/dL	9–30 µmol/L
Lactate dehydrogenase, serum	45–90 U/L	45–90 U/L
Luteinizing hormone, serum/ plasma (LH)	Male: 6–23 mIU/mL	6–23 U/L
	Female:	
	Follicular phase, 5–30 mIU/mL	5–30 U/L
	Midcycle, 75–150 mIU/mL	75–150 U/L
	Postmenopause, 30–200 mIU/mL	30–200 U/L
Osmolality, serum	275–295 mOsm/kg	275–295 mOsm/kg
Parathyroid hormone, serum, N-terminal	230–630 pg/mL	230–630 ng/L
Phosphatase (alkaline), serum (p-NPP at 30°C)	20–70 U/L	20–70 U/L
Phosphorus (inorganic), serum	3.0–4.5 mg/dL	1.0–1.5 mmol/L
Prolactin, serum (hPRL)	<20 ng/mL	<20 µg/L
Proteins, serum		
Total (recumbent)	6.0–8.0 g/dL	60–80 g/L
Albumin	3.5–5.5 g/dL	35–55 g/L
Globulin	2.3–3.5 g/dL	23–35 g/L
Thyroid-stimulating hormone, serum or plasma (TSH)	0.5–5.0 µU/mL	0.5–5.0 mU/L
Thyroidal iodine (^{123}I) uptake	8–30% of administered dose/24 hr	0.08–0.30/24 hr
Thyroxine (T_4), serum	4.5–12 µg/dL	58–154 nmol/L
Triglycerides, serum	35–160 mg/dL	0.4–1.81 mmol/L
Triiodothyronine (T_3), serum (RIA)	115–190 ng/dL	1.8–2.9 nmol/L
Triiodothyronine (T_3) resin uptake	25–38%	0.25–0.38
Urea nitrogen, serum (BUN)	7–18 mg/dL	1.2–3.0 mmol urea/L
Uric acid, serum	3.0–8.2 mg/dL	0.18–0.48 mmol/L
Cerebrospinal Fluid		
Cell count	0–5 cells/mm^3	0–5 × 10^6/L
Chloride	118–132 mEq/L	118–132 mmol/L
Gamma globulin	3–12% total proteins	0.03–0.12
Glucose	50–75 mg/dL	2.8–4.2 mmol/L
Pressure	70–180 mm H$_2$O	70–180 mm H$_2$O
Proteins, total	<40 mg/dL	<0.40 g/L
Hematology		
Bleeding time (template)	2–7 min	2–7 min
Erythrocyte count	Male: 4.3–5.9 million/mm^3	4.3–5.9 × 10^{12}/L
	Female: 3.5–5.5 million/mm^3	3.5–5.5 × 10^{12}/L
Erythrocyte sedimentation rate (Westergren)	Male: 0–15 mm/hr	0–15 mm/hr
	Female: 0–20 mm/hr	0–20 mm/hr
Hematocrit (Hct)	Male: 40–54%	0.40–0.54
	Female: 37–47%	0.37–0.47

Test	Conventional Units	SI Units
Hematology—cont'd		
Hemoglobin A$_{IC}$	≤6%	≤ 0.06%
Hemoglobin, blood (Hb)	Male: 13.5–17.5 g/dL	2.09–2.71 mmol/L
	Female: 12.0–16.0 g/dL	1.86–2.48 mmol/L
Hemoglobin, plasma	1–4 mg/dL	0.16–0.62 mmol/L
Leukocyte count and differential		
Leukocyte count	4500–11,000/mm^3	4.5–11.0 × 10^9/L
Segmented neutrophils	54–62%	0.54–0.62
Bands	3–5%	0.03–0.05
Eosinophils	1–3%	0.01–0.03
Basophils	0–0.75%	0–0.0075
Lymphocytes	25–33%	0.25–0.33
Monocytes	3–7%	0.03–0.07
Mean corpuscular hemoglobin (MCH)	25.4–34.6 pg/cell	0.39–0.54 fmol/cell
Mean corpuscular hemoglobin concentration (MCHC)	31–37% Hb/cell	4.81–5.74 mmol Hb/L
Mean corpuscular volume (MCV)	80–100 μm^3	80–100 fl
Partial thromboplastin time (activated) (aPTT)	25–40 sec	25–40 sec
Platelet count	150,000–400,000/mm^3	150–400 × 10^9/L
Prothrombin time (PT)	12–14 sec	12–14 sec
Reticulocyte count	0.5–1.5% of red cells	0.005–0.015
Thrombin time	<2 sec deviation from control	<2 sec deviation from control
Volume		
Plasma	Male: 25–43 mL/kg	0.025–0.043 L/kg
	Female: 28–45 mL/kg	0.028–0.045 L/kg
Red cell	Male: 20–36 mL/kg	0.020–0.036 L/kg
	Female: 19–31 mL/kg	0.019–0.031 L/kg
Sweat		
Chloride	0–35 mmol/L	0–35 mmol/L
Urine		
Calcium	100–300 mg/24 hr	2.5–7.5 mmol/24 hr
Creatinine clearance	Male: 97–137 mL/min	
	Female: 88–128 mL/min	
Estriol, total (in pregnancy)		
30 wk	6–18 mg/24 hr	21–62 μmol/24 hr
35 wk	9–28 mg/24 hr	31–97 μmol/24 hr
40 wk	13–42 mg/24 hr	45–146 μmol/24 hr
17-Hydroxycorticosteroids	Male: 3.0–9.0 mg/24 hr	8.2–25.0 μmol/24 hr
	Female: 2.0–8.0 mg/24 hr	5.5–22.0 μmol/24 hr
17-Ketosteroids, total	Male: 8–22 mg/24 hr	28–76 μmol/24 hr
	Female: 6–15 mg/24 hr	21–52 μmol/24 hr
Osmolality	50–1400 mOsm/kg	
Oxalate	8–40 μg/mL	90–445 μmol/L
Proteins, total	<150 mg/24 hr	<0.15 g/24 hr

questions

DIRECTIONS: Each numbered item or incomplete statement is followed by options arranged in alphabetical or logical order. Select the best answer to each question. Some options may be partially correct, but there is only **ONE BEST** answer.

1. A 50-year-old patient undergoes a gastrectomy. Which of the following agents is most likely to be given to prevent megaloblastic anemia, fatigue, and neurologic problems in this patient?
   A. Ferritin
   B. Ferrous sulfate
   C. Folic acid
   D. Intrinsic factor
   E. Vitamin B_{12}

2. After receiving fibrinolytic therapy, a 48-year-old woman is first given heparin and then switched to warfarin. The dosage of warfarin is calculated on the basis of the patient's prothrombin time (PT) and international normalized ratio (INR). No anticoagulant effect of the drug can be detected, even when the dosage is increased to several times the normal dosage and plasma levels of warfarin are correspondingly high. In this case, the lack of an anticoagulant effect is most likely due to an alteration in which of the following?
   A. Absorption of warfarin
   B. Binding of warfarin to plasma proteins
   C. Metabolism of warfarin by cytochrome P-450
   D. Vitamin K epoxidase
   E. Vitamin K epoxide reductase

3. A 57-year-old man who is brought to the hospital with intense chest pain responds well to treatment with nitroglycerin. Angiography confirms the presence of a coronary obstruction, and he is scheduled to undergo angioplasty. Which of the following agents is a platelet inhibitor that would prevent cardiac ischemic complications during angioplasty in this patient?
   A. Abciximab
   B. Alteplase
   C. Daclizumab
   D. Lepirudin
   E. Urokinase

4. A 41-year-old woman has been taking drugs for many years to control her schizophrenia and has suffered numerous typical adverse effects of treatment, including akathisia, parkinsonism, galactorrhea, and amenorrhea. These effects are caused by blockade of which of the following receptors in this patient?
A. α-Adrenergic receptors
B. Dopamine receptors
C. Muscarinic receptors
D. Nicotinic receptors
E. Serotonin receptors

5. A 43-year-old man has a bipolar disorder characterized by recurring episodes of mania and depression. He is being treated with lithium. Which of the following is the most common early sign of lithium toxicity in this patient?
A. Cardiac arrhythmias
B. Changes in personality
C. Gastrointestinal upset
D. Hallucinations
E. Renal shutdown

6. After threatening to jump from a bridge 40 feet tall, a 43-year-old man is given an extensive psychiatric evaluation and diagnosed with schizophrenia. Which of the following drugs is the most appropriate treatment for this patient?
A. Bupropion
B. Carbamazepine
C. Lamotrigine
D. Sertraline
E. Risperidone

7. A 57-year-old woman has a history of insomnia. She says that since she has been having trouble keeping a good-paying job, she has started to have more frequent episodes of sleeplessness. She also complains that she does not have enough money to pay for medicine. Which of the following low-cost non-benzodiazepine drugs would be most useful in the treatment of insomnia in this patient?
A. Buspirone
B. Diphenhydramine
C. Eszopiclone
D. Triazolam
E. Zolpidem

8. A 27-year-old man has a seizure disorder characterized by a 3-Hz spike-and-wave pattern on the EEG. Which of the following drugs is most appropriate for treatment of this patient?
A. Carbamazepine
B. Lorazepam
C. Phenytoin
D. Tiagabine
E. Valproate

9. A 55-year-old man is scheduled to undergo reconstructive surgery with isoflurane as the anesthetic. Before selecting this anesthetic, the possibility of drug interactions must be taken into account. Which of the following drugs would be expected to increase the neuromuscular blocking effects of isoflurane in this patient?
A. Bumetanide
B. Clopidogrel
C. Fluphenazine
D. Midazolam
E. Tobramycin

10. A 43-year-old man who is a heavy smoker is scheduled to undergo bronchoscopy in evaluation of his pulmonary function. He is given an intravenous injection of midazolam because of its anxiolytic and amnestic actions. Which of the following is the molecular site of action for the anxiolytic and amnestic actions of this drug?
A. Calcium channel
B. Cyclic adenosine monophosphate (cAMP) pathway
C. GABA-chloride ionophore
D. *N*-methyl-D-aspartate (NMDA) receptor
E. Sodium channel

11. A 29-year-old woman is scheduled to undergo reconstructive surgery. Administering general anesthesia with which of the following inhalational anesthetics would most likely cause the greatest depression of respiration?
A. Desflurane
B. Halothane
C. Isoflurane
D. Nitrous oxide
E. Sevoflurane

12. A 25-year-old woman seeks medical help to overcome her addiction to heroin. Which of the following agents is most likely to be used for this patient?
A. Clonidine
B. Codeine
C. Meperidine
D. Methadone
E. Pentazocine

13. A 47-year-old woman who is known to have idiopathic systemic lupus erythematosus (SLE) requires therapeutic treatment for a cardiovascular disorder. Which of the following drugs should be used cautiously in this patient with a history of SLE?
A. Hydrochlorothiazide
B. Lisinopril
C. Procainamide
D. Quinidine
E. Verapamil

14. A 51-year-old man with congestive heart failure has been effectively managed for 4 years with furosemide and enalapril therapy. Because of recent worsening of his condition, digoxin is added to his therapeutic regimen. Which of the following is the molecular target for the beneficial actions of digoxin in this patient?
   A. Angiotensin-converting enzyme (ACE)
   B. β-Adrenergic receptors
   C. Na^+/K^+-ATPase
   D. $Na^+/K^+/2Cl^-$ cotransport system
   E. Phosphodiesterase

15. A 57-year-old woman has a total cholesterol level of 280 mg/dL and a low-density lipoprotein (LDL) level of 180 mg/dL. She begins treatment with an antihyperlipidemic agent and experiences severe flushing of the skin. Which of the following agents is most likely responsible for this adverse effect in this patient?
   A. Colesevelam
   B. Cholestyramine
   C. Gemfibrozil
   D. Lovastatin
   E. Niacin

16. This table shows five sets of laboratory data. Which set of values (A, B, C, D, or E) reflects changes that are expected to occur when patients with congestive heart failure are treated with digoxin?

	Cardiac Output	Stroke Volume	Heart Rate	Peripheral Vascular Resistance
A	↑	↑	↓	↑
B	↑	↓	↑	↓
C	↔	↑	↓	↑
D	↓	↓	↑	↓
E	↑	↑	↓	↓

17. A 43-year-old woman has had several attacks of paroxysmal supraventricular tachycardia (PSVT) during the past few years, and now her attacks are occurring more frequently. Which of the following drugs is most appropriate for prophylactic therapy in this patient?
   A. Esmolol
   B. Lidocaine
   C. Nifedipine
   D. Procainamide
   E. Verapamil

18. A 58-year-old man experiences chest pain when he exercises strenuously. He is instructed to take nitroglycerin sublingually when episodes of pain occur. Which of the following is the most common side effect found in patients who use sublingual nitroglycerin for the relief of acute anginal attacks?
A. Bradycardia
B. Diuresis
C. Headache
D. Marked sedation
E. Vomiting

19. A 33-year-old woman begins doxycycline treatment for *Chlamydia trachomatis* infection. One week later, she develops severe oropharyngeal candidiasis. Which of the following antifungal agents that acts by binding to ergosterol would be appropriate to use as an oral lozenge to treat this patient?
A. Flucytosine
B. Miconazole
C. Metronidazole
D. Nystatin
E. Terbinafine

20. A 27-year-old man is infected with HIV and has a CD4$^+$ cell count of less than 40/mm^3. Which of the following drugs should be prescribed to prevent the development of *Mycobacterium avium-intracellulare* complex (MAC) disease in this patient?
A. Azithromycin
B. Ceftriaxone
C. Ciprofloxacin
D. Fosfomycin
E. Meropenem

21. A 14-month-old girl who has an earache is taken to a pediatric clinic, and ampicillin is prescribed. Five days after she begins taking the drug, her condition worsens, and she has a temperature as high as 39.4ºC (103ºF). The pediatrician reexamines the child and notes that meningeal irritation is present. The child is hospitalized and diagnosed with meningitis caused by a β-lactamase–positive strain of *Haemophilus influenzae*. Which of the following drugs is most likely to provide effective treatment for this patient?
A. Benzathine penicillin G
B. Ceftriaxone
C. Erythromycin
D. Penicillin V
E. Ticarcillin

22. A 16-year-old boy who is being treated for leukemia develops a fever. He begins treatment with antibacterial, antiviral, and antifungal agents and 2 days later develops acute renal failure. Which of the following drugs is most likely responsible for this adverse effect in this patient?
   A. Acyclovir
   B. Amphotericin B
   C. Ampicillin
   D. Ceftazidime
   E. Vancomycin

23. A 29-year-old African-American man who is working as a Peace Corps volunteer in Africa receives a blood transfusion after a surgical procedure. He subsequently develops symptoms of malaria, and laboratory studies show that he is infected with *Plasmodium vivax*. His symptoms are controlled with chloroquine. Which of the following drugs would be the most effective against the exoerythrocytic form of *P. vivax* in this patient?
   A. Chloroquine
   B. Mefloquine
   C. Primaquine
   D. Pyrimethamine-sulfadoxine
   E. Quinine

24. An 8-year-old boy develops osteomyelitis of the left distal femur after being kicked during a touch football game. The infection is treated with subtherapeutic doses of nafcillin, and he develops adjacent septic arthritis in the left knee. The knee is surgically drained, and antibiotic therapy is prescribed. Which of the following antibiotics is most appropriate at this time for the treatment of this boy?
   A. Cefazolin
   B. Ciprofloxacin
   C. Clindamycin
   D. Doxycycline
   E. Gentamicin

25. A 46-year-old man suffering from insomnia, memory loss, irritability, depression, shyness, and tremor, visits a primary care clinic. Additional findings include mild symptoms of gingivitis, stomatitis, and excess salivation. Chronic exposure to which of the following metals is most likely responsible for these findings in this patient?
   A. Arsenic
   B. Cadmium
   C. Lead
   D. Mercury
   E. Thallium

26. A 39-year-old man sprays his fruit orchard with parathion. Later in the day, he notes an increase in salivation, lacrimation, and urination, and has diarrhea. Which of the following would be the drug of choice for treating these symptoms of poisoning?
A. Amyl nitrite
B. Atropine
C. Dimercaprol
D. Disulfiram
E. Edetate calcium disodium

27. A 23-year-old woman is found unconscious in her bedroom, which is located above the garage in which her car is still running. Which of the following is most appropriate for the immediate treatment of this patient?
A. Acetylcysteine
B. Hydroxocobalamin
C. 100% oxygen
D. Sodium bicarbonate
E. Sodium nitrite

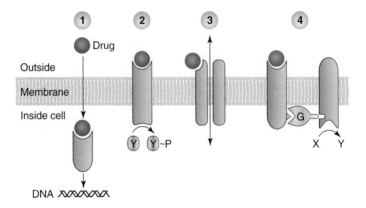

28. The accompanying figure depicts four different transmembrane signaling mechanisms for drugs and hormones. Which of the following agents acts via mechanism 1 to produce its pharmacologic effects?
A. Acetylcholine
B. Dopamine
C. Epinephrine
D. Glucocorticoids
E. Pituitary hormones

29. A 78-year-old man is given an infusion of lidocaine for the control of ventricular tachycardia. A dose adjustment is required. Which of the following parameters would be the most important in selecting a new infusion rate that is therapeutically effective but nontoxic?
A. Bioavailability
B. Clearance
C. Glomerular filtration rate (GFR)
D. Plasma protein binding
E. Volume of distribution

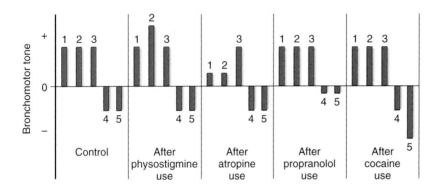

30. In the accompanying figure, changes in bronchomotor tone in experimental subjects are depicted in terms of constriction (+) or relaxation (−). The first panel of the figure (control) shows changes that were elicited by five different procedures (numbered 1 through 5), each of which was performed alone. The remaining panels show changes that were elicited by the same five procedures, each of which was performed after pretreatment with a different drug. Based on the results, procedure 1 is most likely:
A. Administration of bethanechol
B. Administration of histamine
C. Administration of isoproterenol
D. Stimulation of sympathetic nerves
E. Stimulation of the vagus nerve

31. The accompanying table shows cardiovascular changes induced by drug treatment in experimental subjects. Which of the following drugs is most likely to cause the changes shown in profile 4?
A. Amphetamine
B. Clonidine
C. Epinephrine
D. Isoproterenol
E. Tyramine

Profile	Mean Blood Pressure	Systolic Blood Pressure	Diastolic Blood Pressure	Heart Rate
1	↑	↑	↑	↓
2	↑↑	↑	↓	↑↑
3	↓	Slight ↑	↓	↑↑
4	↓	↓	↓	↓

32. While undergoing a routine eye examination, a 58-year-old woman is found to have 20/70 visual acuity in the right eye and 20/60 in the left eye without correction. Tonometry shows an intraocular pressure of 39 mm Hg in both eyes; ophthalmoscopy shows physiologic cupping of the optic disks of both eyes; and a visual field examination shows a nerve fiber bundle defect. Treatment with echothiophate is prescribed. This drug exerts its beneficial effects by inhibiting which of the following enzymes in this patient?
A. Acetylcholinesterase (AChE)
B. Carbonic anhydrase (CA)
C. Catechol-O-methyltransferase (COMT)
D. Choline acetyltransferase (CAT)
E. Tyrosine hydroxylase (TH)

33. Despite treatment, a 5-year-old boy with asthma has been suffering from wheezing attacks for 2 years. He is referred to a pulmonary clinic and begins therapy with fluticasone/salmeterol (Advair Diskus) given twice a day and an albuterol nebulizer used as needed. Fluticasone reduces lung inflammation by which of the following mechanisms in this patient?
A. Blockade of phospholipid breakdown
B. Blockade of triglyceride breakdown
C. Inhibition of cyclooxygenase
D. Inhibition of lipoxygenase
E. Inhibition of phosphodiesterase

34. A 7-year-old boy with acute lymphoblastic leukemia is treated with oral prednisone daily and weekly injections of vincristine during the induction phase of therapy. Which of the following toxicities is associated with vincristine in the treatment of this patient?
A. Cardiotoxicity
B. Hepatotoxicity
C. Neurotoxicity
D. Pulmonary toxicity
E. Renal toxicity

35. A 47-year-old woman has a metastatic carcinoma. When an anticancer drug is used to treat metastatic tumors, it is often difficult to achieve maximal beneficial effects with minimal adverse effects. This is also true with drugs that must be bioactivated before they become cytotoxic. Which of the following is an example of a prodrug that requires bioactivation and may be beneficial in the treatment of metastatic carcinoma in this patient?
A. Busulfan
B. Carmustine
C. Cyclophosphamide
D. Mechlorethamine
E. Methotrexate

36. A 33-year-old man with testicular carcinoma is being treated with multiple antineoplastic agents. Which of the following agents acts by inhibiting topoisomerase and is most likely to be included in his treatment regimen?
A. Bleomycin
B. Cisplatin
C. Etoposide
D. Paclitaxel
E. Vincristine

37. Three weeks after an 11-year-old boy has a viral illness, he complains of continual thirst and excessive urination. He develops nausea, vomiting, dehydration, and heavy breathing. He subsequently lapses into a coma and is admitted to the hospital. Clinical and laboratory findings include severe dehydration, tachycardia with deep and rapid respirations, a blood glucose level of 800 mg/dL, ketonemia, ketonuria, and serious metabolic acidosis. Which of the following is the agent of choice for the immediate treatment of this patient?
A. Glucagon
B. Glyburide
C. Metformin
D. Regular insulin
E. Ultralente insulin

38. The accompanying table shows five sets of laboratory values. The first set shows the normal ranges, and the other four sets show abnormal values. Which set (A, B, C, or D) reflects values that would be expected to occur in a 47-year-old woman who has systemic lupus erythematosus and is being treated with prednisone?

	Serum Glucose (mg/dL)	Plasma ACTH (pg/mL)	Serum Sodium (mEq/L)	Serum Cortisol (μg/dL)
Normal	70–110	10–80	136–145	6–23
A	60	250	137	1
B	160	1	132	0.5
C	175	250	150	60
D	50	400	120	1

ACTH, adrenocorticotropic hormone.

39. A 33-year-old woman develops excessive hair growth on her face, chest, and back. Laboratory studies do not indicate any increase in androgen hormone production. Which of the following drugs may improve her condition?
A. Aldosterone
B. Clomiphene
C. Ethinyl estradiol
D. Spironolactone
E. Triamcinolone

40. A 49-year-old woman has a syndrome characterized by severe gastric hyperacidity, peptic ulcer disease, and gastrinomas. Which of the following is the most effective drug for treating this syndrome in this patient?
A. Famotidine
B. Mesalamine
C. Misoprostol
D. Omeprazole
E. Sucralfate

41. A 57-year-old woman complains of inflamed, stiff, and painful joints and is treated with daily oral prednisone therapy. Prednisone acts by which of the following mechanisms to ameliorate these symptoms of rheumatoid arthritis in this patient?
A. Activates phospholipase A_2
B. Decreases intracellular concentrations of lipocortin
C. Inhibits cyclooxygenase-1 (COX-1)
D. Inhibits lipoxygenase
E. Reduces the expression of cyclooxygenase-2 (COX-2)

42. A 68-year-old man with gout is prescribed probenecid. He later develops a severe rash and stops taking the drug. Several days later, he begins monotherapy with allopurinol and experiences an acute attack of gouty arthritis. The allopurinol-induced attack in this patient could have been avoided by concurrent treatment with allopurinol and which of the following drugs?
A. Aspirin
B. Colchicine
C. Hydroxychloroquine
D. Ibuprofen
E. Sulfinpyrazone

43. A 47-year-old woman has a lengthy history of rheumatoid arthritis but is otherwise in good health. Although the drug that she is currently taking has controlled her symptoms reasonably well, it has also caused significant gastrointestinal side effects. Which of the following agents would be most appropriate for treatment of her rheumatoid arthritis in this patient with minimal gastrointestinal side effects?
A. Acetaminophen
B. Celecoxib
C. Naproxen
D. Sulindac
E. Tolmetin

44. A 16-year-old girl has severe cramping pain that begins a few hours before the start of her menstrual flow. She says that the pain has occurred monthly for the past 10 months. She also complains of headaches and of being very tired during her menstrual period. Which of the following is the most appropriate medication to relieve the severe cramping associated with this girl's menstrual period?
A. Acetaminophen
B. Dexamethasone
C. Ibuprofen
D. Indomethacin
E. Valdecoxib

45. In experimental studies, when anesthetized subjects are treated intravenously with drug X, they exhibit a marked decrease in mean blood pressure and a large reflex increase in heart rate. Pretreatment of the subjects with either atropine or propranolol fails to block the decrease in blood pressure. Drug X is most likely to be which of the following agents?
A. Acetylcholine
B. Epinephrine
C. Histamine
D. Isoproterenol
E. Norepinephrine

46. A 57-year-old man with non-Hodgkin's lymphoma is scheduled to begin combination cancer chemotherapy. To prevent chemotherapy-induced nausea and vomiting, his oncologist prescribes a drug that acts as a selective 5-HT_3 receptor antagonist. Which of the following drugs is most likely prescribed for this patient?
A. Diphenhydramine
B. Dronabinol
C. Metoclopramide
D. Ondansetron
E. Prochlorperazine

47. For 6 months, a 39-year-old woman has been experiencing severe left-sided pulsatile headaches. Before each headache attack, she feels disoriented and sees bilateral flashes of light. The pain is always unilateral and is often associated with nausea, vomiting, and photophobia. Which of the following is the most appropriate drug to administer intranasally for the termination of severe headaches in this patient?
A. Acetaminophen
B. Amitriptyline
C. Dihydroergotamine
D. Ibuprofen
E. Propranolol

48. A 19-year-old female fashion model who has been taking illicit dexfenfluramine as an appetite depressant to lose weight develops pulmonary hypertension. Which of the following drugs can be used to lower pulmonary vascular resistance in this patient?
A. Alprostadil
B. Dinoprostone
C. Epoprostenol
D. Latanoprost
E. Misprostol

49. A 13-year-old girl has severe, frequently recurring asthmatic attacks. During the attacks, she becomes cyanotic, dyspneic, and agitated. Which of the following drugs would be expected to provide immediate relief with the fewest adverse effects in controlling asthmatic attacks in this patient?
A. Albuterol
B. Atropine
C. Cromolyn sodium
D. Ephedrine
E. Epinephrine

50. A 71-year-old man with acute angle-closure glaucoma is brought to the emergency department because he is experiencing extreme pain in his left eye, is seeing halos around lights, and has an intensely red left eye and a steamy-appearing cornea. Which of the following drugs would be considered appropriate medical treatment for this disorder?
A. Atropine
B. Edrophonium
C. Furosemide
D. Pilocarpine
E. Timolol

answers

1. **E** (vitamin B_{12}) is correct. Gastric mucosal cells are required for the production of intrinsic factor, and intrinsic factor is required for the absorption of vitamin B_{12}. Because gastrectomy eliminates mucosal cells, patients who have undergone this procedure suffer from a vitamin B_{12} deficiency. Treatment with vitamin B_{12} (cyanocobalamin) can prevent megaloblastic anemia, fatigue, and neurologic problems in these patients.

    A (ferritin) is incorrect. Ferritin is the major iron storage–binding protein in the body. The depletion of iron stores can lead to microcytic anemia. Ferrous sulfate is used to treat microcytic anemia in patients with iron deficiency.

    B (ferrous sulfate) is incorrect. The depletion of iron stores can lead to microcytic anemia. Ferrous sulfate is used to treat microcytic anemia in patients with iron deficiency.

    C (folic acid) is incorrect. Although folic acid would reverse the anemia associated with vitamin B_{12} deficiency, neurologic problems would ensue because vitamin B_{12} is also required for myelin synthesis.

    D (intrinsic factor) is incorrect. Although the patient is deficient in intrinsic factor, it is a glycoprotein that is not available as a drug, and therefore, a patient who cannot produce intrinsic factor is given an injection of vitamin B_{12} monthly.

2. **E** (vitamin K epoxide reductase) is correct. Because the patient's plasma levels of warfarin were high, the lack of an anticoagulant effect cannot be attributed to pharmacokinetics. Therefore, it must be attributed to pharmacodynamics. The most common pharmacodynamic cause of resistance to warfarin is an alteration in vitamin K epoxide reductase, the enzyme normally inhibited by warfarin. An alteration in vitamin K epoxide reductase renders it insensitive to the inhibitory effects of warfarin without interfering with the synthesis of vitamin K–dependent clotting factors.

    A (absorption of warfarin) is incorrect. Because the plasma levels of warfarin were high, the lack of an anticoagulant effect cannot be attributed to pharmacokinetic parameters, such as lack of absorption, displacement from plasma proteins, or induced metabolism. However, lipid lowering resins such as cholestyramine can bind warfarin in the gastrointestinal tract and lead to low levels of warfarin.

B (binding of warfarin to plasma proteins) is incorrect. Because the plasma levels of warfarin were high, the lack of an anticoagulant effect cannot be attributed to a pharmacokinetic parameter, such as displacement from plasma protein binding. Under normal circumstances, more than 95% of warfarin is bound to plasma proteins. Binding can be reduced by displacement with other drugs such as salicylates or sulfonamides, but this would enhance, rather than diminish, warfarin's anticoagulant effect.

C (metabolism of warfarin by cytochrome P-450) is incorrect. Because the plasma levels of warfarin were high, the lack of an anticoagulant effect cannot be attributed to a pharmacokinetic parameter, such as increased metabolism. The anticoagulant effect can be diminished by concomitant therapy with cytochrome P-450 inducers that accelerate the hepatic metabolism of warfarin. However, under such circumstances, the circulating levels of warfarin would be reduced, not elevated.

D (vitamin K epoxidase) is incorrect. Vitamin K epoxidase is not the site of action of warfarin, however, *vitamin K epoxide reductase* is the enzyme inhibited by warfarin.

3. **A** (abciximab) is correct. Abciximab is a platelet inhibitor that acts by binding to glycoprotein IIb/IIIa receptors. The drug is given in combination with other agents to prevent cardiac ischemic complications in patients undergoing percutaneous transluminal coronary angioplasty. The drug also shows promise for use in the treatment of thrombotic arterial disease.

B (alteplase) is incorrect. Alteplase acts as a fibrinolytic drug, rather than an antiplatelet drug. Alteplase, a biosynthetic form of human tissue plasminogen activator (tPA), is used to dissolve clots in cases of acute pulmonary thromboembolism or acute coronary arterial thromboembolism associated with evolving transmural myocardial infarction (MI).

C (daclizumab) is incorrect. Daclizumab is a monoclonal antibody against the interleukin 2 receptor. It is used to prevent organ rejection after transplantation.

D (lepirudin) is incorrect. Lepirudin is a recombinant form of hirudin, a highly specific direct inhibitor of thrombin found in leeches. It is the first drug approved in the United States for treatment of patients with heparin-induced thrombocytopenia (HIT).

E (urokinase) is incorrect. Urokinase acts as a fibrinolytic drug, rather than an antiplatelet drug. Urokinase is an enzyme obtained from tissue cultures of human kidney cells that has fibrinolytic actions. It produces less hypersensitivity reactions than streptokinase, although streptokinase is considerably less expensive than urokinase. Urokinase is used to lyse pulmonary emboli, to lyse coronary arterial thrombi associated with evolving transmural myocardial infarction, and to manage occluded intravenous catheters.

4. **B** (dopamine receptors) is correct. Most antipsychotic agents are potent dopamine receptor antagonists. Inhibition of the dopamine receptors causes the side effects described in the patient.

A (α-adrenergic receptors) is incorrect. Side effects associated with the use of antipsychotic drugs such as orthostatic hypotension, impotence, and failure to ejaculate are caused by the blockade of α-adrenergic receptors. These side effects are prominent with the older drugs such as chlorpromazine or mesoridazine.

C (muscarinic receptors) is incorrect. Side effects associated with the use of antipsychotic drugs such as dry mouth, loss of accommodation, constipation, and difficulty urinating are caused by the blockade of muscarinic receptors; these side effects are highest with thioridazine and clozapine.

D (nicotinic receptors) is incorrect. Antipsychotic drugs do not typically inhibit nicotinic receptors.

E (serotonin receptors) is incorrect. Risperidone is a widely used antipsychotic agent that acts as a selective monoamine inhibitor and has a high affinity for serotonin 5-HT$_2$ receptors and dopamine D$_2$ receptors. It is also a potent α$_1$-adrenergic receptor antagonist and can produce hypotension. Orthostatic hypotension is most likely to occur during the initiation of therapy and may be accompanied by dizziness, sinus tachycardia, or syncope. The newer agents, sometimes referred to a "atypical agents," have a higher affinity for the serotonin 5-HT$_2$ than dopamine D$_2$ receptors. They include clozapine, olanzapine, quetiapine, and ziprazidone.

5. **C** (gastrointestinal upset) is correct. Lithium regularly causes several adverse reactions, even at therapeutic serum concentrations. These reactions include a fine hand tremor, weight gain, xerostomia, polydipsia, polyuria, mild nausea and vomiting, diarrhea, and a decrease in libido. Gastrointestinal effects often resolve with continued therapy and can be alleviated by taking divided doses with meals.

A (cardiac arrhythmias) is incorrect. Although electrocardiographic abnormalities are noted in up to 30% of patients receiving lithium, they are usually limited to reversible ST-T wave changes (T wave depression and, rarely, T wave inversion). At therapeutic dosages, lithium rarely causes conduction and rhythm abnormalities of the heart; if these abnormalities occur, they may be secondary to an underlying cardiac disease.

B (changes in personality) is incorrect. Lithium therapy is not associated with causing personality changes.

D (hallucinations) is incorrect. Lithium therapy is not associated with causing hallucinations.

E (renal shutdown) is incorrect. Lithium therapy is not associated with renal shutdown. If patients experience polydipsia with polyuria, it is usually during the first few weeks of treatment and soon disappears. Polyuria may recur unexpectedly as diabetes insipidus. In this case, a nephrogenic diabetes insipidus–like syndrome can develop, with constant thirst and a large output of extremely dilute urine.

6. E (risperidone) is correct. Risperidone is an antipsychotic agent that, along with other atypical agents, is deemed to be the standard of care for schizophrenia and related disorders, and with the exception of clozapine, may be considered as first-line treatment options for the management of psychosis. Psychotic disorders, including acute and chronic schizophrenic psychoses, and affective symptoms associated with schizophrenia have responded to treatment with risperidone. Selected data suggest advantages of atypical antipsychotics over typical antipsychotic agents (e.g., phenothiazines) such as a possible reduction in the negative symptoms of schizophrenia and a reduced incidence of extrapyramidal symptoms. Unlike clozapine, the first serotonin-dopamine blocking agent marketed, risperidone is not associated with agranulocytosis. Risperidone has been effective in patients with acute mania or with refractory bipolar disorder.

A (bupropion) is incorrect. Bupropion is not used in the treatment of schizophrenia. Bupropion is a second-generation antidepressant drug that selectively inhibits the neuronal reuptake of dopamine. It is not a tricyclic antidepressant (TCA) and is well tolerated in patients who experience orthostatic hypotension when taking TCAs. However, bupropion has a greater potential for causing seizures than do other antidepressants. A sustained-release oral form is approved for the management of smoking cessation.

B (carbamazepine) is incorrect. Carbamazepine is not used in the treatment of schizophrenia. Carbamazepine is an orally administered anticonvulsant drug that is structurally similar to TCAs. It is used in the treatment of partial seizures and tonic-clonic seizures. In children, carbamazepine use is preferable to phenobarbital use because it is associated with fewer adverse effects on behavior and alertness. It is also effective in treating chonic pain of neurologic origin, such as trigeminal neuralgia.

C (lamotrigine) is incorrect. Lamotrigine is not used in the treatment of schizophrenia. Lamotrigine is an orally administered anticonvulsant agent that has some antifolate activity. The drug acts at voltage-sensitive sodium channels to stabilize neuronal membranes. Blocking the sodium channels decreases the release of glutamate, and this decreases the frequency of seizures. Lamotrigine is also now approved for the long-term maintenance treatment of bipolar disorders.

D (sertraline) is incorrect. Sertraline is not used in the treatment of schizophrenia. Sertraline is an orally administered antidepressant drug. Like fluoxetine, paroxetine, citalopram, and escitalopram, it acts as a selective serotonin reuptake inhibitor (SSRI).

7. **B** (diphenhydramine) is correct. Diphenhydramine is a first-generation antihistamine that has significant sedative properties and is used in low-cost over-the-counter sleep aids.

A (buspirone) is incorrect. Buspirone is an antianxiety agent that has minimal sedative properties and is not used to induce sleep.

C (eszopiclone) is incorrect. Eszopiclone is a non-benzodiazepine sedative-hypnotic that is indicated for chronic treatment of insomnia. However, it is a new drug that is not inexpensive. Although eszopiclone is chemically unrelated to the benzodiazepines, it nonselectively binds to all three $GABA_A$ receptor subtypes. It is the S-isomer of racemic zopiclone, and it appears that the (S)-zopiclone isomer is primarily responsible for the drug's sedative and hypnotic actions. Flumazenil, a benzodiazepine antagonist, antagonizes its sedative actions.

D (triazolam) is incorrect. Triazolam is used to treat insomnia, but it is a benzodiazepine. Flumazenil, a benzodiazepine antagonist, antagonizes its sedative actions.

E (zolpidem) is incorrect. Zolpidem is a non-benzodiazepine sedative-hypnotic that is used for the short-term treatment of insomnia. However, as a relatively new drug it is not inexpensive. Unlike the benzodiazepines, which nonselectively interact with all three known benzodiazepine-receptor subtypes; zolpidem preferentially binds to the benzodiazepine-1 (BZ-1) receptor. Flumazenil, a benzodiazepine antagonist, antagonizes its sedative actions.

8. **E** (valproate) is correct. The patient's EEG pattern is typical of generalized absence (petit mal) seizures. In adults with seizures of this type, valproate and ethosuximide are considered the drugs of choice. In children ethosuximide is usually preferred. Valproate is also effective for use in the treatment of partial seizures, generalized tonic-clonic (grand mal) seizures, and generalized myoclonic seizures.

A (carbamazepine) is incorrect. The patient's seizures are generalized absence seizures. Carbamazepine is used to treat partial seizures and generalized tonic-clonic seizures but not petit mal seizures. It is also effective in the management of pain of neurologic origin (such as trigeminal neuralgia) and in the treatment of some psychiatric disorders (such as bipolar disorders and intermittent explosive disorder).

B (lorazepam) is incorrect. The patient's seizures are generalized absence seizures. Lorazepam is a benzodiazepine administered both orally and by injection for the treatment of anxiety and status epilepticus, respectively. It is not used for the treatment of petit mal seizures; however, clonazepam is an oral benzodiazepine that is sometimes used for the short-term management of refractory petit mal seizures.

C (phenytoin) is incorrect. The patient's seizures are generalized absence seizures. Phenytoin is an antiepileptic drug that can be used alone or in combination with other anticonvulsants to prevent tonic-clonic seizures and partial seizures with complex symptomatology (psychomotor seizures). It is not used in the treatment of petit mal seizures.

D (tiagabine) is incorrect. Tiagabine is an anticonvulsant used as adjunctive treatment of partial seizures. It inhibits neuronal and glial uptake of gamma aminobutyric acid (GABA) by binding to recognition sites associated with the GABA uptake carrier. It is not used in the treatment of petit mal seizures.

9. E (tobramycin) is correct. The concurrent use of isoflurane with parenterally administered tobramycin (an aminoglycoside) or polymyxin B, or with nondepolarizing neuromuscular blockers (tubocurarine type) can result in an additive neuromuscular blockade.

A (bumetanide) is incorrect. Bumetanide, a loop diuretic, is used in the management of edema associated with congestive heart failure, cirrhosis, and renal diseases. Bumetanide would not increase the neuromuscular blocking actions of isoflurane.

B (clopidogrel) is incorrect. Clopidogrel would not increase the neuromuscular blocking actions of isoflurane. Clopidogrel, whose active metabolite selectively and irreversibly inhibits ADP (adenosine diphosphate)-induced platelet aggregation, is an alternative to aspirin as an antiplatelet drug.

C (fluphenazine) is incorrect. Fluphenazine, a phenothiazine derivative, would not increase the neuromuscular blocking actions of isoflurane. It is used in the treatment of schizophrenia.

D (midazolam) is incorrect. Midazolam, a benzodiazepine that is used in the treatment of insomnia, would not increase the neuromuscular blocking actions of isoflurane; however, it would increase the anesthetic efficacy of isoflurane.

10. C (GABA-chloride ionophore) is correct. Midazolam and other benzodiazepines bind to the GABA-chloride ionophore and facilitate GABA-driven passage of chloride through the chloride ion channel. This results in hyperpolarization or suppression of electrical activity in the brain.

A (calcium channel) is incorrect. As discussed in option C, midazolam acts by binding to the GABA-chloride ionophore; it does not bind to calcium channels. When calcium channels in the membranes of myocardial and vascular smooth muscle cells are open, they allow for a slow, inward calcium flow that contributes to excitation-contraction coupling and electrical discharge. Calcium channels can be blocked by dihydropyridines (e.g., nifedipine), verapamil, or diltiazem.

B (cyclic adenosine monophosphate pathway) is incorrect. As discussed for option C, midazolam acts by binding to the GABA-chloride ionophore; it does not act via the cAMP pathway. Isoproterenol and other beta-adrenergic receptor agonists are examples of drugs that act via the cAMP pathway.

D (*N*-methyl-D-aspartate receptor) is incorrect. Midazolam does not bind to NMDA receptors. When glutamate binds to these receptors, a calcium channel is opened.

E (sodium channel) is incorrect. As discussed in option C, midazolam acts by binding to the GABA-chloride ionophore; it does not bind to sodium channels. When sodium channels are open, they allow sodium to flow down its concentration gradient into cells, thereby producing a localized excitatory postsynaptic potential (a depolarization). Sodium channels are opened, for example, when acetylcholine binds to nicotinic receptors. Several of the anticonvulsants exert their actions by blocking sodium channels (e.g., phenytoin and carbamazepine).

11. **C** (isoflurane) is correct. Desflurane, halothane, isoflurane, and sevoflurane are examples of halogenated anesthetics. Nitrous oxide is a nonhalogenated anesthetic. All of these inhalational anesthetics cause a dose-dependent suppression of respiration. At equal levels of anesthesia, however, isoflurane causes the greatest, and nitrous oxide the least, depression of respiration.

A (desflurane) is incorrect. Refer to the explanation for option C. Desflurane and nitrous oxide have the lowest blood to gas partition coefficients and, thus, the most rapid onset of action and recovery from anesthesia.

B (halothane) is incorrect. Refer to the explanation for option C. Multiple exposures to halothane have been associated with hepatotoxicity. Halothane is sometimes still used in children because it has a less pungent odor than most other halogenated anesthetics.

D (nitrous oxide) is incorrect. Refer to the explanation for option C. Nitrous oxide is a colorless, odorless, tasteless, nonflammable, nonirritating, volatile gas used for general anesthesia. It is a powerful analgesic with relatively weak inhalational anesthetic activity and usually must be supplemented with other agents if general anesthesia is desired. It is also used in low doses to provide analgesia in obstetrics and during procedures that do not require unconsciousness.

E (sevoflurane) is incorrect. Refer to the explanation for option C. It is easier to adjust the depth of anesthesia with sevoflurane than with enflurane, halothane, or isoflurane. Induction and recovery from anesthesia is also relatively rapid and cardiorespiratory depression is minimal which makes it generally safe in patients with coronary artery disease.

12. **D** (methadone) is correct. Methadone is a synthetic opioid agonist. Its major use today is the detoxification of patients who are addicted to heroin or other opioids. Methadone can be given orally and has a relatively long half-life; it does *not* cause the dramatic "highs" and "lows" associated with more rapidly acting drugs, such as heroin, morphine, or meperidine.

    A (clonidine) is incorrect. Methadone is the agent used most commonly in opioid detoxification programs. However, clonidine has been used in some cases to reduce the symptoms of withdrawal from opioids. Clonidine also has some value for patients going through withdrawal from nicotine or alcohol.

    B (codeine) is incorrect. Codeine is not used in the management of opioid withdrawal. It is a weak opioid agonist used as a single agent or in combination with acetaminophen or other non-narcotic analgesics for the treatment of mild to moderate pain. It is also widely used as a cough suppressant.

    C (meperidine) is incorrect. Meperidine is not used in the management of opioid withdrawal. It is a synthetic opioid agonist belonging to the phenylpiperidine class which includes alfentanil, diphenoxylate, fentanyl, loperamide, and sufentanil. Meperidine is considered a second-line agent for the treatment of acute pain. It is metabolized to normeperidine, a compound capable of inducing seizures at high concentrations, and therefore, it is not recommended for the treatment of chronic pain because of the risk of seizures with repetitive dosing. Moreover, meperidine's short duration of action and abuse potential are other reasons for not using this drug.

    E (pentazocine) is incorrect. Pentazocine is not used in the management of opioid withdrawal. Pentazocine, a mixed agonist/antagonist at opioid receptors, is used to treat moderate to severe pain. Because it is less active at the μ receptor, it produces less respiratory depression and may pose a lower risk of physical dependence than morphine.

13. **C** (procainamide) is correct. Long-term treatment with procainamide can precipitate a lupus-like syndrome. However, in the absence of reasonable alternatives, it is probably safe to use the drug with caution in patients who have a history of idiopathic SLE. Procainamide is a class Ia antiarrhythmic agent that is used in the treatment of atrial fibrillation, atrial flutter, paroxysmal atrial tachycardia, and ventricular tachycardia. Procainamide and hydralazine are the two cardiovascular drugs associated with producing an SLE-like syndrome.

    A (hydrochlorothiazide) is incorrect. Hydrochlorothiazide is a thiazide diuretic used in the management of edema and hypertension. It does not precipitate a lupus-like syndrome.

B (lisinopril) is incorrect. Lisinopril is an angiotensin-converting enzyme (ACE) inhibitor used in the management of hypertension, congestive heart failure, post-myocardial infarction, and diabetic nephropathy or retinopathy. It does not precipitate a lupus-like syndrome. Its use has been associated with producing dry cough, angioneurotic edema, and hyperkalemia.

D (quinidine) is incorrect. Although quinidine therapy will not precipitate a lupus-like syndrome, this therapy has been associated with a variety of adverse hematologic effects. These include hemolysis, which can produce hemolytic anemia (especially in patients with glucose-6-phosphate dehydrogenase deficiency); aplastic anemia; leukopenia; agranulocytosis; thrombocytopenia; and thrombocytopenic purpura. Quinidine is also a class Ia antiarrhythmic drug used for the treatment of atrial flutter and fibrillation, paroxysmal supraventricular tachycardia, paroxysmal atrioventricular junctional rhythm, premature atrial contractions, atrial tachycardia, and ventricular tachycardia.

E (verapamil) is incorrect. Verapamil is a calcium channel blocker used for the treatment of angina, hypertension, and supraventricular tachyarrhythmias. It does not precipitate a lupus-like syndrome.

14. **C** (Na^+/K^+-ATPase) is correct. Digoxin is a digitalis glycoside that inhibits Na^+/K^+-ATPase. This causes an increase in intracellular sodium, which in turn causes an increase in intracellular calcium. The intracellular calcium then stimulates the actin-myosin complex and thereby causes a decrease in cardiac fiber length. Even though digoxin has been used for many years in patients with heart failure, ACE inhibitors have replaced it as first-line therapy for heart failure due to systolic dysfunction, but digoxin still continues to be used as adjunctive therapy for late stage heart failure disease.

A [angiotensin-converting enzyme (ACE)] is incorrect. Digoxin does not inhibit ACE. Lisinopril is an ACE inhibitor used in the treatment of hypertension, congestive heart failure, post-myocardial infarction, and diabetic nephropathy or retinopathy.

B (β-adrenergic receptors) is incorrect. Digoxin does not interact with β-adrenergic receptors. Dobutamine is an example of a cardiotonic drug that stimulates β-adrenergic receptors.

D ($Na^+/K^+/2Cl^-$ cotransport system) is incorrect. Digoxin does not inhibit the $Na^+/K^+/2Cl^-$ cotransport system. Furosemide, a loop diuretic that inhibits the the $Na^+/K^+/2Cl^-$ cotransport system, is used in the management of edema associated with congestive heart failure, cirrhosis, and renal disease, including the nephrotic syndrome.

E (phosphodiesterase) is incorrect. Digoxin does not inhibit phosphodiesterase. Inamrinone and milrinone are examples of inotropic agents that inhibit type III phosphodiesterase.

15. **E** (niacin) is correct. Niacin, or nicotinic acid, is a B-complex vitamin. The mechanism of its lipid-lowering effect is unknown but is unrelated to its biochemical role as a vitamin. Proposed mechanisms of action include decreased hepatic synthesis of LDL and very low density lipoprotein (VLDL), inhibition of free fatty acid release from adipose tissue, and inhibition of lipolysis. Studies suggest that women have a greater hypolipidemic response to niacin therapy than do men when the drug is given in equivalent doses. Large doses act on the peripheral circulation, producing dilation of cutaneous blood vessels and an increase in blood flow, mainly in the face, neck, and chest. This flushing may be related to the release of prostacyclin and can be minimized by pretreatment with aspirin.

   A (colesevelam) is incorrect. Colesevelam is a bile acid–binding resin that acts like cholestyramine and colestipol (refer to option B). However, in contrast to cholestryramine and colestipol, colesevelam has less potential to reduce the bioavailability of other drugs.

   B (cholestyramine) is incorrect. Cholestyramine is a bile acid–binding resin that is administered orally. Cholestyramine was originally used to treat pruritus secondary to cholestasis, but its main use today is to treat hypercholesterolemia with concomitant hypertriglyceridemia. Because cholestyramine is not absorbed orally, it has a better toxicity profile than do other classes of antilipidemic drugs and is the drug of choice for treating hyperlipidemia in pregnant women and children. Flushing is not associated with cholestyramine treatment.

   C (gemfibrozil) is incorrect. Gemfibrozil is a fibric acid derivative. It reduces VLDL levels and increases the activity of lipoprotein lipases. It does not cause flushing.

   D (lovastatin) is incorrect. Lovastatin was the first of a class of lipid-lowering agents called HMG-CoA reductase inhibitors. It was also the first HMG-CoA reductase inhibitor demonstrated to slow coronary atherosclerosis. Lovastatin is a prodrug that has little or no inherent activity but is hydrolyzed in vivo to mevinolinic acid. Mevinolinic acid is structurally similar to hydroxymethylglutaryl-coenzyme A (HMG-CoA). Interference with the activity of the reductase enzyme reduces the quantity of mevalonic acid, a precursor of cholesterol. Other drugs in this class are atorvastatin, fluvastatin, pravastatin, rousvastatin, and simvastatin. Lovastatin and other HMG-CoA reductase inhibitors do not cause flushing. Note the common ending statin.

16. **E** (set E) is correct. In patients with congestive heart failure (CHF), digoxin restores contractility of the heart muscle and stimulates the vagus nerve. These actions cause an increase in cardiac output and stroke volume and cause a decrease in the heart rate and peripheral vascular resistance. Digoxin also increases the responsiveness of the baroreceptor reflex; this is *not* due predominantly to a direct inotropic effect of the drugs, but rather to important additional mechanisms contributing to the efficacy of the drugs used in the treatment of heart failure. A patient with CHF has high sympathetic tone contributing to tachycardia and increased peripheral vascular resistance. The increased cardiac output associated with the inotropic effects of digoxin results in a withdrawal of sympathetic tone contributing to the decrease in heart rate and decrease in peripheral vascular resistance.

A (set A) is incorrect. Refer to the explanation for options C and E.

B (set B) is incorrect. Refer to the explanation for options C and E.

C (set C) is incorrect. Set C describes the effects of digoxin in a patient with normal heart function. Digoxin still causes an increase in stroke volume as well as a decrease in heart rate due to stimulation of the vagus nerve. However, the patient with normal heart function has low symptathetic tone, and thus, there is not a withdrawal of sympathetic activity. Moreover, the direct effect of digoxin on the vasculature is vasoconstriction leading to an increase in peripheral vascular resistance. Therefore, the heart is pumping against an increased peripheral vascular resistance and consequently cardiac output is not increased.

D (set D) is incorrect. Refer to the explanation for options C and E.

17. **E** (verapamil) is correct. Verapamil is a calcium channel blocker that has a selective depressing action on the atrioventricular (AV) node tissue. It is effective in both the short-term treatment and the long-term prophylaxis of PSVT.

A (esmolol) is incorrect. Esmolol, a short-acting β-adrenergic receptor blocker, is used for the short-term control of supraventricular tachyarrhythmias, including sinus tachycardia and PSVT. It is also used to control the ventricular rate in patients with atrial fibrillation or atrial flutter. However, it is not appropriate for PSVT prophylaxis because it has to be given by continuous intravenous infusion.

B (lidocaine) is incorrect. Lidocaine is administered intravenously and has a short half-life, so it is not suitable for prophylactic therapy.

C (nifedipine) is incorrect. Nifedipine has more prominent effects on vasodilation and coronary blood flow than do diltiazem and verapamil. Unlike both diltiazem and verapamil, however, nifedipine has negligible effects on AV node conduction.

D (procainamide) is incorrect. Procainamide is effective for use in the treatment of atrial and ventricular arrhythmias. However, its long-term use is not advised, because of the need for frequent dosing and the common occurrence of lupus-related effects.

18. **C** (headache) is correct. Nitroglycerin is frequently prescribed for patients with typical angina pectoris, a form of angina in which chest pain occurs with exercise. A persistent, throbbing headache often occurs with nitroglycerin administration. These nitrate-induced headaches usually diminish quickly; however, sometimes aspirin or other NSAIDs may be given to alleviate the pain. Transient cutaneous vasodilation and flushing of the head and neck region can also occur with nitroglycerin. Hypotension and reflex tachycardia, common side effects of nitroglycerin and other nitrates, are due to dilation of arteries and veins.

A (bradycardia) is incorrect. Nitrates are not associated with bradycardia. They may cause an increase in heart rate as a result of autonomic reflex mechanisms.

B (diuresis) is incorrect. Nitrates do not produce diuresis. In fact, by prolonging vasodilation, they cause water retention.

D (marked sedation) is incorrect. Nitrates do not cause sedation, but they often cause severe headaches.

E (vomiting) is incorrect. Nitrates are not typically associated with vomiting.

19. **D** (nystatin) is correct. Topical preparations of nystatin or amphotericin B are effective when used in the treatment of oropharyngeal candidiasis because they are not absorbed and exert local effects only. Nystatin binds to sterols in the cell membranes of both fungal and human cells. The drug is fungistatic in low concentrations, but it exhibits fungicidal activity in high concentrations or when used against extremely susceptible organisms. It is used either as an oral lozenge or as a swish for the treatment of oropharyngeal candidiasis.

A (flucytosine) is incorrect. Flucytosine is not indicated for use in the treatment of superficial *Candida* infections. It is used to treat systemic and subcutaneous mycoses. After flucytosine penetrates fungal cells, it is converted to fluorouracil by the fungal enzyme cytosine deaminase. Mammalian cells do not convert flucytosine to fluorouracil. Acting as an antimetabolite, fluorouracil competes with uracil, interferes with pyrimidine metabolism, and eventually disrupts both RNA and protein synthesis in fungal cells.

B (miconazole) is incorrect. Miconazole is not indicated for the treatment of oropharyngeal candidiasis, nor does it act by binding to ergosterol in fungal cells. It is used topically or intravaginally for the treatment of various fungal infections. Miconazole inhibits ergosterol synthesis by inhibiting 14α-demethylase, a cytochrome P-450 enzyme required for the conversion of lanosterol to ergosterol, an essential component of the fungal cell membrane.

C (metronidazole) is incorrect. Metronidazole is an antibacterial and antiprotozoal agent that has no antifungal activity.

E (terbinafine) is incorrect. Terbinafine is not indicated for the treatment of oropharyngeal candidiasis, nor does it act by binding to ergosterol in fungal cells. Terbinafine can be administered either orally or topically, and it is highly effective for treating onychomycosis because of its fungicidal activity and ability to concentrate within the nail. Terbinafine exerts its antifungal activity by interfering with fungal sterol biosynthesis by inhibiting the enzyme squalene monooxygenase, a key enzyme in sterol biosynthesis in the fungal membrane.

20. **A** (azithromycin) is correct. Azithromycin is a macrolide antibiotic that is used to prevent MAC disease in HIV-positive individuals who have a low $CD4^+$ cell count. The structure of azithromycin is similar to that of erythromycin. In comparison with erythromycin, however, azithromycin has a longer half-life (and therefore can be given once daily), has less inhibitory effect on the P-450 system, and produces less gastrointestinal intolerance. Azithromycin also reaches higher intracellular concentrations, and this increases its efficacy and duration of action.

B (ceftriaxone) is incorrect. Ceftriaxone is a parenteral third-generation cephalosporin. It has significant activity against many gram-negative organisms, and it is able to achieve high enough concentrations in cerebrospinal fluid to make it useful in the treatment of meningitis. Ceftriaxone is not helpful in the prevention of MAC disease.

C (ciprofloxacin) is incorrect. Ciprofloxacin is a fluoroquinolone and a broad-spectrum antibacterial that is most active against aerobic gram-negative organisms, including enteric pathogens. Ciprofloxacin is particularly useful as an oral agent in the treatment of serious gram-negative infections. It is not helpful for the prevention of MAC disease.

D (fosfomycin) is incorrect. Fosfomycin inhibits bacterial cell wall synthesis by blocking one of the steps in the synthesis of peptidoglycan. The drug is approved for single-dose treatment of uncomplicated urinary tract infections; however, it appears to be less efficacious than single-dose treatment with a fluoroquinolone or with trimethoprim-sulfamethoxazole. Fosfomycin is not helpful for the prevention of MAC disease.

E (meropenem) is incorrect. Meropenem is a semisynthetic carbapenem antibiotic that is administered intravenously. Meropenem is similar to imipenem, but it does not require concomitant administration of a renal enzyme inhibitor (such as cilastatin). Meropenem is not helpful for the prevention of MAC disease.

21. **B** (ceftriaxone) is correct. Like other third-generation cephalosporins, ceftriaxone has significant activity against gram-negative organisms and is able to penetrate the cerebrospinal fluid (CSF) in concentrations that make it useful in the treatment of β-lactamase-negative and β-lactamase-positive meningitis.

A (benzathine penicillin G) is incorrect. Benzathine is only administered intramuscularly. Serum concentrations of penicillin G can be detected for up to 30 days following the administration of benzathine penicillin G. Penicillin penetrates inflamed meninges; however, only minimal CSF levels are attained after administration of benzathine penicillin G. Thus, this drug is unacceptable for use in the treatment of *H. influenzae* meningitis.

C (erythromycin) is incorrect. Because only small amounts of erythromycin penetrate the CSF, this drug would not be used to treat *H. influenzae* meningitis.

D (penicillin V) is incorrect. Although all the antibiotics listed as options may be effective against *H. influenzae,* only ceftriaxone is able to penetrate the blood-brain barrier and reach CSF concentrations that are effective for use in the treatment of meningitis. Moreover, penicillins G and V are not effective against β-lactamase-producing bacteria. Penicillin V is preferable to penicillin G when oral administration is desired, because penicillin V has better gastric acid stability and therefore reaches higher plasma levels.

E (ticarcillin) is incorrect. Ticarcillin is not used for the treatment of meningitis caused by *H. influenza.* Ticarcillin is a semisynthetic, extended-spectrum carboxypenicillin used mainly in the treatment of infections caused by gram-negative bacteria and in combination with an aminoglycoside to treat systemic *Pseudomonas* infections. It is given by injection for the treatment of intra-abdominal infections, respiratory and urinary tract infections, skin and soft tissue infections, and other infections caused by susceptible organisms.

22. **B** (amphotericin B) is correct. Nephrotoxicity occurs in more than 80% of patients treated with large cumulative doses of amphotericin B. Patients with nephrotoxicity may suffer from azotemia, hypokalemia, hyposthenuria, nephrocalcinosis, renal tubular acidosis, or frank renal failure. Renal tubular acidosis may be present without concurrent systemic acidosis and is attributable in part to renal tubular necrosis following the lysis of cholesterol-rich lysosomal membranes of renal tubular cells.

A (acyclovir) is incorrect. Acyclovir can cause nephrotoxicity, but it is less likely than amphotericin B to do so. In addition, acute renal failure usually does not develop so rapidly with this agent. Acyclovir-induced nephrotoxicity appears to result from crystallization of the drug within the nephron. Acyclovir, a synthetic deoxyguanosine analogue, is used for the management of herpesviruses (e.g., herpes simplex virus and varicella-zoster virus).

C (ampicillin) is incorrect. Adverse effects on the kidney are very rare with ampicillin use. Ampicillin, an extended-spectrum penicillin, is primarily given by injection for treating serious infections caused by penicillin-susceptible organisms, including anaerobes, enteroccocci, *Listeria monocytogenes,* and susceptible strains of gram-negative cocci and bacilli.

D (ceftazidime) is incorrect. Adverse effects on the kidney are not associated with ceftazidime use. Ceftazidime, a parenteral third-generation cephalosporin, is commonly used in the empiric treatment of fever in neutropenic patients.

E (vancomycin) is incorrect. Vancomycin can cause nephrotoxicity, but it is less likely than amphotericin B to do so. In addition, acute renal failure usually does not develop so rapidly with this agent. Vancomycin, a bactericidal inhibitor of cell wall synthesis, is used primarily for the treatment of infections caused by methicillin-resistant *Staphylococcus aureus* (MRSA), gram-positive infections due to susceptible organism(s), and for streptococcal and enterococcal infections in patients who are allergic to penicillin and other β-lactam antibiotics.

23. **C** (primaquine) is correct. *P. vivax* and *P. ovale* are *Plasmodium* species that have a persistent exoerythrocytic (hepatic) form. If this form is not eradicated, relapses will occur. Primaquine is the only antimalarial drug that blocks exoerythrocytic schizogony; other antimalarial agents block erythrocytic schizogony. In patients infected with *P. vivax* or *P. ovale,* primaquine is given in combination with a blood schizonticidal agent, such as chloroquine. Patients with reduced glucose-6-phosphate dehydrogenase levels are at increased risk for acute hemolytic anemia when they are treated with primaquine. The degree of hemolysis in these patients is dependent on ethnic origin and dosage level. In patients of African descent, the degree of hemolysis is often mild and possibly self-limiting. In those of Asian or Mediterranean descent, hemolysis can be severe. Primaquine use should be discontinued at the first signs of hemolytic anemia.

A (chloroquine) is incorrect. As discussed in option C, chloroquine is not effective against the exoerythrocytic form of *P. vivax* or *P. ovale;* therefore, it must be given in combination with primaquine to treat patients infected with these forms of malaria. Chloroquine can be used alone to treat patients with malaria that is caused by *P. malariae* or a chloroquine-sensitive strain of *P. falciparum.*

B (mefloquine) is incorrect. Mefloquine acts as blood schizonticides. It is not effective against the exoerythrocytic form of *P. vivax* or *P. ovale*. Mefloquine is given orally for the prevention or treatment of malaria caused by chloroquine-resistant strains of *P. falciparum* or by other *Plasmodium* species.

D (pyrimethamine-sulfadoxine) is incorrect. Pyrimethamine-sulfadoxine (Fansidar) is not effective against the exoerythrocytic form of *P. vivax* or *P. ovale*. Pyrimethamine and sulfadoxine have been used together in an oral preparation to treat or prevent malaria; however, the combination is no longer recommended for malaria prophylaxis, because it places individuals at risk for fatal toxic epidermal necrolysis. Pyrimethamine inhibits parasitic dihydrofolate reductase, whereas sulfadoxine antagonizes parasitic *p*-aminobenzoic acid (PABA). When given together, the drugs have a synergistic effect on folic acid–dependent biochemical pathways.

E (quinine) is incorrect. Quinine acts as blood schizonticides. It is not effective against the exoerythrocytic form of *P. vivax* or *P. ovale*. Quinine can be given orally or parenterally to treat chloroquine-resistant malaria.

24. **A** (cefazolin) is correct. *Staphylococcus aureus* is the most common cause of osteomyelitis in children. Nafcillin treatment is effective only if doses are high enough to achieve therapeutic concentrations in the bone. After the patient's knee is drained, an appropriate dosage of parenterally administered cefazolin would be effective in the management of this patient. Therapy may later be changed to oral cephalexin.

B (ciprofloxacin) is incorrect. Children should not be treated with ciprofloxacin and other fluoroquinolones, because these drugs may damage their cartilage.

C (clindamycin) is incorrect. If the patient is allergic to penicillins or cephalosporins, clindamycin can be used as an alternative to cefazolin. Clindamycin is used to treat infections with anaerobic bacteria. It is also used in combination with pyrimethamine to treat *Toxoplasma* encephalitis in patients with AIDS.

D (doxycycline) is incorrect. Children should not be treated with doxycycline and other tetracyclines because these drugs may damage their teeth and bones.

E (gentamicin) is incorrect. Gentamicin is an aminoglycoside antibiotic and it is most active against aerobic gram-negative rods. Although gentamicin is not the drug of choice to treat an infection caused by *S. aureus*, it is sometimes used in combination with other antibiotics to treat infections caused by *S. aureus* or by some species of *Streptococcus*.

25. **D** (mercury) is correct. The patient's clinical manifestations are consistent with the diagnosis of chronic poisoning from the inhalation of mercury vapor. Treatment consists of eliminating the exposure. Dimercaprol is used to treat acute inorganic mercury poisoning; however, it should not be used to treat chronic inhalational mercury poisoning, because it may redistribute mercury to the brain.

A (arsenic) is incorrect. Chronic exposure to arsenic dust or fumes causes irritation to the skin, mucous membranes, and respiratory tract. Systemic effects from chronic arsenic exposure include anorexia, nausea, vomiting, diarrhea, weakness, peripheral sensory neuropathy, hepatitis, and loss of hair. Hyperpigmentation of the skin along with transverse white lines of the nails (Mees' lines) is characteristic of chronic arsenic exposure. Lung and skin cancer have been associated with chronic arsenic exposure.

B (cadmium) is incorrect. The kidney is the main target of chronic cadmium exposure, but the lungs, bones, and cardiovascular system are also affected. Cadmium is a carcinogen.

C (lead) is incorrect. Characteristic findings in patients with chronic lead poisoning include abdominal pain, constipation, anorexia, headache, irritability, and fatigue. Other findings may include microcytic anemia (with or without basophilic stippling) and signs of peripheral neuropathy, such as wristdrop and footdrop.

E (thallium) is incorrect. Thallium is used as a rodenticide. In humans, thallium toxicity affects the gastrointestinal tract, cardiovascular system, brain, liver, and kidney. Characteristic signs of thallium poisoning are alopecia and reddening of the skin.

26. **B** (atropine) is correct. Atropine is indicated for use in the treatment of a cholinergic crisis caused by poisoning with an organophosphate, such as parathion. The principal effects of atropine treatment are a reduction in salivary, bronchial, and sweat gland secretions; mydriasis; cycloplegia; changes in heart rate; contraction of sphincter muscles in the bladder and gastrointestinal tract; decreased gastric secretion; and decreased gastric motility.

A (amyl nitrite) is incorrect. Amyl nitrite is not used to treat organophosphate poisoning. It is used as an antidote to treat cyanide poisoning. Amyl nitrite oxidizes hemoglobin to form methemoglobin. The methemoglobin binds excess cyanide and forms cyanmethemoglobin, a nontoxic compound.

C (dimercaprol) is incorrect. Dimercaprol is not used to treat organophosphate poisoning. Dimercaprol is a heavy metal chelator used in the treatment of acute arsenic, mercury, gold, or lead poisoning.

D (disulfiram) is incorrect. Disulfiram is not used to treat organophosphate poisoning. It is used in the management of ethanol abuse. Disulfiram competes with nicotinamide adenine dinucleotide (NAD) for binding sites on aldehyde dehydrogenase. This action interferes with the hepatic oxidation of acetaldehyde. The accumulation of acetaldehyde makes the individual very ill and, thus, serves as a deterrent to the consumption of alcohol.

E (edetate calcium disodium) is incorrect. Edetate calcium disodium is not used to treat organophosphate poisoning. Edetate calcium disodium (calcium EDTA, or CaNa$_2$ EDTA) is a parenteral drug used in the treatment of lead toxicity; this agent should not be confused with the non–calcium-containing salt (edetate disodium) that is used in the treatment of hypercalcemia.

27. **C** (100% oxygen) is correct. The woman is suffering from carbon monoxide poisoning. Emergency treatment of carbon monoxide poisoning consists of maintaining the airway, assisting with ventilation, and providing support with 100% oxygen.

A (acetylcysteine) is incorrect. Acetylcysteine is used as an antidote in cases of acetaminophen hepatotoxicity. It is not indicated for use in the treatment of carbon monoxide poisoning.

B (hydroxocobalamin) is incorrect. Hydroxocobalamin is not indicated for use in the treatment of carbon monoxide poisoning. Hydroxocobalamin (vitamin B$_{12}$) can be used to treat or prevent cyanide toxicity associated with sodium nitroprusside therapy. The vitamin combines with cyanide to form cyanocobalamin, which is nontoxic and excreted in the urine.

D (sodium bicarbonate) is incorrect. Sodium bicarbonate is not indicated for use in the treatment of carbon monoxide poisoning. Sodium bicarbonate is used to treat overdoses of tricyclic antidepressants or other cardiodepressant agents.

E (sodium nitrite) is incorrect. Sodium nitrite is not indicated for use in the treatment of carbon monoxide poisoning. Sodium nitrite is used as an antidote in cases of cyanide poisoning. Sodium nitrite oxidizes hemoglobin to methemoglobin. The methemoglobin then binds to cyanide and forms cyanmethemoglobin, a nontoxic compound.

28. **D** (glucocorticoids) is correct. Glucocorticoids act by binding to intracellular receptors that regulate gene expression (mechanism 1). They do not act via the three other signal mechanisms depicted in the figure: ligand-regulated transmembrane enzymes, such as protein tyrosine kinases (mechanism 2); ligand-gated channels (mechanism 3); and G proteins and second messengers (mechanism 4).

A (acetylcholine) is incorrect. Acetylcholine binds to nicotinic receptors that regulate ligand-gated channels (mechanism 3), and it also binds to muscarinic receptors that act via G proteins and second messengers (mechanism 4).

B (dopamine) is incorrect. Dopamine exerts all of its actions via mechanism 4. Dopamine acts on D_1 and D_5 dopamine receptors to couple via G_s to increase intracellular cAMP levels and on D_2, D_3, and D_4 dopamine receptors to couple via G_i to decrease intracellular cAMP levels or to open K^+ channels or to close Ca^{2+} channels.

C (epinephrine) is incorrect. Epinephrine exerts all of its actions via mechanism 4. Epinephrine's action at α_1-adrenergic receptors is coupled via G_q to increases phospholipase C activity to increase the formation of diacylglycerol (DAG) and inositol trisphosphate (IP_3). Its action at all β-adrenergic receptors is via G_s and its action on α_2-adrenergic receptors is via G_i to increase and decrease intracellular cAMP levels, respectively.

E (pituitary hormones) is incorrect. Pituitary hormones all act via G-protein–coupled mechanisms (mechanism 4).

29. **B** (clearance) is correct. The steady-state concentration (C_{ss}) of a drug is equal to input divided by output. Input is the rate of infusion (R_0), and output is clearance (CL). $C_{ss} = R_0/CL$. Thus, clearance is the most important factor for determining the rate of infusion.

A (bioavailability) is incorrect. Bioavailability is not a factor if drugs are given by intravenous infusion. Lidocaine must be given by intravenous infusion because it is subject to a high first-pass effect (i.e., it is highly metabolized during its first pass through the liver).

C (glomerular filtration rate) is incorrect. Because lidocaine is mainly cleared by metabolism, the GFR is not important.

D (plasma protein binding) is incorrect. As discussed in option B, clearance (CL) is the most important factor for determining the rate of infusion. However, plasma protein binding and the volume of distribution (V_d) have some impact. This is because CL is equal to the V_d multiplied by the rate constant for drug elimination from the body (k_e). $CL = V_d \times k_e$. Plasma protein binding affects the V_d and thus affects the CL.

E (volume of distribution) is incorrect. As discussed in option B, clearance (CL) is the most important factor for determining the rate of infusion. However, plasma protein binding and the volume of distribution (V_d) have some impact. This is because CL is equal to the V_d multiplied by the rate constant for drug elimination from the body (k_e). $CL = V_d \times k_e$. Plasma protein binding affects the V_d and thus affects the CL.

30. **A** (administration of bethanechol) is correct. When given alone, bethanechol causes bronchoconstriction. The drug is resistant to cholinesterase, so its effects are not potentiated by physostigmine. Bethanechol exerts its effects by binding to muscarinic receptors, so its response is markedly attenuated by atropine.

B (administration of histamine) is incorrect. The results of procedure 3 are consistent with the administration of histamine. When given alone, histamine causes bronchoconstriction. This effect is not blocked by atropine.

C (administration of isoproterenol) is incorrect. The results of procedure 4 are consistent with the administration of isoproterenol. When given alone, isoproterenol causes bronchodilation. The drug is not taken up into the nerve terminal (uptake 1), so its effects are not potentiated by cocaine.

D (stimulation of sympathetic nerves) is incorrect. Sympathetic nerve stimulation does not cause bronchoconstriction.

E (stimulation of the vagus nerve) is incorrect. The results of procedure 2 are consistent with stimulation of the vagus nerve. The effects of vagal nerve stimulation are potentiated by physostigmine, a cholinesterase inhibitor.

31. B (clonidine) is correct. Clonidine acts centrally to decrease sympathetic outflow from the brain. This results in decreases in the mean, systolic, and diastolic blood pressures, and it also decreases the heart rate (profile 4).

A (amphetamine) and E (tyramine) are incorrect. Amphetamine and tyramine are indirect-acting sympathomimetic amines. These agents cause the release of norepinephrine from nerve terminals, so their cardiovascular effects are similar to those of norepinephrine. The effects include an increase in the mean, systolic, and diastolic blood pressures and a decrease (a reflex effect) in the heart rate (profile 1).

C (epinephrine) is incorrect. Epinephrine increases the mean and systolic blood pressure (an α_1-adrenergic receptor effect), decreases the diastolic blood pressure (a β_2-adrenergic receptor effect), and increases the heart rate (a β_1-adrenergic receptor effect) (profile 2).

D (isoproterenol) is incorrect. Isoproterenol increases the cardiac output, and this may lead to a slight increase in the systolic blood pressure. By causing vasodilation (a β_2-adrenergic receptor effect) and stimulating β_1-adrenergic receptors, isoproterenol decreases the diastolic and mean blood pressure and increases the heart rate (profile 3).

32. A (acetylcholinesterase) is correct. The patient's ophthalmologic findings are consistent with the diagnosis of open-angle glaucoma. Echothiophate is an indirect-acting cholinergic receptor agonist that inhibits AChE and thereby potentiates the action of acetylcholine on the parasympathomimetic receptors. The drug is used as a miotic in diagnostic tests, to decrease intraocular pressure in patients with glaucoma, and to treat strabismus.

B (carbonic anhydrase) is incorrect. Echothiophate does not inhibit CA. An example of a CA inhibitor is acetazolamide, a drug that is used to prevent and treat altitude sickness and is also used as an adjunct in the treatment of glaucoma and epilepsy.

C (catechol-*O*-methyltransferase) is incorrect. Echothiophate does not inhibit COMT. Examples of COMT inhibitors are tolcapone and entacapone, drugs that are given orally and are used as an adjunct to levodopa-carbidopa in the treatment of Parkinson's disease.

D (choline acetyltransferase) is incorrect. Echothiophate does not inhibit CAT. There is no known selective and specific inhibitor of CAT used as a pharmacologic drug.

E (tyrosine hydroxylase) is incorrect. Echothiophate does not inhibit TH. TH is the rate-limiting step in catecholamine synthesis. Methyltyrosine inhibits TH, but its use is limited to the treatment of pheochromocytoma.

33. **A** (blockade of phospholipid breakdown) is correct. Fluticasone and other glucocorticoids exert their anti-inflammatory effects by stimulating the synthesis of lipocortins. Lipocortins are agents that inhibit phospholipase A_2 and thereby prevent the breakdown of phospholipids to yield arachidonic which is the substrate for cyclooxygenase and lipoxygenase.

B (blockade of triglyceride breakdown) is incorrect. Glucocorticoids do not block triglyceride breakdown.

C (inhibition of cyclooxygenase) is incorrect. Glucocorticoids do not directly inhibit cyclooxygenase. All nonsteroidal anti-inflammatory drugs (NSAIDs) inhibit cyclooxygenase, and some of them (e.g., indomethacin and ketoprofen) also inhibit lipoxygenase. Cyclooxygenase inhibitors are not used in the treatment of asthma.

D (inhibition of lipoxygenase) is incorrect. Glucocorticoids do not directly inhibit lipoxygenase. Zileuton is an inhibitor lipoxygenase that was used in the treatment of asthma, but the manufacturer no longer supplies this drug.

E (inhibition of phosphodiesterase) is incorrect. Glucocorticoids do not inhibit phosphodiesterase. Theophylline inhibits type III and type IV phosphodiesterases, which are responsible for breaking down cAMP in smooth muscle cells, and this mechanism may contribute in part to its beneficial effects in asthma.

34. **C** (neurotoxicity) is correct. Neurotoxicity is a characteristic toxicity associated with vincristine use. In fact, it is the dose-limiting adverse effect of vincristine therapy. Initially, vincristine-induced neurotoxicity presents as sensory impairment and paresthesias and then progresses to neuropathic pain and decreased motor skills. Clinical manifestations are peripheral neuropathy, peripheral paresthesias, neuritis, numbness, hyporeflexia, neuropathic pain, and tingling ("stocking-and-glove" pattern).

A (cardiotoxicity) is incorrect. Several of the antineoplastic drugs have unique or characteristic toxicities. Doxorubicin and daunorubicin cause cardiotoxicity. This type of toxicity is not associated with vincristine.

B (hepatotoxicity) is incorrect. Several of the antineoplastic drugs have unique or characteristic toxicities. Methotrexate causes hepatotoxicity. This type of toxicity is not associated with vincristine.

D (pulmonary toxicity) is incorrect. Several of the antineoplastic drugs have unique or characteristic toxicities. Bleomycin and busulfan cause pulmonary toxicity. This type of toxicity is not associated with vincristine.

E (renal toxicity) is incorrect. Several of the antineoplastic drugs have unique or characteristic toxicities. Cisplatin causes renal toxicity. This type of toxicity is not associated with vincristine.

35. **C** (cyclophosphamide) is correct. Cyclophosphamide is a prodrug that must be activated by the cytochrome P-450 system in order to become cytotoxic. The hepatic microsomal system converts cyclophosphamide to aldophosphamide and 4-hydroxycyclophosphamide. These are further converted to acrolein and phosphoramide mustard. The mustard compound is a potent alkylator of DNA. Once DNA-DNA interstrand cross-links are formed, DNA processing stops and cell death ensues. Cyclophosphamide is used in the treatment of several types of carcinoma.

A (busulfan) is incorrect. Busulfan does not require bioactivation. Busulfan is a sufonate-type alkylating agent that reacts more readily with thiol groups of amino acids and proteins than do nitrogen mustards, but it also binds to DNA at the N-7 position of guanine. Busulfan is used to treat chronic myelogenous leukemia in patients who are not candidates for interferon therapy or bone marrow transplantation.

B (carmustine) is incorrect. Carmustine does not require bioactivation. Carmustine has two chloroethyl groups that alkylate nucleic acids and cell proteins and form DNA-DNA or DNA-protein cross-links. During carmustine decomposition, isocyanates are also formed and can react by carbamoylating the lysine residues of proteins. Carmustine is a nitrosourea that crosses the blood-brain barrier, so it is often used in the treatment of brain tumors such as glioblastoma, brainstem glioma, medulloblastoma, astrocytoma, ependymoma, and metastatic brain cancer. It is also used in the treatment of multiple myeloma, Hodgkin's disease, and non-Hodgkin's lymphoma.

D (mechlorethamine) is incorrect. Mechlorethamine does not require bioactivation. It is a bifunctional alkylating agent that exerts its chemotherapeutic effects by substituting alkyl groups for hydrogen ions in a number of organic compounds. Mechlorethamine reacts readily with phosphate, amino, hydroxyl, sulfhydryl, carboxyl, and imidazole groups on amino acids. When these reactions occur, DNA-DNA interstrand cross-linking and DNA-protein cross-linking take place. This leads to DNA strand breakage and interferes with DNA replication, RNA transcription, and nucleic acid function. Mechlorethamine is used to treat Hodgkin's disease, non-Hodgkin's lymphoma, and cutaneous T-cell lymphoma (mycosis fungoides).

E (methotrexate) is incorrect. Methotrexate does not require bioactivation. It acts by inhibiting dihydrofolate reductase. Methotrexate is used in the treatment of various malignancies including osteosarcoma, non-Hodgkin's lymphoma, Hodgkin's disease, childhood acute lymphocytic leukemia, cutaneous T cell lymphoma (mycosis fungoides), head and neck cancer, lung cancer, and breast cancer.

36. **C** (etoposide) is correct. Etoposide is a cell cycle–specific (CCS) antineoplastic drug that acts by inhibiting topoisomerase II, an enzyme involved in the coiling and uncoiling of DNA. Etoposide is used in the treatment of a wide array of solid tumors and hematologic cancers. In the treatment of testicular carcinoma, it is given in combination with bleomycin and cisplatin.

A (bleomycin) is incorrect. As discussed in option C, bleomycin does not act by inhibiting topoisomerase. Bleomycin is a CCS drug that acts by causing scission of single- and double-stranded DNA. This scission occurs when free radicals are formed via the interaction of bleomycin, iron, and oxygen.

B (cisplatin) is incorrect. As discussed in option C, cisplatin does not act by inhibiting topoisomerase. Cisplatin is a cell cycle–nonspecific (CCNS) drug that acts as a DNA alkylating agent.

D (paclitaxel) is incorrect. Paclitaxel does not act by inhibiting topoisomerase. Both paclitaxel and the vinca alkaloids act by blocking mitosis, but they do so in different ways. Mitosis is characterized by the assembly and disassembly of microtubules, a process that requires the polymerization and depolymerization of tubulin. When vinca alkaloids bind to tubulin, they inhibit assembly. In contrast, when paclitaxel binds to tubulin, it inhibits disassembly. The combination of paclitaxel and cisplatin is considered the treatment of choice for stage III and stage IV ovarian cancer. Paclitaxel is being studied for use as a single agent and in combination with other chemotherapeutic agents in the treatment of many other solid tumors, including breast, lung, and head and neck cancers.

E (vincristine) is incorrect. Vincristine does not act by inhibiting topoisomerase. Both the vinca alkaloids (vincristine and vinblastine) and paclitaxel act by blocking mitosis, but they do so in different ways. Mitosis is characterized by the assembly and disassembly of microtubules, a process that requires the polymerization and depolymerization of tubulin. When vincristine binds to tubulin, it inhibits assembly. In contrast, when paclitaxel binds to tubulin, it inhibits disassembly. Vincristine is used in the treatment of a variety of cancers, including acute lymphoblastic leukemia, breast carcinoma, Hodgkin's disease, non-Hodgkin's lymphoma, multiple myeloma, soft tissue sarcoma, osteogenic sarcoma, and brain tumors.

37. **D** (regular insulin) is correct. The clinical and laboratory findings are consistent with the diagnosis of diabetic ketoacidosis in a patient with type 1 (insulin-dependent) diabetes mellitus. Intravenous administration of regular insulin should be started immediately to counteract the patient's severe hyperglycemic condition.

A (glucagon) is incorrect. Glucagon is an endogenous hormone synthesized by the A (alpha) cells of the pancreatic islets of Langerhans. The actions of glucagon counteract hypoglycemia, rather than hyperglycemia.

B (glyburide) is incorrect. Glyburide is an oral antidiabetic drug that is used only in the treatment of type 2 diabetes mellitus. Glyburide is a potent second-generation sulfonylurea that acts primarily by increasing the secretion of insulin and thereby lowering the blood glucose level.

C (metformin) is incorrect. Metformin is an oral antidiabetic drug that is used only in the treatment of type 2 diabetes mellitus. Metformin decreases hepatic gluconeogenesis and appears to improve utilization of glucose in skeletal muscle and adipose tissue by facilitating the binding of insulin to insulin receptors and thereby increasing cell membrane glucose transport.

E (ultralente insulin) is incorrect. Ultralente insulin, or extended insulin zinc suspension, is a long-acting preparation. Although it would not be helpful for the immediate treatment of the patient described in this question, it could be used as part of his long-term insulin maintenance therapy when he is released from the hospital.

38. **B** (set B) is correct. Prednisone has significant glucocorticoid activity and would markedly increase blood glucose levels. It suppresses the pituitary-adrenal axis, so levels of ACTH and cortisol would be low. Because prednisone has weaker mineralocorticoid activity than cortisol, the sodium level would be slightly below normal.

A (set A) is incorrect. The laboratory values in set A suggest the presence of congenital adrenal hyperplasia caused by a deficiency of 11β-hydroxylase. Because there is an excess of 11-deoxycorticosterone (DOC), there is no hyponatremia.

C (set C) is incorrect. The laboratory values in set C suggest the presence of Cushing's disease.

D (set D) is incorrect. The laboratory values in set D suggest the presence of Addison's disease.

39. **D** (spironolactone) is correct. The patient's clinical and laboratory findings are consistent with the diagnosis of female hirsutism. This disorder is sometimes treated with spironolactone. By inhibiting the effects of aldosterone on the distal renal tubules, spironolactone causes an increase in the excretion of sodium, chloride, and water and causes a decrease in the excretion of potassium, ammonium, and phosphate. In patients with severe heart failure, spironolactone reduces the number of hospitalizations and improves the overall survival rate when used with conventional therapy, such as angiotensin-converting enzyme (ACE) inhibitors, loop diuretics, or digoxin.

A (aldosterone) is incorrect. Aldosterone is not used in the treatment of hirsutism. In fact, aldosterone is not available as a drug.

B (clomiphene) is incorrect. Clomiphene is not used in the treatment of hirsutism. Clomiphene, a selective-estrogen receptor-modulator (SERM) because of its ability to compete with estradiol for estrogen receptors in the hypothalamus, is used to induce ovulation in women, including those with polycystic ovary syndrome.

C (ethinyl estradiol) is incorrect. Ethinyl estradiol is not used in the treatment of hirsutism. It is the estrogenic component of many oral combination contraceptives.

E (triamcinolone) is incorrect. Triamcinolone is not used in the treatment of hirsutism. Triamcinolone is a synthetic glucocorticoid used as anti-inflammatory and immunosuppressive agent.

40. **D** (omeprazole) is correct. The patient's manifestations are consistent with the diagnosis of Zollinger-Ellison syndrome. This syndrome is usually a fatal disorder in which hypersecretion of gastric acid is caused by gastrin-secreting tumors (gastrinomas). The most effective drug for treating Zollinger-Ellison syndrome is omeprazole, an orally administered agent that suppresses gastric acid secretion by inhibiting the proton pump (H^+,K^+-ATPase) in parietal cells. Omeprazole is also used in the short-term treatment of gastroesophageal reflux disease and in treating gastric and duodenal ulcers. Other proton pump inhibitors in this class are esomeprazole, lansoprazole, pantoprazole, and rabeprazole. Note the common ending prazole.

A (famotidine) is incorrect. Famotidine, cimetidine, ranitidine, and nizatidine are orally or parenterally administered agents that reduce basal and nocturnal gastric acid secretions by competitively inhibiting the binding of histamine to H_2 receptors on the gastric basolateral membrane of parietal cells. Although these H_2-receptor antagonists can be used to treat Zollinger-Ellison syndrome, they are not as effective as omeprazole and other proton pump inhibitors. Note the common ending tidine.

B (mesalamine) is incorrect. Sulfasalazine is a prodrug used in the treatment of ulcerative colitis. Sulfasalazine is cleaved by intestinal bacteria to yield sulfapyridine and mesalamine (5-aminosalicylic acid, or 5-ASA). Mesalamine has anti-inflammatory effects. Although its exact mechanisms of action are unknown, it is believed to act at least in part by blocking cyclooxygenase and thereby inhibiting prostaglandin production in the bowel mucosa.

C (misoprostol) is incorrect. Misoprostol is an orally administered synthetic prostaglandin E_1 analogue. It is primarily used to prevent gastric ulcers in patients who are taking nonsteroidal anti-inflammatory drugs (NSAIDs) on a long-term basis.

E (sucralfate) is incorrect. Sucralfate is an orally administered drug that is effective for use in the treatment of active duodenal ulcers and for maintenance therapy following the resolution of these ulcers. The efficacy of sucralfate for use in the treatment of gastric ulcers is comparable to the efficacy of cimetidine. Sucralfate reacts with hydrochloric acid in the stomach to form an adherent, paste-like substance capable of acting as an acid buffer.

41. **E** (reduces the expression of cyclooxygenase-2) is correct. Prednisone and other adrenal steroids have two major effects that contribute to their anti-inflammatory actions. The first effect is an increase in the synthesis of lipocortin, a protein that inhibits phospholipase A_2 and thereby inhibits the cleavage of arachidonic acid from membrane phospholipids. The second effect is a reduction in the expression of COX-2, an enzyme that converts arachidonic acid into inflammatory prostanoids.

A (activates phospholipase A_2) is incorrect. As described in option E, prednisone and other adrenal steroids increase the synthesis of lipocortin, so intracellular concentrations of lipocortin are increased, rather than decreased. Lipocortin does not activate phospholipase A_2; it inhibits it.

B (decreases intracellular concentrations of lipocortin) is incorrect. As described in option E, prednisone and other adrenal steroids increase the synthesis of lipocortin, so intracellular concentrations of lipocortin are increased, rather than decreased. Lipocortin does not activate phospholipase A_2; it inhibits it.

C (inhibits cyclooxygenase-1) is incorrect. Prednisone and other adrenal steroids do not inhibit COX-1. However, they decrease the concentration of arachidonic acid, which is the substrate for COX-1 and lipoxygenase.

D (inhibits lipoxygenase) is incorrect. Prednisone and other adrenal steroids do not inhibit lipoxygenase. However, they decrease the concentration of arachidonic acid, which is the substrate for COX-1 and lipoxygenase.

42. **B** (colchicine) is correct. When allopurinol treatment is initiated, an acute attack of gouty arthritis sometimes occurs. The attack is due to the resorption of uric acid from tissues. To avoid this effect, colchicine can be given early in the course of allopurinol treatment.

A (aspirin) is incorrect. Aspirin is not used to treat gout. In fact, low doses of aspirin increase the plasma levels of uric acid.

C (hydroxychloroquine) is incorrect. Hydroxychloroquine is not used to treat gouty arthritis but is used to treat rheumatoid arthritis and lupus erythematosus.

D (ibuprofen) is incorrect. Nonsteroidal anti-inflammatory drugs (NSAIDs) can be used on a short-term basis to control acute gouty arthritis. Indomethacin is the NSAID most frequently used for this purpose, but ibuprofen is sometimes used. An allopurinol-induced attack cannot be avoided by concurrent treatment with allopurinol and ibuprofen.

E (sulfinpyrazone) is incorrect. Sulfinpyrazone is not the drug of choice to treat an acute attack of gouty arthritis. Furthermore, the use of sulfinpyrazone during the early course of allopurinol treatment increases the risk of forming renal calculi. Sulfinpyrazone is a uricosuric agent that acts similar to probenecid.

43. **B** (celecoxib) is correct. Celecoxib is a nonsteroidal anti-inflammatory drug (NSAID) that acts by selectively inhibiting cyclooxygenase-2 (COX-2). It is able to relieve the symptoms of rheumatoid arthritis and osteoarthritis without causing gastropathy. Note that the Food and Drug Administration issued a public health advisory that the COX-2 inhibitors may be associated with an increased risk of serious cardiovascular events (heart attack and stroke), especially when used chronically or in very high risk settings (e.g., after open heart surgery). Since then, rofecoxib (Vioxx) and valdecoxib (Bextra) have been removed from the market. Patients who are at a high risk of gastrointestinal (GI) bleeding, have a history of intolerance to nonselective NSAIDs, or are not doing well on nonselective NSAIDs may still be appropriate candidates for celecoxib therapy.

A (acetaminophen) is incorrect. Acetaminophen does not have sufficient anti-inflammatory activity to relieve the symptoms of severe rheumatoid arthritis.

C (naproxen) is incorrect. Naproxen is an NSAID that inhibits both COX-1 and COX-2. Inhibition of COX-1 is responsible for gastrointestinal and renal toxicity.

D (sulindac) is incorrect. Sulindac is an NSAID that inhibits both COX-1 and COX-2. Inhibition of COX-1 is responsible for gastrointestinal and renal toxicity.

E (tolmetin) is incorrect. Tolmetin is an NSAID that inhibits both COX-1 and COX-2. Inhibition of COX-1 is responsible for gastrointestinal and renal toxicity.

44. C (ibuprofen) is correct. The patient's clinical manifestations are consistent with the diagnosis of primary dysmenorrhea caused by increased endometrial synthesis of PGE_2 and $PGF_{2\alpha}$ during menstruation, producing uterine contraction and ischemic pain. Ibuprofen is a nonsteroidal anti-inflammatory drug (NSAID) that is used to treat dysmenorrhea as well as rheumatoid arthritis and osteoarthritis.

A (acetaminophen) is incorrect. Acetaminophen is a central acting cyclooxygenase (COX) inhibitor that has only weak anti-inflammatory actions; thus, it would not be very effective in treating the symptoms of severe dysmenorrhea.

B (dexamethasone) is incorrect. Dexamethasone is a glucocorticoid that is used as an anti-inflammatory or immunosuppressive agent. It is not recommended for use in the treatment of dysmenorrhea.

D (indomethacin) is incorrect. Indomethacin is a nonselective cyclooxygenase (COX) inhibitor that has strong anti-inflammatory actions and would be effective in treating the symptoms of dysmenorrhea; however, less toxic NSAIDs, such as ibuprofen, would be preferred.

B (valdecoxib) is incorrect. Valdecoxib is a selective COX-2 inhibitor that exhibits anti-inflammatory, analgesic, and antipyretic activities but does not inhibit platelet aggregation. It was indicated for the management of dysmenorrhea, osteoarthritis, and rheumatoid arthritis. However in 2005, the manufacturer voluntarily removed it from the market when studies indicated that the COX-2 inhibitors may be associated with an increased risk of serious cardiovascular events (heart attack and stroke), especially when used chronically or in very high risk settings (e.g., after open heart surgery).

45. C (histamine) is correct. Histamine acts at H_1 receptors on endothelial cells to cause the formation of nitric oxide (NO), which activates guanylyl cyclase to increase cGMP in the vasculature to cause vasodilation. The subsequent decrease in mean blood pressure is accompanied by reflex tachycardia. Neither atropine (a muscarinic receptor antagonist) nor propranolol (a β-adrenergic receptor antagonist) will block the decrease in blood pressure. Propranolol will block the reflex tachycardia.

A (acetylcholine) is incorrect. Acetylcholine would cause a decrease in blood pressure, with reflex tachycardia. However, the effects of acetylcholine would be blocked by atropine.

B (epinephrine) is incorrect. Epinephrine would increase the blood pressure and heart rate.

D (isoproterenol) is incorrect. Isoproterenol would cause a decrease in blood pressure, with reflex tachycardia. However, the effects of isoproterenol would be blocked by propranolol.

E (norepinephrine) is incorrect. Norepinephrine would cause an increase in blood pressure and a reflex decrease in heart rate.

46. **D** (ondansetron) is correct. Ondansetron is the first selective serotonin receptor antagonist to be used as an antiemetic. The drug acts by blocking 5-HT_3 receptors found centrally in the chemoreceptor trigger zone (CTZ) and peripherally at vagus nerve terminals in the intestines. Ondansetron can be administered orally or parenterally and is safe and highly effective. Its use has made it easier for cancer patients to tolerate chemotherapy and has improved their quality of life. Other antiemetic agents in this class include dolasetron, granisetron, and palonosetron; note the common ending–setron.

A (diphenhydramine) is incorrect. Diphenhydramine is a histamine H_1 receptor antagonist that is primarily used to treat allergies. Because of its anticholinergic properties, however, diphenhydramine is effective in the relief of nausea, vomiting, and vertigo associated with motion sickness. Diphenhydramine has significant antimuscarinic activity and produces marked sedation in most patients. The drug's gastrointestinal side effects are minimal.

B (dronabinol) is incorrect. Dronabinol is a synthetic preparation of Δ^9-tetrahydrocannabinol (THC), one of the many cannabinoids found in *Cannabis sativa*. Dronabinol is taken orally and is indicated for the relief of chemotherapy-induced nausea and vomiting in patients who have failed to respond to other antiemetics. It is also used as an appetite stimulant in patients with cancer or AIDS.

C (metoclopramide) is incorrect. Metoclopramide is a drug that enhances gastrointestinal motility and is an effective antiemetic. Metoclopramide, prochlorperazine, and many other antiemetics act by blocking dopamine D_2 receptors in the CTZ.

E (prochlorperazine) is incorrect. Prochlorperazine, a piperazine phenothiazine, is an effective antiemetic and antipsychotic agent. Metoclopramide, prochlorperazine, and many other antiemetics act by blocking dopamine D_2 receptors in the CTZ.

47. **C** (dihydroergotamine) is correct. The patient's symptoms are consistent with the diagnosis of migraine headache disorder. Dihydroergotamine is an ergot alkaloid that is administered parenterally or intranasally to terminate migraine headaches. Dihydroergotamine is a more potent α-adrenergic receptor agonist than ergonovine and is a less potent dopamine receptor agonist than bromocriptine. Dihydroergotamine reduces extracranial blood flow, decreases pulsations in the cranial arteries, and decreases hypoperfusion of the basilar artery territory.

A (acetaminophen) is incorrect. Acetaminophen is a non-narcotic analgesic that is often used to provide relief of pain caused by vascular headaches; however, it is usually ineffective for use in the treatment of severe migraine headaches, such as those described in this case.

B (amitriptyline) is incorrect. Amitriptyline is not used to terminate migraine headaches, but it is sometimes used to prevent migraine headaches. Timolol, valproic acid, and methysergide are also approved for migraine prophylaxis.

D (ibuprofen) is incorrect. Ibuprofen is a non-narcotic analgesic that is often used to provide relief of pain caused by vascular headaches; however, it is usually ineffective for use in the treatment of severe migraine headaches, such as those described in this case.

E (propranolol) is incorrect. Propranolol is not used to terminate migraine headaches, but it is sometimes used to prevent migraine headaches. Timolol, valproic acid, and methysergide are also approved for migraine prophylaxis.

48. **C** (epoprostenol) is correct: Dexfenfluramine, which exerts its anorectant effect by increasing neuronal synaptic concentrations of serotonin by stimulating serotonin release and inhibiting serotonin reuptake, has been discontinued in the United States when it became apparent that there was an unacceptable risk of cardiac valvulopathy with the use of this drug. Epoprostenol (prostacyclin; PGI_2) is a vasodilator and an inhibitor of platelet aggregation. Intravenous epoprostenol is used for the treatment of primary pulmonary hypertension caused by dexfenfluramine.

A (alprostadil) is incorrect. Alprostatil is not used to treat pulmonary hypertension. Alprostadil, a naturally occurring PGE_1 compound, is used to treat impotence in adult males and to maintain the patency of the ductus arteriosus in neonates up until the time of corrective surgery.

B (dinoprostone) is incorrect. Dinoprostone is not used to treat pulmonary hypertension. Dinoprostone, a PGE_2 compound, is administered vaginally as an oxytocic agent for cervical ripening induction in women at or near term for labor induction and to induce abortion in the second trimester of pregnancy and to evacuate the contents of the uterus following intrauterine fetal death, missed abortion, or benign hydatidiform mole.

D (latanoprost) is incorrect. Latanoprost is not used to treat pulmonary hypertension. Latanoprost, a $PGF_{2\alpha}$ analogue, is a prodrug used for the treatment of elevated intraocular pressure.

E (misoprostol) is incorrect. Misoprostol is not used to treat pulmonary hypertension. Misoprostol, a synthetic, oral PGE_1 analogue, is used for the prevention of gastric and duodenal ulcers secondary to use of nonsteroidal anti-inflammatory drugs (NSAIDs).

49. **A** (albuterol) is correct. Albuterol is a bronchodilator that acts fairly selectively on β_2-adrenergic receptors and is therefore relatively free of adverse cardiac effects.

B (atropine) is incorrect. Atropine has bronchodilator action, but it is usually not adequate to provide relief from an asthmatic attack. Moreover, atropine has an extensive profile of adverse effects caused by the generalized inhibition of muscarinic receptors. Ipratropium bromide is structurally similar to atropine, except that it is a quaternary ammonium compound that does not cross the blood-brain barrier. Ipratropium bromide is given by oral inhalation or nasal spray as a bronchodilator in the management of bronchospasm associated with chronic obstructive pulmonary disease.

C (cromolyn sodium) is incorrect. Cromolyn sodium is not appropriate for use in the treatment of asthmatic attacks. Cromolyn is used as a prophylactic agent in the treatment of mild to moderate asthma, as a nasal inhaler to treat seasonal allergic rhinitis, as an ophthalmic solution to treat allergic or vernal conjunctivitis, and orally to treat systemic mastocytosis and ulcerative colitis. It acts at the surface of the mast cell to inhibit degranulation.

D (ephedrine) is incorrect. Ephedrine releases endogenous norepinephrine from its storage sites and thereby causes an indirect sympathomimetic effect. Although ephedrine has been used to treat bronchospasms, the more specific β_2-adrenergic receptor agonists are preferred.

E (epinephrine) is incorrect. Epinephrine is a nonselective β-adrenergic receptor agonist. Although it is effective in the treatment of acute asthmatic attacks, its use is associated with an array of potentially dangerous adverse effects that are not seen with the use of selective β_2-adrenergic receptor agonists.

50. **D** (pilocarpine) is correct. A topical ophthalmic preparation of pilocarpine is used in the treatment of acute angle-closure glaucoma as well as in the treatment of chronic open-angle glaucoma.

A (atropine) is incorrect. In patients with acute angle-closure glaucoma, atropine is contraindicated because it can induce cycloplegia and mydriasis and thereby increase intraocular pressure.

B (edrophonium) is incorrect. Edrophonium is not used in the treatment of glaucoma. It is a rapid-acting, short-duration cholinesterase inhibitor that is used in the diagnosis of myasthenia gravis.

C (furosemide) is incorrect. Furosemide is not used in the treatment of glaucoma. It is a loop diuretic that is used in the treatment of hypertension and heart failure.

E (timolol) is incorrect. Timolol is not used in the treatment of acute angle-closure glaucoma. Topical preparations of timolol are used in the treatment of chronic open-angle glaucoma and ocular hypertension.

questions

DIRECTIONS: Each numbered item or incomplete statement is followed by options arranged in alphabetical or logical order. Select the best answer to each question. Some options may be partially correct, but there is only **ONE BEST** answer.

1. A 61-year-old diabetic man receives a kidney transplant. He begins immunosuppressive therapy and is told that he must continue this therapy for the rest of his life. Which of the following drugs interferes with T-cell function by binding to immunophilins and would be appropriate to prevent kidney rejection in this patient?
   A. Cyclophosphamide
   B. Cyclosporine
   C. Daclizumab
   D. Leflunomide
   E. Prednisone

2. A 61-year-old man with renal failure and generally poor health begins dialysis treatment. One year later, he complains of increased shortness of breath while walking. Laboratory findings establish that he has normocytic anemia. Which of the following factors is this patient most lacking and is responsible for his normocytic anemia?
   A. Erythropoietin
   B. Folic acid
   C. Intrinsic factor
   D. Iron
   E. Vitamin B_{12}

3. A 41-year-old woman is being treated for promyelocytic leukemia. She develops septicemia and suffers from widespread ecchymoses and profuse bleeding. Laboratory results confirm the diagnosis of disseminated intravascular coagulation (DIC). In addition to administering fresh frozen plasma and antibiotics, treating the patient with which of the following agents might also be useful?
   A. Abciximab
   B. Bivalirudin
   C. Heparin
   D. Vitamin K
   E. Warfarin

4. A 51-year-old woman was brought to the emergency department with multiple injuries encountered in an automobile accident. She also has other significant health issues. Which of the following conditions would be a relative contraindication for the administration of morphine to this patient to alleviate pain?
A. Acute pulmonary edema
B. Broken ribs
C. Diabetes mellitus
D. Severe head injury and concussion
E. Terminal cancer

5. A 42-year-old woman who has recently been promoted to a managerial position is suffering from anxiety and has trouble sleeping. Which of the following drugs would be expected to alleviate her insomnia with minimal daytime sedative effects?
A. Diazepam
B. Flumazenil
C. Flurazepam
D. Phenobarbital
E. Zaleplon

6. A 73-year-old woman is being treated with levodopa (L-dopa) to alleviate the symptoms of Parkinson's disease. To potentiate the effects of levodopa, the physician begins concurrent treatment with a drug that decreases the metabolism of dopamine without producing life-threatening side effects. Which of the following drugs is most likely prescribed to potentiate the effects of levodopa by decreasing the oxidative metabolism of dopamine in this patient?
A. Amantadine
B. Carbidopa
C. Entacapone
D. Phenelzine
E. Selegiline

7. A 62-year-old man has been treated several years for schizophrenia. He now has developed benign prostatic hyperplasia (BPH) and experiences chronic constipation and urinary retention when taking his antipsychotic medications. Which of the following antipsychotic agents is now most appropriate to control the symptoms of schizophrenia in this patient while producing minimal constipation and urinary retention?
A. Chlorpromazine
B. Clozapine
C. Olanzapine
D. Risperidone
E. Thioridazine

8. A 32-year-old man is being treated with phenelzine for a major depressive disorder. He is brought to the emergency department by his wife, who says that her husband has a history of peptic ulcer disease. He has recently begun complaining of insomnia and flu-like symptoms and appears to be suicidal. The patient is admitted for overnight observation and is treated for his symptoms. Early the next morning, he becomes delirious, hyperpyretic, and comatose. Which of the following medications is most likely responsible for the reaction observed in this patient?

A. Acetaminophen

B. Codeine

C. Fluoxetine

D. Ranitidine

E. Zolpidem

9. A 31-year-old woman complains of severe burning pain that involves the right maxillary region of her face and sometimes spreads over the right jaw. She speaks slowly, as if she cannot find the right words, and has a motionless mask-like face with a sad, suffering expression in her eyes. Which of the following treatments is most appropriate to provide relief of symptoms in this patient?

A. Alprazolam

B. Amitriptyline

C. Cyclobenzaprine

D. Naproxen

E. Oxycodone

10. A 6-year-old boy exhibits multiple types of disruptive behavior in his home and in the classroom and has not been progressing at the educational rate of his peers. He is tested and found to have attention-deficit hyperactivity disorder (ADHD). Which of the following stimulant drugs, that in part acts by blocking dopamine uptake in central adrenergic neurons, is most appropriate for the treatment of ADHD in this young boy?

A. Amphetamine

B. Atomoxetine

C. Bupropion

D. Methylphenidate

E. Modafinil

11. An 11-year-old boy is scheduled to undergo surgery to repair an inguinal hernia. His anesthesiologist plans to concurrently administer a general anesthetic and pancuronium as a nondepolarizing muscle relaxant. Which general anesthetic is most likely to potentiate the muscle relaxant effects of pancuronium in this boy?

A. Etomidate

B. Fentanyl

C. Isoflurane

D. Propofol

E. Thiopental

12. A 48-year-old woman has a long history of alcohol abuse. Laboratory studies show no increase in her levels of hepatic enzymes (serum transaminases and alkaline phosphatase) or bilirubin. Although the patient has tried many times to quit drinking, she has been unsuccessful in her attempts. Which of the following agents is most likely to help her abstain from drinking alcohol in the future?

A. Chlorpromazine
B. Codeine
C. Haloperidol
D. Naltrexone
E. Phenobarbital

13. A 78-year-old woman is admitted to the hospital after suffering a severe myocardial infarction. Findings include pulmonary congestion, ventricular tachyarrhythmia, episodes of ventricular fibrillation requiring cardioversion, and a myocardial ejection fraction of 25%. Which of the following drugs would be considered the first drug of choice for suppressing ventricular arrhythmias in this patient?

A. Amiodarone
B. Esmolol
C. Lidocaine
D. Nifedipine
E. Quinidine

14. This table shows five sets of laboratory data. Which set of values (A, B, C, D, or E) reflects changes that are expected to occur when patients with hypertension are treated with diltiazem?

	Peripheral Vascular Resistance	Atrioventricular Node Conduction Velocity	Sinoatrial Node Discharge	Coronary Blood Flow
A	↓	↑	↑	↑
B	↑	↑	↓	↑↑
C	↓	↓	↓	↑
D	↑	↓	↑	↓
E	↓	↑	↓	↓

15. A 78-year-old man who has been treated with an antihypertensive drug for many years and has recently gained about 9 kg (20 pounds) is admitted to the hospital with the chief complaint of increasing shortness of breath. Clinical findings include dyspnea, cyanosis, tachycardia, pulse of 99 bpm, blood pressure of 159/99 mm Hg, and pitting edema of the extremities and sacral region. Digoxin is given for cardiac failure, and treatment with an antihypertensive drug is continued. Which of the following cardiovascular drugs causes hypokalemia and could potentiate the toxicity of digoxin in this patient?
A. Hydrochlorothiazide
B. Lisinopril
C. Metoprolol
D. Quinidine
E. Verapamil

16. This table shows five sets of effects. Which set (A, B, C, D, or E) is produced by acetazolamide?

	Tubular Bicarbonate Concentration	Ammonia Excretion	Urine pH	Urinary Potassium Excretion
A	↑	↓	↑	↑
B	↑	↑	↓	↓
C	↑	↓	↑	↓
D	↓	↑	↓	↑
E	↓	↓	↑	↑

17. In the accompanying figure, curves X, Y, and Z represent changes in the action potential of the cardiac muscle in response to the administration of various antiarrhythmic agents. Which of the following agents would be most likely to produce the changes depicted in curve X?
A. Adenosine
B. Pindolol
C. Propranolol
D. Sotalol
E. Verapamil

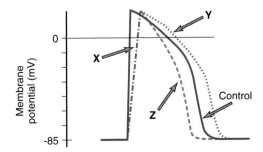

18. A 69-year-old man suffers a heart attack and is treated prophylactically with warfarin. Later, his physician decides to add an antihyperlipoproteinemic agent to the treatment regimen. Which of the following agents is most likely to potentiate the anticoagulant effect of warfarin upon addition to this patient's drug therapy regimen?
A. Colesevelam
B. Cholestyramine
C. Ezetimibe
D. Gemfibrozil
E. Pravastatin

19. An 18-year-old sexually active woman has recurring herpes genitalis. Which of the following drugs would be most appropriate for treatment of recurrent herpes genitalis in this patient?
A. Acyclovir
B. Amantadine
C. Indinavir
D. Rifampin
E. Zidovudine

20. A 39-year-old woman is diagnosed with *Pseudomonas aeruginosa* infection. A fourth-generation cephalosporin is prescribed. Which of the following is the molecular target where a fourth-generation cephalosporin exerts its actions against the bacteria harbored in this patient?
A. Cell wall synthesis
B. DNA synthesis
C. Mitochondria
D. Plasma membrane
E. Protein synthesis

21. A 25-year-old noncompliant woman has within the past 3 days had sexual activity with individuals infected with *Treponema pallidum, Neisseria gonorrhoeae,* and *Chlamydia trachomatis.* Which of the following drugs, in a single dose, would provide protection against all three of these sexually transmitted microorganisms in this patient?
A. Azithromycin
B. Ceftriaxone
C. Doxycycline
D. Ofloxacin
E. Penicillin G; benzathine

22. A 42-year-old man visits a clinic because he has had a persistent fever and pain in his right knee for 1 week. Examination shows extensive swelling of the knee and decreased mobility of the joint. Aspirated synovial fluid contains a large number of leukocytes. A Gram stain and culture of the fluid show the presence of *Staphylococcus aureus,* and sensitivity tests show that the organism is resistant to penicillin G but sensitive to methicillin. The patient says that when he was treated with penicillin in the past, he had a severe anaphylactic reaction. Which of the following drugs would be most appropriate to treat the infection in this patient?
A. Aztreonam
B. Cefazolin
C. Doxycycline
D. Erythromycin
E. Vancomycin

23. A 39-year-old man is taken to the emergency department because he is suffering from fever, night sweats, and increasing fatigue. Blood studies show a white blood cell (WBC) count of 145,000/mm³, with a differential blood count of more than 90% leukemic blast cells; platelet count of 35,000/mm³; and hematocrit of 28%. A bone marrow aspirate confirms the diagnosis of acute nonlymphocytic leukemia. Twenty-four hours after chemotherapy is initiated, an infection occurs. Empiric antibiotic therapy is given. Six days later, the patient develops a fever. Cultures for bacteria are negative, so a fungal infection is suspected. Which of the following drugs would be the most appropriate for treating a fungal infection in this patient?
A. Amphotericin B
B. Flucytosine
C. Ketoconazole
D. Pentamidine
E. Terbinafine

24. A 69-year-old man is taken to the emergency department after suffering for 2 days from a fever, chills, chest pain, and an increasing shortness of breath. His sputum is rust-colored. Chest x-ray and a Gram stain of the sputum suggest the diagnosis of pneumonia due to *Streptococcus pneumoniae.* Blood culture results are pending, and therapy must be initiated immediately. Which of the following would be the drug of choice, based on its activity and low potential for adverse effects, to treat the infection in this patient?
A. Cefepime
B. Clindamycin
C. Penicillin G
D. Polymyxin B
E. Vancomycin

25. A 31-year-old man with tuberculosis is being treated on a long-term basis with appropriate multidrug therapy. Because his treatment regimen includes isoniazid, he is routinely being monitored for hepatotoxicity. Which other adverse effect associated with isoniazid therapy should be included in the monitoring of this patient?
A. Optic neuritis
B. Ototoxicity
C. Peripheral neuropathy
D. Red discoloration of body secretions
E. Renal toxicity

26. An 8-year-old boy presents at the pediatric clinic with symptoms that include gastrointestinal discomfort, central nervous system disturbances, "wristdrop" and "footdrop," a black line (Burton's line) on the gums, microcytic anemia, and the presence of stippled red blood cells. Chronic exposure to which of the following environmental substances is most likely responsible for the clinical presentation of this young boy?
A. Carbon monoxide
B. Chlorinated hydrocarbon insecticide
C. Inorganic lead
D. Inorganic mercury
E. Organic phosphate ester

27. A 44-year-old woman who attempted suicide by taking a drug overdose is rushed to the hospital in a coma. Findings include dilated pupils, dry skin and mucous membranes, hypertension, pulmonary edema, and sinus tachycardia, with a prolonged QRS interval resembling ventricular tachycardia. Three hours after hospitalization, the patient begins to experience seizures. In addition to supportive therapy, she is treated with activated charcoal, followed by gastric lavage, sodium bicarbonate, diazepam, and pancuronium. Which of the following drugs would be expected to cause the symptoms observed in this patient when consumed in excess?
A. Acetaminophen
B. Amitriptyline
C. Isoniazid
D. Lithium
E. Salicylate

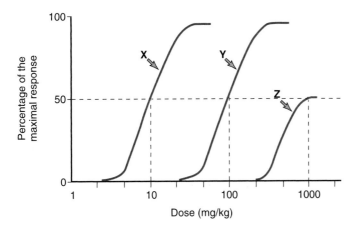

28. The accompanying figure depicts dose-response curves for drugs X, Y, and Z.
A comparison of the curves shows that drug X
A. Has greater efficacy than drug Y
B. Has lesser efficacy than drug Y
C. Has the same potency as drug Y
D. Is more potent than drug Y
E. Is safer than drug Y or drug Z

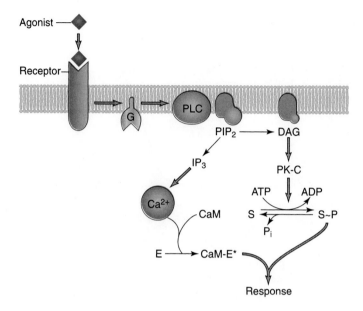

G, G protein; PLC, phospholipase C; PIP$_2$,
phosphatidylinositol 4,5-bisphosphate; DAG, diacylglycerol;
IP$_3$, inositol triphosphate; CaM, calmodulin; E, calmodulin-
binding enzyme; CaM-E*, activated state; PK-C, protein kinase C;
ATP, adenosine triphosphate; ADP, adenosine diphosphate;
S, substrate for protein kinase C; S~P, phosphorylated substrate;
and P$_i$, inorganic phosphate.

29. The accompanying figure depicts the polyphosphoinositide signaling pathway. Which molecule in this signaling pathway is referred to as a second messenger?
A. Calmodulin (CaM)
B. G protein (G)
C. Inositol triphosphate (IP$_3$)
D. Phospholipase C (PLC)
E. Protein kinase C (PK-C)

30. Drug X has a half-life of 7 hours and is eliminated from the body by first-order kinetics. A single intravenous dose provides a therapeutic level of the drug for 14 hours. Doubling the dose would provide a therapeutic level for a total of how many hours?
A. 14 hours
B. 21 hours
C. 28 hours
D. 35 hours
E. 28 to 35 hours

31. A 42-year-old man requires emergency tracheal intubation and is given
succinylcholine. Which of the following best describes the molecular action
of succinylcholine as a neuromuscular blocker in this patient?
A. Acetylcholinesterase inhibitor
B. Muscarinic receptor agonist
C. Muscarinic receptor antagonist
D. Nicotinic receptor agonist
E. Nicotinic receptor antagonist

32. In experimental studies when anesthetized subjects are treated intravenously with
an agonist (drug X), they have an increase in their blood glucose level and in the
force of ventricular contraction, and a pronounced decrease in peripheral
resistance. Pretreatment of the subjects with an antagonist (drug Y) almost
completely blocks all of these effects. Drug Y is most likely to be which of the
following agents?
A. Atenolol
B. Atropine
C. Guanethidine
D. Phentolamine
E. Propranolol

33. This table shows cardiovascular changes induced by drug treatment in
experimental subjects. Which of the following drugs is most likely to cause the
changes shown in profile 3?
A. Clonidine
B. Epinephrine
C. Isoproterenol
D. Norepinephrine
E. Propranolol

Profile	Mean Blood Pressure	Systolic Blood Pressure	Diastolic Blood Pressure	Heart Rate
1	↑	↑	↑	↓
2	↑	↑	↓	↑
3	↓	Slight ↑	↓	↑
4	↓	↓	↓	↓

34. In experimental studies when anesthetized subjects are treated intravenously with drug X, they show a marked increase in both diastolic and systolic blood pressure and a pronounced slowing of the heart. However, if they are pretreated with prazosin, they show a modest increase in the systolic blood pressure and heart rate. Drug X is most likely to be which of the following agents?

A. Acetylcholine
B. Epinephrine
C. Histamine
D. Isoproterenol
E. Norepinephrine

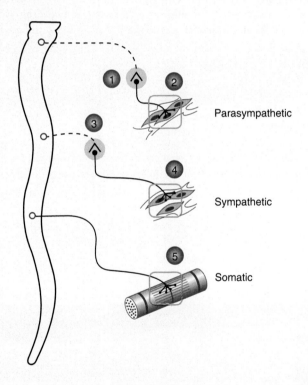

35. The accompanying figure depicts nerves in the autonomic and somatic nervous system. Five sites are labeled with the numbers 1 through 5. Muscarinic receptors are commonly associated with which site?

A. Site 1
B. Site 2
C. Site 3
D. Site 4
E. Site 5

36. An 11-year-old girl frequently experiences severe asthmatic attacks and becomes cyanotic, dyspneic, and agitated when playing outdoors. Which of the following agents has no bronchodilator activity but may prevent symptoms in this girl by inhibiting antigen-induced release of mediators that cause bronchospasms?
A. Albuterol
B. Cromolyn sodium
C. Ipratropium
D. Tiotropium
E. Zafirlukast

37. A 77-year-old man undergoes surgery for colorectal cancer. He has stage III disease with regional lymph node involvement; therefore, he is subsequently treated with a combination of irinotecan, fluorouracil, and leucovorin (IFL protocol). Which of the following adverse effects is most likely to occur in this patient from the fluorouracil component of the drug protocol?
A. Cardiotoxicity
B. Exfoliative dermatitis
C. Gastrointestinal ulceration
D. Nephrotoxicity
E. Pancreatitis

38. A 58-year-old man suffers from increasing inability to use his right arm and leg and complains of severe headaches that do not respond to conventional analgesics. CT scan shows a tumor located on the left side of the brain in the high parietal region. The tumor is removed, and biopsy shows a highly malignant glioblastoma. Which of the following drugs when administered systemically is most likely to slow the regrowth of this tumor in this patient?
A. Busulfan
B. Carmustine
C. Methotrexate
D. Prednisone
E. Streptozocin

39. A 67-year-old man suffers from back pain, fatigue, recurrent infections, and gingival bleeding. His bone marrow is found to contain nests of plasma cells. Diagnosis of multiple myeloma is confirmed. Which of the following drugs is most likely to be effective in treating this disease in this patient?
A. Aldesleukin
B. Azathioprine
C. Cyclosporine
D. Melphalan
E. Methotrexate

40. A 32-year-old man has had episodes of watery diarrhea and abdominal pain for the past year. He has been defecating as many as 10 times a day during the past week, and he has lost about 10 kg (22 pounds) during the past 3 months. His temperature is 38.3° C (101° F). Laboratory studies and sigmoidoscopy findings are consistent with the diagnosis of severe acute ulcerative colitis. The patient's symptoms are significantly alleviated by an initial course of parenteral treatment with hydrocortisone and are then successfully controlled by oral treatment with prednisone. As the prednisone treatment is gradually withdrawn, the patient will be given a drug to maintain remission of the disease. Which of the following drugs is most appropriate to maintain this patient's disease in a state of remission?
A. Amoxicillin
B. Bismuth subsalicylate
C. Cyclosporine
D. Metronidazole
E. Sulfasalazine

41. A 51-year-old man complains of increasing anxiety, restlessness, and palpitations. Physical examination shows tachycardia, tremor, and the presence of a 2.5-cm nodule on his thyroid gland. Which of the following drugs could be prescribed as short-term therapy to diminish this patient's symptoms?
A. Amiodarone
B. Finasteride
C. Procainamide
D. Propranolol
E. Spironolactone

42. This table compares the pharmacologic properties of five adrenal steroids (drugs A, B, C, D, and E) with the properties of cortisol. Which adrenal steroid is dexamethasone?

	Mineralocorticoid (Salt-Retaining) Potency	Glucocorticoid (Anti-inflammatory) Potency	Duration of Action
Cortisol	1	1	Short
A	0	5	Medium
B	20	0	Short
C	0.3	5	Short
D	0	30	Long
E	250	10	Short

43. A 45-year-old moderately obese man is diagnosed with type 2 diabetes mellitus. Dietary modifications and exercise fail to control his glucose levels. Which oral antidiabetic agent would most likely improve glucose tolerance and lower basal and postprandial plasma glucose in this patient without producing episodes of hypoglycemia while helping him lose weight?
A. Acarbose
B. Glipizide
C. Metformin
D. Pioglitazone
E. Repaglinide

44. A 49-year-old woman with rheumatoid arthritis is initially treated with aspirin for 3 months. She stops taking aspirin and is subsequently treated with other nonsteroidal anti-inflammatory drugs (NSAIDs) for about 1 year. In spite of adequate dosing and meticulous patient compliance, the patient's inflammation and erosive bone changes are still evident and appear to be getting worse. Which of the following disease-modifying antirheumatic drugs (DMARDs) that targets purine and pyrimidine biosynthesis would be most appropriate to add to the therapeutic regimen to reduce the persistent and active arthritis in this patient?
A. Auranofin
B. Hydroxychloroquine
C. Infliximab
D. Leflunomide
E. Methotrexate

45. A 59-year-old woman with osteoarthritis and histories of cardiovascular disease and sulfonamide-hypersensitivity has been taking high doses of aspirin for 3 years. She has now developed an aspirin-induced peptic ulcer. Which of the following medications would be most appropriate for the control of pain in this patient?
A. Acetaminophen
B. Celecoxib
C. Naproxen
D. Oxycodone
E. Rofecoxib

46. A 55-year-old man complains that he has attacks of excruciating pain in his big toe. Examination of the foot shows that the first metatarsophalangeal joint is swollen, hot, red, and tender. Laboratory findings include a serum uric acid level of 16.1 mg/dL. His renal creatinine clearance is 40 mL/min. Which of the following is the most appropriate medication to prevent future attacks of gouty arthritis in this patient?
A. Allopurinol
B. Colchicine
C. Indomethacin
D. Probenecid
E. Salicylates

47. This table shows five sets of effects. Which set (A, B, C, D, or E) is produced by histamine?

	Gastric Secretion	Blood Pressure	Heart Rate	Capillary Permeability
A	↑	↓	↑	↑
B	↑	↑	↓	↓
C	↑	↓	↑	↓
D	↓	↑	↓	↑
E	↓	↓	↑	↑

48. A 33-year-old man complains that he has been having left-sided pulsatile headaches for the past year. The headaches are preceded by bilateral flashes of light and a sensation of lightheadedness. Ergotamine is prescribed. When this proves ineffective, the physician stops ergotamine treatment and begins treatment with a relatively selective serotonin 5-HT$_{1D}$ receptor agonist. Which of the following drugs is this patient most likely to be given at this time?
A. Buspirone
B. Dihydroergotamine
C. Metoclopramide
D. Ondansetron
E. Sumatriptan

49. A 55-year-old woman complains of sneezing attacks, congestion, runny nose, and red and itchy eyes. She says that her symptoms do not have a seasonal pattern and that they disappear when she is on vacation. Which of the following treatments is most likely to alleviate this patient's symptoms?
A. Cimetidine
B. Desensitization
C. Fexofenadine
D. Fluticasone
E. Naphazoline

50. A 23-year-old woman has polymorphic, erythematous, and well-circumscribed edematous papules (wheals) over her entire body. She says that the lesions (1) cause intense itching; (2) appeared overnight; and (3) have been present for 3 days. She has driven her automobile to the appointment and needs to drive herself home. Which of the following is the most appropriate medication for this patient?
A. Chlorpheniramine
B. Desloratadine
C. Famotidine
D. Prednisone
E. Triamcinolone cream

answers

1. **B** (cyclosporine) is correct. Cyclosporine binds cyclophilin (an immunophilin) and the cyclosporine-cyclophilin complex then binds to and inhibits calcineurin (a calcium-calmodulin activated phosphatase). Calcineurin catalyzes critical dephosphorylation reactions necessary for early cytokine gene transcription, and subsequent early activation of T cells. Calcineurin inhibition blocks the signal transduction produced by the nuclear receptor referred to as the nuclear factor of activated T cells (NF-AT), resulting in a failure to activate NF-AT regulated genes. Some NF-AT activated genes are required for B-cell activation (IL-4 and CD40 ligand) and for T-cell activation (IL-2 and interferon gamma). Cyclosporine does not affect suppressor T cells or T-cell independent, antibody-mediated immunity. Cyclosporine is used almost exclusively for immunosuppressive therapy. It is used primarily to prevent allograft rejection, but it is also given to treat autoimmune conditions such as uveitis, psoriasis, rheumatoid arthritis, inflammatory bowel disease, and certain nephropathies.

   A (cyclophosphamide) is incorrect. Cyclophosphamide does not bind to an immunophilin. It is a cell cycle–nonspecific (CCNS) antineoplastic agent that is also used as an immunosuppressant agent in the management of various immunologic disorders, including nephrotic syndrome, Wegener's granulomatosis, rheumatoid arthritis, graft-versus-host disease, and graft rejection.

   C (daclizumab) is incorrect. Daclizumab does not bind to an immunophilin. Daclizumab and basiliximab are monoclonal antibodies that bind specifically to the alpha subunit of the IL-2 receptor expressed on T cells. This prevents the activation of T cells by IL-2. These monoclonal antibodies are used as part of an immunosuppressive regimen that usually includes cyclosporine and corticosteroids for kidney transplant rejection prophylaxis.

   D (leflunomide) is incorrect. Leflunomide does not bind to an immunophilin. Leflunomide is converted to an active metabolite that inhibits dihydroorotate dehydrogenase, an enzyme located in mitochondria that catalyzes a key step in *de novo* pyrimidine synthesis. It arrests lymphocytes in the G_1 phase of the cell cycle. Leflunomide is not used for kidney transplant rejection prophylaxis but for the treatment of rheumatoid arthritis.

E (prednisone) is incorrect. Prednisone does not bind to an immunophilin. It is a glucocorticoid that affects protein synthesis resulting in immunosuppressive and anti-inflammatory effects. Prednisone is used to prevent allograft rejection and to treat asthma, systemic lupus erythematosus, and many other inflammatory disorders. It is also used in induction therapy for acute lymphoblastic leukemia.

2. **A** (erythropoietin) is correct. Erythropoietin is a glycoprotein that is synthesized in the kidney and stimulates red blood cell production. In patients with renal failure, the lack of erythropoietin synthesis results in normocytic anemia.

B (folic acid) is incorrect. A deficiency of folic acid would cause macrocytic megaloblastic anemia. Prolonged renal dialysis could contribute to folic acid deficiency.

C (intrinsic factor) is incorrect. A decrease in the production of intrinsic factor by the gastric mucosal cells leads to pernicious anemia. Intrinsic factor is required for vitamin B_{12} absorption, so eventually a patient with intrinsic factor deficiency will develop a vitamin B_{12} deficiency, and this will result in macrocytic megaloblastic anemia.

D (iron) is incorrect. A deficiency of iron is usually due to excessive bleeding and will lead to microcytic anemia.

E (vitamin B_{12}) is incorrect. A deficiency of vitamin B_{12} will cause macrocytic megaloblastic anemia.

3. **C** (heparin) is correct. Heparin therapy, administered in a dosage lower than that used in patients with venous thrombosis, may be useful for increasing the neutralization of thrombin. This is particularly true in patients who have DIC associated with promyelocytic leukemia.

A (abciximab) is incorrect. Abciximab is not indicated for use in the treatment of DIC. It is an antiplatelet drug that acts by binding to glycoprotein IIb/IIIa receptors.

B (bivalirudin) is incorrect. Bivalirudin is not indicated for use in the treatment of DIC. Bivalirudin, a bivalent analogue of hirudin found in leeches, is a specific and reversible direct thrombin inhibitor. It is approved for use in the treatment of (1) unstable angina in patients undergoing percutaneous transluminal coronary angioplasty; (2) percutaneous coronary intervention with glycoprotein IIb/IIIa blockade; (3) acute myocardial infarction in combination with streptokinase; and (4) deep venous thrombosis prophylaxis.

D (vitamin K) is incorrect. Vitamin K is not indicated for use in the treatment of DIC. Vitamin K promotes blood clotting by increasing the formation of the vitamin K–dependent clotting factors.

E (warfarin) is incorrect. Warfarin is not indicated for use in the treatment of DIC. Like heparin, warfarin is an anticoagulant; however, warfarin has not been found to be effective for use in the treatment of DIC.

4. **D** (severe head injury and concussion) is correct. Morphine and other opioid agonists are contraindicated in patients with head trauma or increased intracranial pressure. This is because opioids can interfere with the evaluation of neurologic parameters. Opioids can also cause hypoventilation, thereby producing cerebral hypoxia and raising the intracranial pressure.

A (acute pulmonary edema) is incorrect. Morphine is used as an adjunct in the treatment of acute pulmonary edema. It reduces anxiety, reduces the perception of shortness of breath, and reduces cardiac preload and afterload.

B (broken ribs) is incorrect. Morphine should not be withheld from patients with severe pain. Morphine or a related opioid agonist is the drug of choice for pain relief in a patient with broken ribs.

C (diabetes mellitus) is incorrect. Opioid analgesics are not contraindicated for patients with diabetes mellitus.

E (terminal cancer) is incorrect. Morphine should not be withheld from patients with severe pain. Morphine or a related opioid agonist is often used for pain relief in terminal cancer patients. In many cases, patients are allowed to determine when they need the next injection. This is referred to as patient-controlled analgesia (PCA).

5. **E** (Zaleplon) is correct. Zaleplon, a short-acting, non-benzodiazepine sedative-hypnotic, decreases the time to sleep without tolerance and has minimal withdrawal-emergent adverse effects. Compared to zolpidem, it has a faster onset of action and a shorter terminal elimination half-life. Both have been reported not to be associated with early morning awakening. These drugs are referred to as BZ_1 (type 1 benzodiazepine) receptor agonists. They act on the $GABA_A$/chloride-ion channel complex and their sedative effects are reversed by flumazenil, a benzodiazepine antagonist.

A (diazepam) is incorrect. Diazepam, a long-acting benzodiazepine, is similar to chlordiazepoxide and clorazepate in that all three generate the same active metabolite. Diazepam is administered orally for the short-term management of anxiety disorders and acute alcohol withdrawal. It is also used as a skeletal muscle relaxant. Its active metabolites accumulate in the body contributing to daytime sedation and tolerance.

B (flumazenil) is incorrect. Flumazenil, a parenteral benzodiazepine antagonist, is used to treat benzodiazepine overdoses and to reverse benzodiazepine sedation during anesthesia. It will also reverse the sedative actions of zolpidem and ezopiclone but not the actions of barbiturates, opioid agonists, or tricyclic antidepressants.

C (flurazepam) is incorrect. Flurazepam is an oral benzodiazepine that is used as a hypnotic agent in the short-term management of insomnia. The prolonged use of flurazepam is less likely to cause rebound insomnia and tolerance to the hypnotic effect than is the prolonged use of a benzodiazepine with a shorter half-life (such as triazolam or oxazepam); however, flurazepam is more likely to cause central nervous system depressant effects in the daytime.

D (phenobarbital) is incorrect. Phenobarbital is a barbiturate with sedative-hypnotic properties. It is currently *not* being used as a hypnotic. Barbiturates augment GABA responses by promoting the binding of GABA to the receptor and increasing the length of time that chloride channels are open in contrast to benzodiazepines, which increase the frequency of channel openings.

6. **E** (selegiline) is correct. Selegiline decreases the metabolism of dopamine by inhibiting monoamine oxidase type B (MAO-B) but not type A (MAO-A). Dopamine is primarily oxidized by MAO-B, whereas norepinephrine and serotonin are mainly metabolized by MAO-A. In the treatment of idiopathic Parkinson's disease, selegiline is used in combination with levodopa or in combination with both levodopa and carbidopa. Because of its selectivity for MAO-B, selegiline is purported to increase dopamine levels while causing fewer drug interactions and having a decreased risk of hypertension than do nonselective MAO inhibitors, such as phenelzine.

A (amantadine) is incorrect. Amantadine is useful in the treatment of Parkinson's disease but it does not decrease the oxidative metabolism of dopamine. It potentiates dopaminergic responses in the central nervous system (CNS) by causing the release of dopamine and norepinephrine from storage sites and inhibiting the reuptake of dopamine and norepinephrine.

B (carbidopa) is incorrect. Carbidopa would most likely be used with levodopa in the treatment of Parkinson's disease in this patient, but it does not decrease the oxidative metabolism of dopamine. Carbidopa inhibits the decarboxylation of peripheral levodopa, and this allows lower doses of levodopa to be used in the treatment of Parkinson's disease.

C (entacapone) is incorrect. Entacapone, a reversible inhibitor of peripheral catechol-*O*-methyltransferase (COMT), is used as an adjunct to levodopa/carbidopa therapy in the treatment of Parkinson's disease, but it does not inhibit the oxidative metabolism of dopamine.

D (phenelzine) is incorrect. Unlike selegiline (discussed in option E), phenelzine inhibits both MAO-A and MAO-B. Because of serious adverse reactions associated with the use of phenelzine, it is considered as a second-line treatment for depression. However, it is effective for several refractory anxiety disorders, especially when phobic reactions are part of the symptoms or associated with mixed anxiety-depressive states.

7. **D** (risperidone) is correct. The major side effects of antipsychotic agents are sedation and neurologic, cardiovascular, and antimuscarinic effects; however, the agents differ in the significance of each of these adverse effects. Because this patient has BPH and constipation, it would be inappropriate to use agents that have significant anticholinergic properties. Risperidone, haloperidol, fluphenazine, quetiapine, thiothixene, and ziprasidone have the lowest antimuscarinic activity and are effective for use in the treatment of schizophrenia.

A (chlorpromazine) is incorrect. Chlorpromazine has significant antimuscarinic side effects and would be inappropriate to use in a patient with BPH and constipation.

B (clozapine) is incorrect. Clozapine has significant antimuscarinic side effects and would be inappropriate to use in a patient with BPH and constipation. Clozapine also requires special monitoring because it causes fatal agranulocytosis in about 1% of treated patients per year.

C (olanzapine) is incorrect. Olanzapine has significant antimuscarinic side effects and would be inappropriate to use in a patient with BPH and constipation.

E (thioridazine) is incorrect. Thioridazine has significant antimuscarinic side effects and would be inappropriate to use in a patient with BPH and constipation. Thioridazine and clozapine have the greatest anticholinergic activity of the currently used antipsychotic drugs. Thioridazine is the phenothiazine most noted for causing pigmentary retinopathy. Thioridazine is also used to treat anxiety associated with major depression, dementia in the elderly, and severe behavioral problems in children because it has the fewest extrapyramidal symptoms of any typical phenothiazine-type antipsychotic drug. However, like other phenothiazines, it can produce a variety of cardiovascular adverse reactions including dose-related effects on ventricular repolarization that may lead to QT interval prolongation and development of torsades de pointes. Therefore, the use of thioridazine should be reserved for patients who have failed to respond to adequate courses of other antipsychotic drugs, either because of inadequate response or intolerable side effects.

8. **C** (fluoxetine) is correct. The patient was being treated with phenelzine, a drug that inhibits monoamine oxidase (MAO) and increases serotonin levels in the brain. The concurrent use of fluoxetine, a selective serotonin reuptake inhibitor (SSRI), could cause him to have a serious drug reaction, called the serotonin syndrome, and may include confusion, seizures, hypepyrexia, and severe hypertension, as well as less severe symptoms. An MAO inhibitor (such as phenelzine, or tranylcypromine) should not be used concurrently with an SSRI (such as fluoxetine). Fluoxetine should also be used cautiously with weak MAO inhibitors such as isoniazid, furazolidone, linezolid (antibiotic), and procarbazine (chemotherapy agent).

A (acetaminophen) is incorrect. Acetaminophen is not known to interact with phenelzine and other MAO inhibitors.

B (codeine) is incorrect. Codeine is not known to interact with phenelzine and other MAO inhibitors. However, meperidine (which is also an opioid agonist) should not be used concurrently with MAO inhibitors because meperidine's major metabolite normeperidine blocks the neuronal reuptake of serotonin. This can cause the accumulation of serotonin and lead to life-threatening reactions, including excitation, sweating, muscle rigidity, hypertension, severe respiratory depression, coma, and vascular collapse.

D (ranitidine) is incorrect. Ranitidine, an H_2-receptor antagonist used in the treatment of various gastrointestinal disorders, is not known to interact with phenelzine and other MAO inhibitors.

E (zolpidem) is incorrect. Zolpidem, a non-benzodiazepine sedative-hypnotic used for the short-term treatment of insomnia, is not known to interact with phenelzine and other MAO inhibitors.

9. **B** (amitriptyline) is correct. The patient's complaints and appearance suggest the diagnosis of atypical facial pain, a disorder that is often caused by chronic depression. Administration of a tricyclic antidepressant, such as amitriptyline, may relieve the symptoms and should be tried first in the treatment of this patient.

A (alprazolam) is incorrect. Benzodiazepines such as alprazolam may relieve the patient's anxiety associated with debilitating pain. However, it would not reduce the pain, and long-term use could lead to dependence.

C (cyclobenzaprine) is incorrect. Cyclobenzaprine, a skeletal muscle relaxant, is used for the relief of muscle spasm associated with acute, painful musculoskeletal conditions, but it is not useful for chronic pain with an affective component such as experienced by this patient.

D (naproxen) is incorrect. Naproxen, a nonsteroidal anti-inflammatory drug (NSAID) with antipyretic and analgesic properties, is not very useful for chronic pain with an affective component such as experienced by this patient.

E (oxycodone) is incorrect. Opioids, such as oxycodone, would reduce the patient's pain without treating her underlying problem, and long-term use could lead to opioid dependence. Opioids would be the treatment of last resort for atypical facial pain and depression in a young patient.

10. **D** (methylphenidate) is correct. Methylphenidate is a central nervous system stimulant that is used in the treatment of ADHD in children. Methylphenidate exerts many of its effects through the blockade of dopamine uptake in the central dopaminergic neurons, in contrast to the amphetamines and cocaine that increase catecholamine release as a primary mechanism.

A (amphetamine) is incorrect. Amphetamine and dextroamphetamine are often used in combination as an oral preparation to treat ADHD or narcolepsy. They are non-catecholamine sympathomimetic agents that mainly stimulate the release of norepinephrine and other biologic amines from central adrenergic nerve endings.

B (atomoxetine) is incorrect. Atomoxetine, a selective norepinephrine reuptake inhibitor, is the first nonstimulant drug approved for the treatment of ADHD.

C (bupropion) is incorrect. Bupropion does selectively inhibit the neuronal reuptake of dopamine and is used off-label for the treatment of multiple neurologic/psychological illnesses, including ADHD and neuropathic pain. However, it is used as an alternative to stimulants or as adjunctive treatment of ADHD, but it is not recommended for children younger than 6 years of age.

E (modafinil) is incorrect. Modafinil is a new psychostimulant medication for narcolepsy with a proposed military application as an alternative to amphetamines to fight fatigue during prolonged combat missions. Clinical studies are in progress to study its efficacy in treating ADHD. Modafinil-induced wakefulness is attenuated by prazosin (α_1-adrenergic antagonist), suggesting that it stimulates the central α_1-adrenergic system. It also increases excitatory glutaminergic transmission in the thalamus and hippocampus. In contrast to the amphetamines and other CNS stimulants, modafinil does not appear to affect dopaminergic systems.

11. C (isoflurane) is correct. All the anesthetics listed in the options are intravenous anesthetics except isoflurane. All the inhalational anesthetics potentiate the effects of nondepolarizing muscle relaxants such as pancuronium. Ketamine is the only intravenous anesthetic that may potentiate to some extent the effects of nondepolarizing muscle relaxants.

A (etomidate) is incorrect. Etomidate, a short-acting, intravenous sedative/hypnotic, does not potentiate the muscle relaxant activity of the nondepolarizing muscle relaxants. It has no analgesic activity but is used for the induction and maintenance of general anesthesia during short procedures. Etomidate does not release histamine. The hemodynamic effects of etomidate are similar to thiopental, except for less increase in heart rate; thus, it is useful in patients with compromised cardiopulmonary function.

B (fentanyl) is incorrect. Fentanyl, an opioid agonist, does not potentiate the muscle relaxant activity of the nondepolarizing muscle relaxants. It is used to aid induction and maintenance of general anesthesia and to supplement regional and spinal analgesia.

D (propofol) is incorrect. Propofol, an intravenous, nonbarbiturate anesthetic, does not potentiate the muscle relaxant activity of the nondepolarizing muscle relaxants. It is used to induce anesthesia that can be maintained by continuous intravenous propofol infusion or with inhalation anesthetics. Propofol induces anesthesia as rapidly as thiopental, but emergence from anesthesia is 10 times more rapid than with thiopental. It has no analgesic activity and causes sedation at a lower dose than those needed for anesthesia. In contrast to other general anesthetics, propofol possesses antiemetic activity.

E (thiopental) is incorrect. Thiopental, an intravenous, ultra-short-acting nonbarbiturate anesthetic, does not potentiate the muscle relaxant activity of the nondepolarizing muscle relaxants. It can be used alone as an anesthetic for short procedures, as an inducing agent, or as an adjunct to regional anesthesia. Thiopental is also used in narcoanalysis in psychiatric disorders, control of status epilepticus, and treatment of increased intracranial pressure.

12. **D** (naltrexone) is correct. In the treatment of alcoholism, naltrexone is purported to interrupt a positive feedback mechanism mediated by endogenous opioids. Naltrexone treatment is not a form of aversion therapy; thus, it will not produce a disulfiram-like reaction if ethanol or opioids are ingested by patients undergoing treatment.

A (chlorpromazine) is incorrect. Chlorpromazine is not used in the treatment of alcoholism. Chlorpromazine, a prototypic aliphatic phenothiazine, is not often used today as an antipsychotic medication. It is used mainly as an antiemetic and for treating hiccups. It is occasionally used for relief of presurgical anxiety; for acute intermittent porphyria; and as an adjunct in the treatment of tetanus; or to treat severe behavioral problems in children.

B (codeine) is incorrect. Codeine is not used in the treatment of alcoholism. Codeine, a low-potency opioid agonist, is used as a single agent and in combination with acetaminophen or aspirin to control moderate pain. It is also widely used as a cough suppressant due to its adequate oral bioavailability and low incidence of side effects at antitussive doses.

C (haloperidol) is incorrect. Haloperidol, a high-potency antipsychotic agent, is not used in the treatment of alcoholism; however, it is used to treat alcoholic hallucinations. It is also used to control tics and vocal utterances of patients with Tourette's syndrome, and for the treatment of severe behavioral problems in children, manifested as impulsive, combative, or explosive hyperexcitability, that are unresponsive to behavioral or counseling therapy.

E (phenobarbital) is incorrect. Phenobarbital is not used in the treatment of alcoholism. It is available as an oral and parenteral barbiturate for the treatment of all seizure disorders except absence (petit mal) seizures. In children, it often is used alone, whereas in adults, it usually is administered in combination with other agents.

13. **A** (amiodarone) is correct. Amiodarone, a class III antiarrhythmic agent, is now considered to be the drug of first choice in treatment of refractory life-threatening ventricular arrhythmias. The 2000 ECC/AHA guidelines suggest that intravenous amiodarone be selected prior to administration of lidocaine in patients requiring advanced cardiac life support for ventricular fibrillation/pulseless ventricular tachycardia. Amiodarone does possess many adverse effects, some of which are severe and potentially fatal (e.g., pulmonary fibrosis), but it is less proarrhythmic than other antiarrhythmic drugs.

 B (esmolol) is incorrect. Esmolol, a short-acting intravenous class II antiarrhythmic drug, would be contraindicated because it blocks β-adrenergic receptors and would further depress the patient's myocardial performance.

 C (lidocaine) is incorrect. Lidocaine, a class IB antiarrhythmic drug, has historically been used as a first-line antiarrhythmic agent for treatment of ventricular arrhythmias for several years. However, lidocaine is now considered a second choice after amiodarone for treatment of ventricular arrhythmias. Lidocaine has been shown to be ineffective for prophylaxis of arrhythmias in patients who have had myocardial infarction.

 D (nifedipine) is incorrect. Nifedipine is a dihydropyridine that acts as a calcium channel blocker. Its use would cause marked hypotension and might worsen the patient's condition.

 E (quinidine) is incorrect. Quinidine is a class IA antiarrhythmic drug. Although it can be used to treat ventricular arrhythmias, amiodarone is preferable to quinidine for use in treating patients with ventricular fibrillation. The ACLS algorithms also include procainamide as an alternative antiarrhythmic for the treatment of ventricular tachycardias during cardiopulmonary resuscitation. Procainamide or amiodarone are currently recommended ahead of lidocaine and adenosine in the revised ACLS algorithm for hemodynamically stable wide-complex tachycardia.

14. **C** (set C) is correct. Diltiazem inhibits the influx of extracellular calcium across both the myocardial and vascular smooth muscle cell membranes. The resultant decrease in intracellular calcium inhibits the contractile processes of the smooth muscle cells. This causes dilation of the coronary and systemic arteries and leads to an improvement in oxygen delivery to the myocardial tissue. In addition, diltiazem decreases the total peripheral vascular resistance, slows the atrioventricular node conduction velocity, decreases the activity of the sinoatrial node, and increases the coronary blood flow.

 A (set A), **B** (set B), **D** (set D), and **E** (set E) are incorrect. Refer to the explanation for option C.

15. **A** (hydrochlorothiazide) is correct. Hydrochlorothiazide-induced electrolyte disturbances (such as hypokalemia, hypomagnesemia, and hypercalcemia) predispose patients to digoxin toxicity and can cause life-threatening arrhythmias. Electrolyte balance must be corrected prior to initiating digoxin therapy.

B (lisinopril) is incorrect. Lisinopril is an angiotensin-converting enzyme (ACE) inhibitor that is used in the treatment of hypertension and congestive heart failure. By decreasing aldosterone secretion, lisinopril causes small increases in serum potassium levels.

C (metoprolol) is incorrect. Metoprolol is a beta$_1$-selective (cardioselective) adrenergic antagonist that is used for the treatment of patients with angina, hypertension, myocardial infarction, and tremor and the prophylaxis of migraine headaches. Cardioselective beta blockers are also utilized in the management of heart failure. Beta blockers at therapeutic doses do not affect serum potassium but with marked overdose hyperkalemia can occur.

D (quinidine) is incorrect. Quinidine and procainamide are class IA antiarrhythmic agents. Quinidine does not cause hypokalemia, but it does reduce the renal and nonrenal clearance of digoxin.

E (verapamil) is incorrect. Verapamil is a class IV antiarrhythmic agent. Verapamil and digoxin interact pharmacokinetically and pharmacodynamically. Verapamil reduces the renal and nonrenal clearance of digoxin. However, verapamil does not cause hypokalemia. Because both verapamil and digoxin slow conduction through the atrioventricular node, these drugs are sometimes used together for ventricular control in a patient with atrial fibrillation or flutter. Dosages need to be adjusted on the basis of the patient's clinical response, rather than on the basis of digoxin serum concentrations, because serum concentrations may not accurately reflect the clinical effects.

16. **A** (set A) is correct. Acetazolamide is a carbonic anhydrase inhibitor that increases the tubular bicarbonate concentration, decreases ammonia excretion, increases urine pH, and increases the urinary potassium excretion. Inhibition of carbonic anhydrase causes urinary HCO_3^- excretion to rise rapidly to approximately 35% of the filtered load. This, along with inhibition of titratable acid and ammonia secretion in the collecting duct system, causes the pH to rise to about 8 and results in metabolic acidosis. The increased excretion of K^+ is secondary to increased delivery of Na^+ to the distal nephron.

B (set B), **C** (set C), **D** (set D), and **E** (set E) are incorrect. Refer to the explanation for option A.

17. **C** (propranolol) is correct. Propranolol may produce the changes depicted in curve X (a class IA response). Like other β-adrenergic receptor antagonists, propranolol is a class II antiarrhythmic agent. However, because of its quinidine-like properties, propranolol also produces some class IA effects, especially when it is given in high doses.

   A (adenosine) is incorrect. Adenosine is a miscellaneous antiarrhythmic agent that enhances potassium conduction and inhibits cyclic adenosine monophosphate (cAMP)-induced calcium influx.

   B (pindolol) is incorrect. Like other β-adrenergic receptor antagonists, pindolol is a class II antiarrhythmic agent. Unlike propranolol (see the discussion of option C), pindolol does not have quinidine-like (local anesthetic) properties.

   D (sotalol) is incorrect. Like other β-adrenergic receptor antagonists, sotalol has class II antiarrhythmic properties. In addition to its class II properties, sotalol has some class III properties. Because of its ability to block potassium channels, it prolongs the effective refractory period by prolonging the action potential.

   E (verapamil) is incorrect. Verapamil is a class IV antiarrhythmic agent. By blocking calcium channels, it slows conduction and increases the refractory period in calcium-dependent tissues, such the atrioventricular node.

18. **D** (gemfibrozil) is correct. Gemfibrozil can potentiate the effects of warfarin by displacing it from plasma protein–binding sites. While warfarin may be added to the regimen of patients already receiving gemfibrozil, INR prothrombin times should be carefully monitored if gemfibrozil is added to the regimen of patients receiving warfarin.

   A (colesevelam) is incorrect. Colesevelam is a bile acid–binding resin similar to cholestyramine and colestipol. In contrast to cholestyramine, colesevelam has no significant effect on the bioavailability of warfarin in humans. However, it may bind with vitamin K in the diet, impairing vitamin K absorption, which would increase warfarin's hypoprothrombinemic effect; this would take several weeks. To avoid this action, administer vitamin K products at least 1 hour before or at least 4 hours after colesevelam.

   B (cholestyramine) is incorrect. Cholestyramine is a bile acid–binding resin. When it is used concurrently with warfarin, it may either increase or decrease warfarin's hypoprothrombinemic effects. When the resin binds with vitamin K in the diet, it impairs vitamin K absorption, and this in turn can increase warfarin's hypoprothrombinemic effects. When the resin binds with warfarin directly, it impairs warfarin's bioavailability and decreases its hypoprothrombinemic effects. To avoid altering warfarin's pharmacokinetics, a bile acid–binding resin should be taken 4 to 6 hours before or after warfarin is taken.

C (ezetimibe) is incorrect. Ezetimibe is used as monotherapy or in combination with HMG-CoA reductase inhibitors for the treatment of hypercholesterolemia. It selectively inhibits the absorption of cholesterol from the small intestine. Co-administration of ezetimibe with warfarin does not appear to affect warfarin's action, but the manufacturer recommends that if ezetimibe is added to warfarin therapy, the INR should be monitored.

E (pravastatin) is incorrect. Pravastatin and lovastatin are drugs that act by inhibiting HMG-CoA reductase. When lovastatin is added to a stabilized regimen of warfarin therapy, hypoprothrombinemia and clinical bleeding sometimes occur. However, pravastatin does not appear to interact with warfarin; thus, it is the preferred HMG-CoA reductase inhibitor to be used during warfarin therapy.

19. **A** (acyclovir) is correct. Acyclovir is used to treat herpes genitalis and herpes labialis, both of which are caused by herpes simplex virus (HSV), and to treat herpes zoster (shingles), which is caused by varicella-zoster virus (VZV). Acyclovir must be phosphorylated to be active. In virus-infected cells, the drug is converted to the monophosphate by viral thymidine kinases. It is subsequently converted to a diphosphate by cellular guanylyl kinase and is finally converted to a triphosphate by various cellular enzymes. Fully active acyclovir triphosphate competes with the natural substrate, deoxyguanosine triphosphate, for a position in the DNA chain of the herpesvirus. After it is incorporated in the chain, it terminates DNA synthesis.

B (amantadine) is incorrect. Amantadine is not effective for use in the treatment of herpesvirus infections. Amantadine is used to alleviate the symptoms of Parkinson's disease and to prevent influenza. The drug is a synthetic antiviral agent that inhibits viral replication within virus-infected cells by blocking the uncoating of the virus particle and thereby preventing the release of viral nucleic acid into the host cell.

C (indinavir) is incorrect. Indinavir is not active against herpesviruses. It is a protease inhibitor that is used in the treatment of HIV infection.

D (rifampin) is incorrect. Rifampin is not active against herpesviruses. It is used primarily to treat tuberculosis. However, it is also effective for use in the prevention of *Haemophilus influenzae* type B (Hib) infection; in the treatment of asymptomatic carriers of *Neisseria meningitidis;* and in patients with leprosy, legionnaires' disease, atypical mycobacterial infections, and staphylococcal infections.

E (zidovudine) is incorrect. Zidovudine (AZT) is not active against herpesviruses. It is a synthetic dideoxynucleoside that is used not only to treat HIV infection but also to prevent the transmission of HIV from infected pregnant women to their offspring. The viral RNA-directed DNA polymerase (reverse transcriptase) enzyme is the site of action of zidovudine.

20.   **A** (cell wall synthesis) is correct. Cefepime is considered to be a fourth-generation cephalosporin. Like other cephalosporins and penicillins, cefepime inhibits the third and final stage of bacterial cell wall synthesis by preferentially binding to specific penicillin-binding proteins (PBPs) that are located inside the bacterial cell wall. In comparison with third-generation cephalosporins, cefepime has a greater ability to penetrate the outer membrane of the bacterial cell and has a lower rate of hydrolysis by bacterial β-lactamases.

   B (DNA synthesis) is incorrect. Cephalosporins act by inhibiting cell wall synthesis; they do not affect DNA synthesis. Fluoroquinolones are antibacterial agents that act by inhibiting DNA gyrase, an enzyme responsible for counteracting the excessive supercoiling of DNA during replication or transcription.

   C (mitochondria) is incorrect. Mitochondria are not specifically targeted by antibacterial agents.

   D (plasma membrane) is incorrect. Cephalosporins act by inhibiting cell wall synthesis; they do not affect the plasma membrane. Polymyxins and gramicidin are examples of antibacterial agents that affect the plasma membrane.

   E (protein synthesis) is incorrect. Cephalosporins act by inhibiting cell wall synthesis; they do not affect protein synthesis. Aminoglycosides (irreversible 30S inhibitor), tetracyclines (reversible 30S inhibitor), macrolides (reversible 50S inhibitor), clindamycin (reversible 50S inhibitor), and chloramphenicol (reversible 50S inhibitor) are examples of antibacterial agents that inhibit protein synthesis.

21.   **A** (azithromycin) is correct. A single dose of azithromycin is effective for the treatment of STDs due to chlamydia and gonorrhea. Likewise, a single dose of azithromycin has been reported to be effective in preventing the disease in persons recently exposed, through sexual intercourse within the last 30 days, to sexual partners with infectious syphilis except in areas where macrolide resistance in *T. pallidum* has been documented.

   B (ceftriaxone) is incorrect. The Centers for Disease Control (CDC) recommends ceftriaxone (125 mg IM as a single dose) for the treatment of uncomplicated gonococcal infection, including vulvovaginitis, cervicitis, urethritis, proctitis, or pharyngitis; however, azithromycin as a single dose or doxycycline for 7 days should be added if chlamydial infection is not ruled out. Ceftriaxone is not recommended for the treatment of syphilis.

   C (doxycycline) is incorrect. Doxycycline is effective against *T. pallidum* (the agent of syphilis), *N. gonorrhoeae* (the agent of gonorrhea), and *C. trachomatis* (an agent of urethritis, cervicitis, and lymphogranuloma venereum); however, it is not effective as a single dose. Moreover, a second agent, such as ceftriaxone or a fluoroquinolone, should also be used to treat the patient's gonorrhea infection.

D (ofloxacin) is incorrect. The CDC recommends ofloxacin (400 mg PO as a single dose) for the treatment of uncomplicated gonorrhea; however, azithromycin as a single dose or doxycycline for 7 days should be added if a chlamydial infection is not ruled out. Ofloxacin is not recommended for the treatment of syphilis.

E (penicillin G; benzathine) is incorrect. A single dose of penicillin G; benzathine (a depot preparation) is effective in the treatment of susceptible strains of *T. pallidum* but it is ineffective in the treatment of gonorrhea or chlamydia.

22. E (vancomycin) is correct. Of the drugs listed, vancomycin would be the best choice for treating an *S. aureus* infection in a patient who is allergic to penicillin. Most strains of *Staphylococcus aureus* and *S. epidermidis* are susceptible to vancomycin, as are streptococci including enterococci, *Corynebacterium,* and *Clostridium.* Vancomycin is particularly useful against penicillin- and methicillin-resistant staphylococcal infections and for treating gram-positive infections in penicillin-allergic patients. Gram-negative bacteria and mycobacteria are resistant to vancomycin. Synergistic bactericidal effects can be achieved when vancomycin is combined with aminoglycosides against *Streptococcus faecalis* and methicillin-resistant organisms, but this increases possible toxicity.

A (aztreonam) is incorrect. Aztreonam is not used in the treatment of *S. aureus* infections. Aztreonam is used in the treatment of infections with aerobic gram-negative bacteria. Clinically, it is effective against bacteremias, skin and soft tissue infections, urinary tract infections, respiratory tract infections, intra-abdominal infections, and gynecologic infections caused by susceptible microorganisms. Aztreonam can be used with caution in patients with penicillin hypersensitivity; no cross-reactivity has been observed in patients with penicillin hypersensitivity given aztreonam.

B (cefazolin) is incorrect. Cefazolin is a first-generation cephalosporin. There is a 5% to 10% cross-sensitivity between penicillins and cephalosporins. Patients with a history of a mild or temporally distant reaction to penicillin appear to be at low risk of a rash or other allergic reaction following the administration of a cephalosporin. However, cephalosporins should be avoided or used only with great caution in patients who have had a recent severe reaction to a penicillin antibiotic.

C (doxycycline) is incorrect. Doxycycline is not used in the treatment of *S. aureus* infections. Doxycycline can be given once daily and is commonly used to treat nongonococcal urethritis and cervicitis as well as exacerbations of bronchitis in patients with chronic obstructive pulmonary disease (COPD). In patients who have poor renal function, doxycycline is considered the tetracycline of choice because it is not dependent on renal elimination. Doxycycline is a bacteriostatic, reversible inhibitor of protein synthesis by binding to bacterial 30S ribosomal subunits; this blocks the binding of tRNA to mRNA.

D (erythromycin) is incorrect. Erythromycin does not penetrate the synovial fluid, so it would be ineffective in treating the patient described. Erythromycin, a macrolide antibiotic, is often used in the treatment of legionnaires' disease and *Mycoplasma pneumoniae* pneumonia, and as an alternative to β-lactam antibiotics in patients who are allergic to β-lactams. It binds to the 50S ribosomal subunit, thus inhibiting bacterial protein synthesis.

23. **A** (amphotericin B) is correct. Amphotericin B is an antifungal antibiotic that is administered parenterally. Its use is associated with many side effects and toxicities. Although several newer, less toxic antifungal agents of the azole class have been introduced, amphotericin B remains the drug of choice for treating many serious systemic fungal infections. Amphotericin B exerts its antifungal effects and many of its adverse effects by binding to sterols in the cell membranes of both fungal (ergosterol) and human cells (cholesterol).

B (flucytosine) is incorrect. Susceptible fungi readily deaminate flucytosine to its active component, 5-fluorouracil. Resistance develops rapidly, however, if flucytosine is used as a single agent. Therefore, it is never used alone in the treatment of fungal infections.

C (ketoconazole) is incorrect. Ketoconazole inhibits ergosterol synthesis by inhibiting 14α-demethylase, a cytochrome P-450 enzyme that is necessary for the conversion of lanosterol to ergosterol, an essential component of the fungal membrane. It has a broad spectrum of antifungal activity against common fungal pathogens such as *Blastomyces dermatitidis, Candida* species, *Cryptococcus neoformans, Coccidioides immitis, Histoplasma capsulatum, Paracoccidioides brasiliensis,* and *Sporothrix schenckii;* however, it is not as effective against severe systemic antifungal infections as is amphotericin B, especially in immunocompromised patients.

D (pentamidine) is incorrect. Pentamidine is not used to treat fungal infections. It has become an important drug in the prophylaxis and treatment of *Pneumocystis carinii* pneumonia (PCP).

E (terbinafine) is incorrect. Terbinafine is an antifungal agent that is effective for treating onychomycosis because of its fungicidal activity and ability to concentrate within the nail; it has been found to be superior to griseofulvin, the drug formerly used to treat this condition. It exerts its antifungal effect by inhibiting the enzyme squalene monooxygenase, a key enzyme in sterol biosynthesis in the fungal membrane.

24. **C** (penicillin G) is correct. Penicillin G is the drug of choice for treating infections caused by *S. pneumoniae*. Clindamycin can be used as an alternative in patients who are allergic to penicillin. Vancomycin or cefepime can be used as an alternative if the strain of *S. pneumoniae* is resistant to penicillin.

A (cefepime) is incorrect. As discussed for option C, cefepime may sometimes be used to treat *S. pneumoniae* infections, but it is not the drug of choice.

B (clindamycin) is incorrect. As discussed for option C, clindamycin may sometimes be used to treat *S. pneumoniae* infections, but it is not the drug of choice.

D (polymyxin B) is incorrect. Polymyxin B is an older antibiotic that is not effective against streptococci and other gram-positive bacteria. It is effective against only gram-negative bacteria. Today, polymyxin B is rarely used systemically because of its potential for causing nephrotoxicity and neurotoxicity.

E (vancomycin) is incorrect. As discussed for option C, vancomycin may sometimes be used to treat *S. pneumoniae* infections, but it is not the drug of choice.

25. **C** (peripheral neuropathy) is correct. Isoniazid can cause dose-dependent peripheral neuropathy. This adverse effect is due to a pyridoxine (vitamin B$_6$) deficiency and can be prevented or treated with pyridoxine.

A (optic neuritis) is incorrect. Optic neuritis is associated with ethambutol therapy in the treatment of tuberculosis. This adverse effect is not associated with isoniazid treatment.

B (ototoxicity) is incorrect. Ototoxicity and renal toxicity are associated with streptomycin therapy in the treatment of tuberculosis. This adverse effect is not associated with isoniazid treatment.

D (red discoloration of body secretions) is incorrect. Red discoloration of body secretions is associated with rifampin therapy in the treatment of tuberculosis. This adverse effect is not associated with isoniazid treatment.

E (renal toxicity) is incorrect. Renal toxicity and ototoxicity are associated with streptomycin therapy in the treatment of tuberculosis. This adverse effect is not associated with isoniazid treatment.

26. **C** (inorganic lead) is correct. The manifestations described are characteristic findings in patients with chronic lead poisoning. Edetate calcium disodium can be used to treat severe cases of lead poisoning, and oral succimer can be used to treat less severe cases.

A (carbon monoxide) is incorrect. Patients poisoned with carbon monoxide complain of headache, dizziness, and nausea. Administration of 100% oxygen is the typical treatment for carbon monoxide poisoning.

B (chlorinated hydrocarbon insecticide) is incorrect. Long-term exposure to an insecticide containing chlorinated hydrocarbons rarely causes marked symptoms. If the hydrocarbon levels accumulate, then recurrent seizures may occur. Signs of hepatitis or renal injury may also develop. These agents are no longer used in the United States, but they still persist in the environment.

D (inorganic mercury) is incorrect. Chronic inorganic mercury poisoning causes signs of permanent central nervous system toxicity, including irritability, memory loss, shyness, depression, insomnia, and tremor. It can also cause gingivitis, stomatitis, and increased salivation.

E (organic phosphate ester) is incorrect. Organophosphate poisoning causes a cholinergic crisis, characterized by an increase in salivation, lacrimation, urination, and defecation. Atropine is always used for the treatment of poisoning with acetylcholinesterase inhibitors. Pralidoxime (2-PAM) is also used with intoxication with organophosphates depending on the agent and time of elapse from exposure but are never used with carbamate type cholinesterase inhibitor (e.g., carbaryl) intoxication.

27. **B** (amitriptyline) is correct. The patient's clinical manifestations are consistent with the diagnosis of an overdose of amitriptyline or other tricyclic antidepressant (TCA). Treatment for this type of overdose is as described in the question.

A (acetaminophen) is incorrect. The effects of acetaminophen toxicity are dose-dependent. Life-threatening hepatic necrosis is the most serious adverse effect. Renal tubular necrosis, hypoglycemic coma, and thrombocytopenia may also occur. The stomach should be emptied promptly by lavage. Acetylcysteine should be administered as early as possible, preferably within 12 hours of the overdose but at least within 24 hours.

C (isoniazid) is incorrect. Seizures are the signature effects of a massive overdose of isoniazid. Acute isoniazid toxicity is treated with pyridoxine.

D (lithium) is incorrect. Lithium is associated with numerous side effects, even when taken in therapeutic doses. Ataxia, giddiness, tinnitus, blurred vision, and a large output of dilute urine may occur when the serum level of lithium is increased. Blood levels greater than 3.0 mEq/L may produce a complex clinical picture, with toxicity affecting multiple organs and organ systems. Serum lithium levels should not be permitted to exceed 2.0 mEq/L during the initial treatment phase.

E (salicylate) is incorrect. Early symptoms of salicylate overdose are due to central nervous system stimulation and may include vomiting, hyperpnea, hyperactivity, and convulsions. These symptoms are accompanied by severe electrolyte disturbances, and they progress quickly to depression, coma, and respiratory failure. Intensive supportive therapy should be instituted immediately. Plasma salicylate levels should be measured to determine the severity of the poisoning and to provide a guide for therapy. In comatose patients, airway-protected gastric lavage is administered. Activated charcoal and a saline cathartic are also administered.

28. D (is more potent than drug Y) is correct. The drug that exerts its 50% maximal response at the lowest concentration is the most potent drug; this is drug X in the figure. Drug X is more potent than drug Y and drug Z.

  A (has greater efficacy than drug Y) is incorrect. Drug X and drug Y are full agonists and have equal efficacy. Drug Z is a partial agonist, so it is not capable of producing a 100% response. All partial agonists are competitive antagonists to full agonists at some doses.

  B (has lesser efficacy than drug Y) is incorrect. Drug X and drug Y are full agonists and have equal efficacy. Drug Z is a partial agonist, so it is not capable of producing a 100% response. All partial agonists are competitive antagonists to full agonists at some doses.

  C (has the same potency as drug Y) is incorrect. As discussed for option D, drug X is more potent than drug Y.

  E (is safer than drug Y or drug Z) is incorrect. The most potent drug is not necessarily the safest drug, because it may also be the most toxic drug.

29. C (inositol triphosphate) is correct. IP_3 and DAG are both second messengers. IP_3 releases calcium from the endoplasmic reticulum. As shown in the figure, stimulation of the muscarinic receptor leads to G protein–mediated activation of PLC. Activation of PLC causes hydrolysis of PIP_2 (a membrane phospholipid) and leads to the accumulation of DAG and IP_3. DAG activates PK-C, which then phosphorylates a protein substrate. IP_3 releases calcium from the endoplasmic reticulum. When CaM binds to the calcium, this activates an enzyme that participates in the biologic response.

  A (calmodulin) is incorrect. Calmodulin is not a second messenger. It is a calcium-binding protein that acts as a calcium-dependent enzyme activator.

  B (G protein) is incorrect. G proteins are not second messengers. They are a family of guanylyl triphosphate (GTP)-binding signal transduction proteins that mediate many hormone and drug effects. G_q activates PLC.

  D (phospholipase C) is incorrect. Phospholipase C (PLC) is not a second messenger. It is an enzyme that cleaves phosphoglycerides between glycerol and phosphate; in this case, it is the enzyme responsible for cleaving diacylglycerol (DAG) and inositol triphosphate (IP_3) from membrane phospholipids.

  E (protein kinase C) is incorrect. Protein kinase C is not a second messenger. It is the diacylglycerol-activated protein kinase that phosphorylates substrate proteins that participate in signal transduction pathways.

30. B (21 hours) is correct. If the dose were doubled, it would take one half-life (7 hours) to get to the level attained when the original single dose was given. Adding 7 + 14 hours provides a total therapeutic level for 21 hours.

A (14 hours) is incorrect. Refer to the explanation for option B. If the dose is doubled, the therapeutic response would have to be longer than observed with the smaller dose.

C (28 hours) is incorrect. Refer to the explanation for option B.

D (35 hours) is incorrect. Refer to the explanation for option B.

B (28 to 35 hours) is incorrect. Refer to the explanation for option B. If repetitive doses of drug X are given, it takes 4 to 5 half-lives to reach a steady-state concentration. In this case because drug X has a half-life of 7 hours, it would take 28 to 35 hours to reach a steady-state level. *Note that this question deals with single doses of the drug and not with multiple doses when a steady state is attained.*

31. **D** (nicotinic receptor agonist) is correct. Succinylcholine is an ultrashort-acting, depolarizing-type skeletal muscle relaxant for intravenous administration. Because of its rapid onset of action, it is preferred in emergencies requiring rapid intubation. Succinylcholine competes with acetylcholine for the nicotinic cholinergic receptors of the motor end plate; and like acetylcholine, it combines with these receptors to produce depolarization. However, succinylcholine causes more persistent depolarization than acetylcholine because it has a higher affinity for the nicotinic cholinergic receptor and a strong resistance to acetylcholinesterase. Depolarization first causes fasciculation of the skeletal muscles and then causes muscle paralysis; thus, a depolarizing blockade of the neuromuscular junction occurs.

A (acetylcholinesterase inhibitor) is incorrect. Succinylcholine is not an inhibitor of acetylcholinesterase. High doses of acetylcholinesterase inhibitors, such as organophosphates and organocarbamates, can cause a depolarizing blockade of the neuromuscular junction because they prevent the breakdown of acetylcholine and the high levels of acetylcholine produce a desensitization of the nicotinic cholinergic receptor at the neuromuscular junction.

B (muscarinic agonist) is incorrect. Succinylcholine is not a muscarinic agonist. Pilocarpine is an example of an alkaloid that acts as an agonist at muscarinic cholinergic receptors on smooth muscles.

C (muscarinic antagonist) is incorrect. Succinylcholine is not a muscarinic antagonist. Atropine is an example of a muscarinic antagonist that blocks the effects of acetylcholine at muscarinic receptors on smooth muscles.

E (nicotinic antagonist) is incorrect. Succinylcholine is not a nicotinic antagonist. Tubocurarine is an example of a drug that blocks the effects of acetylcholine on nicotinic cholinergic receptors at the neuromuscular junction. Drugs that act like tubocurarine are referred to as nondepolarizing neuromuscular blockers. Hexamethonium is another nicotinic cholinergic receptor that antagonizes the effects of acetylcholine on nicotinic receptors in the autonomic ganglia.

32. **E** (propranolol) is correct. The effects described are the types of effects produced by a nonselective β-adrenergic receptor agonist, such as epinephrine. Therefore, blockade of these effects would require a nonselective β-adrenergic receptor antagonist, such as propranolol or nadalol.

    A (atenolol) is incorrect. Atenolol is a selective $β_1$-adrenergic receptor antagonist. It would not block the $β_2$-adrenergic receptor effects described in the question, which include the increase in blood glucose level and the pronounced decrease in peripheral resistance produced by the nonselective β-adrenergic receptor agonist.

    B (atropine) is incorrect. Atropine is a muscarinic receptor antagonist. It would not block the effects described in the question, which are the types of effects produced by a nonselective β-adrenergic receptor agonist.

    C (guanethidine) is incorrect. Guanethidine is an adrenergic neuronal blocking agent. It causes depletion of norepinephrine in the synapse, thereby reducing total peripheral resistance and blood pressure. Subjects that are pretreated with guanethidine are supersensitive to the effects of nonselective β-adrenergic receptor agonists, such as epinephrine, due to up-regulation of adrenergic receptors. The use of guanethidine as a clinical drug has been discontinued in the United States because of its extensive adverse effects in comparison to widely used antihypertensive medications.

    D (phentolamine) is incorrect. Phentolamine is a nonselective α-adrenergic receptor antagonist. It would not block the effects described in the question, which are the types of effects produced by a nonselective β-adrenergic receptor agonist.

33. **C** (isoproterenol) is correct. Isoproterenol increases the cardiac output, and this may lead to a slight increase in the systolic blood pressure. By causing vasodilation (a $β_2$-adrenergic receptor effect) and stimulating $β_1$-adrenergic receptors, isoproterenol decreases the diastolic and mean blood pressure and increases the heart rate (profile 3).

    A (clonidine) is incorrect. Clonidine, a centrally acting sympatholytic drug, decreases the mean, systolic, and diastolic blood pressure, and it also decreases the heart rate (profile 4).

    B (epinephrine) is incorrect. Epinephrine increases the mean and systolic blood pressure (an $α_1$-adrenergic receptor effect), decreases the diastolic blood pressure (a $β_2$-adrenergic receptor effect), and increases the heart rate (a $β_1$-adrenergic receptor effect) (profile 2).

    D (norepinephrine) is incorrect. Norepinephrine increases (an $α_1$-adrenergic receptor effect) the mean, systolic, and diastolic blood pressure, and it evokes reflex bradycardia (profile 1).

    E (propranolol) is incorrect. Propranolol, a nonselective β-adrenergic receptor antagonist, decreases the mean, systolic, and diastolic blood pressure, and it also decreases the heart rate (profile 4).

34.   **E** (norepinephrine) is correct. Norepinephrine is a strong α- and β_1-adrenergic receptor agonist. It has minimal effects on β_2-adrenergic receptors. Via its actions on α_1-receptors, norepinephrine causes marked vasoconstriction and evokes reflex bradycardia. Its direct effect on the heart is masked by the large increase in parasympathetic activity in response to the elevation in blood pressure. In the presence of prazosin (an α_1-adrenergic receptor antagonist), only the direct effects of norepinephrine on the heart are observed.

A (acetylcholine) is incorrect. Acetylcholine causes a pronounced decrease in blood pressure. It acts on muscarinic receptors on endothelial cells to induce nitric oxide synthase resulting in the formation of endothelial-derived relaxation factor which is nitric oxide. Nitric oxide, in a paracrine fashion, activates guanylyl cyclase in the vascular smooth muscle to produce cyclic quanylyl monophosphate (cGMP), which causes vasodilation. With acetylcholine, there is an indirect (reflex) increase in heart rate; however, with acetylcholine the increase is smaller than with other vasodilators because acetylcholine acts directly to slow the heart rate, and this partially opposes the reflex tachycardia. Prazosin would not markedly alter these responses.

B (epinephrine) is incorrect. Epinephrine stimulates all adrenergic receptors. Its stimulation of α_1-receptors causes an increase in systolic blood pressure and a slight increase in mean blood pressure; its stimulation of β_2-receptors causes a decrease in diastolic pressure; and its stimulation of β_1-receptors causes the heart rate to increase. The pressor response that occurs when epinephrine is given alone is converted to a depressor response when epinephrine is given in the presence of an α_1-adrenergic receptor antagonist, such as prazosin. This phenomenon is referred to as epinephrine reversal.

C (histamine) is incorrect. Histamine causes a pronounced decrease in blood pressure. It acts on histaminergic receptors on endothelial cells to induce nitric oxide synthase resulting in the formation of endothelium-derived relaxation factor, which is nitric oxide. Nitric oxide, in a paracrine fashion, activates guanylyl cyclase in the vascular smooth muscle to produce cyclic quanylyl monophosphate (cGMP), which causes vasodilation. With histamine, there is an indirect (reflex) increase in heart rate. Prazosin would not markedly alter these responses.

D (isoproterenol) is incorrect. Isoproterenol stimulates β-receptors. It causes a decrease in blood pressure and an increase in heart rate. Prazosin would not markedly alter these effects.

35.   **B** (site 2) is correct. Muscarinic receptors are located at the parasympathetic postsynaptic junction (site 2).

A (site 1) and **C** (site 3) are incorrect. Muscarinic receptors are located at site 2. Nicotinic receptors are located at the parasympathetic ganglion (site 1), at the sympathetic ganglion (site 3), and at the somatic neuromuscular junction (site 5).

D (site 4) is incorrect. Muscarinic receptors are located at site 2. The α-adrenergic and β-adrenergic receptors are located at the sympathetic postsynaptic junctions (site 4).

E (site 5) is incorrect. Muscarinic receptors are located at site 2. Nicotinic receptors are located at the parasympathetic ganglion (site 1), at the sympathetic ganglion (site 3), and at the somatic neuromuscular junction (site 5).

36. **B** (cromolyn sodium) is correct. Cromolyn inhibits mast cell degranulation. This in turn prevents the release of histamine, slow-reacting substance of anaphylaxis (SRS-A), and other mediators of type I allergic reactions. Cromolyn is not a bronchodilator, an antihistamine, nor a vasoconstrictor; therefore, it is useful as an agent to prevent, rather than treat, asthmatic attacks.

A (albuterol) is incorrect. Albuterol does not inhibit antigen-induced release of mediators that cause bronchospasms. It is a selective β_2-receptor agonist widely used as a bronchodilator in the management of asthma exacerbations or other chronic obstructive airway diseases.

C (ipratropium) is incorrect. Ipratropium does not inhibit antigen-induced release of mediators that cause bronchospasms. It is a quaternary ammonium derivative of atropine used as a bronchodilator in the management of cholinergic-mediated bronchospasm associated with chronic obstructive pulmonary disease (COPD) or as an adjunct to other bronchodilators in the management of patients with asthma.

D (tiotropium) is incorrect. Tiotropium does not inhibit antigen-induced release of mediators that cause bronchospasms. Tiotropium, a quaternary ammonium derivative similar to ipratropium, is used for the maintenance treatment of chronic obstructive pulmonary disease (COPD). It is administered once daily, a major advantage over ipratropium, which requires administration up to four times per day.

E (zafirlukast) is incorrect. Zafirlukast does not inhibit antigen-induced release of mediators that cause bronchospasms. It is an oral leukotriene receptor antagonist used for the treatment of asthma. Leukotriene receptor antagonists primarily decrease the inflammatory process of asthma, thus reducing asthma symptoms. Zafirlukast is used as monotherapy or in combination with inhaled corticosteroids or beta-agonists. Two leukotriene receptor antagonists (zafirlukast and montelukast) are available; note their common ending -lukast.

37. **C** (gastrointestinal ulceration) is correct. The Food and Drug Administration has recently approved irinotecan as part of a first-line treatment regimen containing fluorouracil and leucovorin for metastatic colorectal cancer. Fluorouracil is also used in the treatment of carcinomas of the esophagus, stomach, colon, rectum, breast, ovary, cervix, bladder, liver, and pancreas. The drug is a fluorinated pyrimidine and acts as an antimetabolite. Adverse gastrointestinal effects are common during fluorouracil therapy. Stomatitis occurs frequently, and gastrointestinal bleeding, esophagitis, and proctitis have also been reported. Irinotecan also produces many gastrointestinal adverse effects.

   A (cardiotoxicity) is incorrect. Cardiotoxicity is not common with fluorouracil treatment. Cardiotoxicity is associated with doxorubicin and daunorubicin treatment.

   B (exfoliative dermatitis) is incorrect. Exfoliative dermatitis is not common with fluorouracil treatment. Exfoliative dermatitis is not unique to or commonly associated with any single anticancer agent.

   D (nephrotoxicity) is incorrect. Nephrotoxicity is not common with fluorouracil treatment. Nephrotoxicity is associated with cisplatin treatment.

   E (pancreatitis) is incorrect. Pancreatitis is not common with fluorouracil treatment. Pancreatitis is not unique to or commonly associated with any single anticancer agent.

38. **B** (carmustine) is correct. Unlike other DNA alkylating agents, carmustine has a high oil-to-water partition coefficient that allows it to cross the blood-brain barrier. The drug is a cell cycle–nonspecific (CCNS) antineoplastic agent that is approved for use in the treatment of malignant brain tumors. The average life expectancy for an individual with a highly malignant glioblastoma is about 17 weeks without postoperative treatment. The expectancy increases to about 62 weeks when cranial radiation and carmustine therapy are given.

   A (busulfan) is incorrect. Like carmustine, busulfan is a CCNS antineoplastic agent that acts as a DNA alkylating agent. Unlike carmustine, it does not cross the blood-brain barrier. Busulfan is used to treat chronic myelogenous leukemia. Because of its selective toxicity against myeloid cells, it is administered to patients who are scheduled to undergo bone marrow transplantation.

   C (methotrexate) is incorrect. Methotrexate can cross the blood-brain barrier to some extent, but drug concentrations in the brain seldom reach therapeutic levels, even after high doses of methotrexate are given intravenously.

D (prednisone) is incorrect. Prednisone may reduce perifocal edema and thereby bring about temporary relief in the patient, but the drug would have no influence on tumor regrowth.

E (streptozocin) is incorrect. Streptozocin is not used in the treatment of brain tumors. The drug is toxic to beta cells of the pancreas and is used almost exclusively to treat islet cell carcinoma of the pancreas.

39. **D** (melphalan) is correct. Melphalan is a cell cycle–nonspecific (CCNS) antineoplastic agent that is used in the treatment of multiple myeloma, testicular seminoma, non-Hodgkin's lymphoma, osteogenic sarcoma, breast cancer, and ovarian carcinoma.

A (aldesleukin) is incorrect. Aldesleukin is not indicated for use in the treatment of multiple myeloma. Aldesleukin (interleukin 2) is an antineoplastic and immunomodulating agent that was developed by using recombinant DNA procedures. It is indicated for use in the treatment of metastatic renal cell carcinoma and is sometimes used in the treatment of acute myelogenous leukemia, non-Hodgkin's lymphoma, HIV infection, and leprosy.

B (azathioprine) is incorrect. Azathioprine is not used in the treatment of cancer. Azathioprine is an immunosuppressive agent that is converted to 6-mercaptopurine. It is commonly used in transplant patients but is also useful in the management of rheumatoid arthritis, lupus nephritis, and psoriatic arthritis.

C (cyclosporine) is incorrect. Cyclosporine is not used in the treatment of cancer. Cyclosporine is an immunosuppressive agent that is mainly used to prevent allograft rejection and to treat various autoimmune conditions, such as uveitis, psoriasis, type 1 diabetes mellitus, rheumatoid arthritis, inflammatory bowel disease, and certain nephropathies.

E (methotrexate) is incorrect. Methotrexate is not indicated for use in the treatment of multiple myeloma. Methotrexate, in large doses, is given as an antineoplastic agent; in small doses, it is given as an immunosuppressive agent for use in the treatment of many non-neoplastic conditions.

40. **E** (sulfasalazine) is correct. Sulfasalazine is used in the treatment of mild or moderate ulcerative colitis. It is particularly valuable for maintaining remission after corticosteroids induce the remission. Sulfasalazine is metabolized by bacteria in the colon to yield sulfapyridine plus 5-aminosalicylic acid (mesalamine). The anti-inflammatory mechanism of mesalamine is due to inhibition of arachidonic acid metabolism in the bowel mucosa by inhibition of cyclooxygenase. This decreases the production of prostaglandins, thereby reducing colonic inflammation. Mesalamine may also inhibit leukotriene synthesis, thereby decreasing the chemotactic stimuli for polymorphonuclear leukocyte accumulation in the bowel.

A (amoxicillin) is incorrect. Amoxicillin is not used to treat ulcerative colitis. Amoxicillin capsules, clarithromycin tablets, and lansoprazole delayed-release capsules are packaged together to improve treatment compliance and eradicate *Helicobacter pylori* infection in patients with duodenal ulcers.

B (bismuth subsalicylate) is incorrect. Bismuth subsalicylate is not used to treat ulcerative colitis. Bismuth subsalicylate, metronidazole, and tetracycline are combined in a "kit" for use in the treatment of active duodenal ulcers.

C (cyclosporine) is incorrect. Cyclosporine has been used in the treatment of severe ulcerative colitis that is unresponsive to corticosteroids. However, it would not be used to maintain remission. Cyclosporine binds to cyclophilin (immunosuppressant-binding protein), and the cyclosporine-cyclophilin complex then binds to and inhibits the calcium-calmodulin activated phosphatase (calcineurin), blocking signal transduction mediated via the nuclear factor of activated T cells (NF-AT) required for B-cell activation (IL-4 and CD40 ligand) and T-cell activation (IL-2 and interferon gamma). Cyclosporine is widely used to prevent allograft rejection and is effective in various autoimmune conditions such as uveitis, psoriasis, type I diabetes mellitus, rheumatoid arthritis, inflammatory bowel disease, and certain nephropathies.

D (metronidazole) is incorrect. Metronidazole is not used to treat ulcerative colitis. Bismuth subsalicylate, metronidazole, and tetracycline are combined in a "kit" for use in the treatment of active duodenal ulcers.

41.   **D** (propranolol) is correct. The patient's clinical manifestations are consistent with the diagnosis of hyperthyroidism. Propranolol is useful for the short-term management of symptoms associated with this disorder.

A (amiodarone) is incorrect. Amiodarone is not used to treat hyperthyroidism. It is a class III antiarrhythmic agent that has a very complex effect on thyroid hormone metabolism. The incidence of amiodarone-induced thyrotoxicosis is reported to be 1% to 23% whereas incidence of hypothyroidism is reported to be 1% to 32%.

B (finasteride) is incorrect. Finasteride is not used to treat hyperthyroidism. Finasteride, a competitive, specific inhibitor of type II 5α-reductase, an enzyme that converts testosterone to 5α-dihydrotestosterone (DHT), is used in the treatment of symptomatic benign prostatic hyperplasia (BPH).

C (procainamide) is incorrect. Procainamide is not used to treat hyperthyroidism. It is a class IA antiarrhythmic agent that is used to treat cardiac arrhythmias, including atrial fibrillation, atrial flutter, paroxysmal atrial tachycardia, and ventricular tachycardia.

E (spironolactone) is incorrect. Spironolactone is not used to treat hyperthyroidism. It is a potassium-sparing diuretic that is used in the management of ascites associated with cirrhosis. Spironolactone is also used in the diagnosis of primary hyperaldosteronism.

42. **D** (drug D) is correct. Dexamethasone is an adrenal steroid that has no mineralocorticoid activity but is a potent glucocorticoid and has a long duration of action. Based on the properties shown in the table, drug A is triamcinolone, drug B is deoxycorticosterone acetate, drug C is prednisolone, drug D is dexamethasone, and drug E is fludrocortisone.

A (drug A) is incorrect. Refer to the explanation for option D. Drug A could be triamcinolone.

B (drug B) is incorrect. Refer to the explanation for option D. Drug B could be deoxycorticosterone acetate.

C (drug C) is incorrect. Refer to the explanation for option D. Drug C could be prednisolone.

E (drug E) is incorrect. Refer to the explanation for option D. Drug E could be fludrocortisone.

43. **C** (metformin) is correct. Insulin resistance is a common pathophysiologic problem in obese patients with type 2 diabetes mellitus. Metformin acts by (1) decreasing hepatic gluconeogenesis production; (2) decreasing intestinal absorption of glucose; and (3) improving insulin sensitivity by increasing peripheral glucose uptake and utilization in these patients. Unlike the sulfonylurea drugs, it rarely causes hypoglycemia, because it does not significantly change insulin concentrations. In contrast to therapy with sulfonylureas or insulin, when patients tend to gain weight, patients taking metformin often lose weight, perhaps as a result of its ability to cause anorexia. Metformin is contraindicated in patients with lactic acidosis or those who may be prone to get lactic acidosis, such as alcoholics or patients with cardiovascular, liver, or kidney disorders.

A (acarbose) is incorrect. Acarbose is an oral antidiabetic agent that inhibits alpha-glucosidases in the brush-border of the enterocytes located in the proximal portion of the small intestine. It lowers postprandial plasma glucose when administered alone or in combination with insulin, metformin, or an oral sulfonylurea. It is a suitable alternative to other oral antidiabetic agents for patients with mild to moderate hyperglycemia or who are at risk for hypoglycemia or lactic acidosis. In contrast to metformin, weight loss, if it occurs, is typically mild. It appears to offset the insulinotropic effects and weight gain associated with sulfonylurea treatment when it is added to sulfonylurea therapy.

B (glipizide) is incorrect. Glipizide is a second-generation sulfonylurea. The sulfonylureas are administered orally to lower blood glucose in patients with type 2 diabetes mellitus. When a sulfonylurea is administered, it binds to adenosine triphosphate (ATP)-sensitive potassium channels on the surface of pancreatic islet cells and thereby reduces potassium conductance and causes membrane depolarization. Depolarization stimulates calcium ion influx through voltage-sensitive calcium channels and increases the intracellular concentration of calcium ions. This in turn induces the secretion, or exocytosis, of insulin. During sulfonylurea therapy, hypoglycemia sometimes occurs and can be severe. Manifestations include hunger, pallor, nausea, fatigue, perspiration, headache, palpitations, numbness of the mouth, tingling in the fingers, tremors, muscle weakness, blurred vision, hypothermia, uncontrolled yawning, irritability, mental confusion, tachycardia, shallow breathing, and loss of consciousness. Patients often tend to gain weight on sulfonylurea therapy. Chlorpropamide and tolbutamide are first-generation sulfonylureas and are not as potent as glipizide and glyburide, which are second-generation sulfonylureas. Chlorpropamide is more likely than the other sulfonylureas to produce a disulfiram-like reaction after ingestion of ethanol. Tolbutamide is the shortest-acting and least potent of the group.

D (pioglitazone) is incorrect. Pioglitazone, an oral antidiabetic agent, specifically targets insulin resistance, which is thought to be central to the pathogenesis of type 2 diabetes as well as dyslipidemia and hypertension in obese patients. Pioglitazone and rosiglitazone are often referred to as "insulin sensitizers." They produce minimal hypoglycemia and when weight gain occurs with "glitazone" therapy, it is usually associated with edema. They should be avoided in patients with liver disorders; the first member of this class, troglitazone, was removed from market due to the risk of idiosyncratic hepatotoxicity.

E (repaglinide) is incorrect. Repaglinide is an oral antidiabetic agent that promotes insulin secretion by a mechanism similar to the sulfonylureas. It is used as an adjunct to diet and exercise in the treatment of type 2 diabetes mellitus and is unique because it has a rapid onset and short duration of action, so when taken just prior to meals, physiologic insulin profiles are produced. It can produce hypoglycemia and promote weight gain. Because it does not have a sulfonamide moiety in its structure it can be used in patients with sulfonamide hypersensitivities, whereas oral sulfonylureas cannot.

44. **E** (methotrexate) is correct. All the listed drugs are DMARDs capable of retarding the progression of bone and articular destruction. However, only methotrexate inhibits the biosynthesis of both purines and pyrimidines. Methotrexate competitively inhibits dihydrofolate reductase, which is the enzyme responsible for converting folic acid to reduced folate cofactors (i.e., tetrahydrofolate). Reduced folates are required for metabolic transfer of 1-carbon units in many biochemical reactions. Some of these reactions influence cell proliferation, including the synthesis of thymidylic acid, DNA nucleotide precursors, and inosinic acid, a purine precursor required for DNA and RNA synthesis. It is effective in treating patients who have degenerative rheumatoid arthritis that cannot be controlled adequately by treatment with aspirin or other NSAIDs alone.

A (auranofin) is incorrect. Auranofin does not inhibit the biosynthesis of both purines and pyrimidines. Auranofin is an oral gold compound that exhibits antiarthritic, anti-inflammatory, and immunomodulating properties. The mechanism of auranofin's antiarthritic effect is unknown, but it may decrease inflammation through inhibition of antigen processing by macrophages or the inhibition of lysosomal enzyme release. It is most effective in the treatment of early active cases of both adult and juvenile types of rheumatoid arthritis unresponsive to NSAIDs but less effective against advanced, chronic cases of rheumatoid arthritis.

B (hydroxychloroquine) is incorrect. Hydroxychloroquine does not inhibit the biosynthesis of both purines and pyrimidines. Its anti-inflammatory actions may result from (1) inhibiting migration of neutrophils and eosinophils; (2) antagonizing histamine and serotonin; or (3) inhibiting prostaglandin synthesis. Hydroxychloroquine is a DMARD that is used to treat mild or moderately severe rheumatoid arthritis. Hydroxychloroquine is also an antimalarial drug; however, it is not used as frequently as chloroquine to treat malaria.

C (infliximab) is incorrect. Infliximab does not inhibit the biosynthesis of both purines and pyrimidines. Infliximab is a monoclonal antibody that targets tumor necrosis factor-alpha (TNF-α). TNF-α has multiple actions: it (1) induces the production of proinflammatory cytokines (IL-1 and IL-6); (2) enhances leukocyte migration by increasing endothelial layer permeability; (3) increases the expression of adhesion molecules by endothelial cells and leukocytes; (4) activates neutrophil and eosinophil functional activity; (5) induces fibroblast proliferation; (6) enhances the synthesis of prostaglandins; and (7) induces the production of acute phase and other liver proteins. Infliximab markedly improves clinical symptoms when given in combination with methotrexate to patients with rheumatoid arthritis. The anti-TNF drugs (infliximab, adalimumab, and etanercept) all increase the risk of tuberculosis and other opportunistic infections. Infliximab is also approved for the treatment of Crohn's disease.

D (leflunomide) is incorrect. Leflunomide inhibits the biosynthesis of pyrimidines but not purines. It is converted to an active metabolite that inhibits dihydroorotate dehydrogenase (DHODH), an enzyme in the mitochondria that catalyzes a key step in *de novo* pyrimidine synthesis. It is the first agent used in the treatment of rheumatoid arthritis that provides both symptomatic improvement and retardation of structural joint damage based on radiographic evidence.

45. **A** (acetaminophen) is correct. Acetaminophen has analgesic and antipyretic activity similar to that of aspirin but it has no peripheral anti-inflammatory activity or effects on platelet function. It is effective in the relief of both acute and chronic pain. The American Geriatrics Society recommends acetaminophen as the analgesic of choice for minor aches and pains in patients older than 50 years of age because of fewer gastrointestinal and renal side effects than nonsteroidal anti-inflammatory drugs (NSAIDs). Acetaminophen is also the preferred analgesic/antipyretic for patients in whom NSAIDs are contraindicated (e.g., a history of gastric ulcer or coagulation disorders). Acetaminophen is effective in the treatment of osteoarthritis but has minimal effects in inflammatory arthritic diseases such as rheumatoid or gouty arthritis.

B (celecoxib) is incorrect. Celecoxib is a selective cyclooxygenase-2 (COX-2) inhibitor with comparable efficacy to other NSAIDs in the treatment of rheumatoid arthritis and osteoarthritis but would be contraindicated for this patient with histories of cardiovascular disease and sulfonamide hypersensitivity. The Food and Drug Administration issued a public health advisory in 2004 that the COX-2 inhibitors may be associated with an increased risk of serious cardiovascular events (heart attack and stroke), especially when used chronically or in very high risk settings (e.g., after open heart surgery).

C (naproxen) is incorrect. Naproxen is an NSAID whose anti-inflammatory actions are due to decreased prostaglandin synthesis via inhibition of COX-1 and COX-2. It is contraindicated for patients with peptic ulcers and should be used with great caution in patients with cardiovascular disease. The Food and Drug Administration issued a public health advisory in 2004 that long-term use of a nonselective NSAID, such as naproxen, may be associated with an increased cardiovascular risk compared to placebo. This effect is likely due to the inhibition of prostaglandin synthesis in the kidney, decreasing renal blood flow leading to acute renal failure and hypertension.

D (oxycodone) is incorrect. Oxycodone is an oral opioid agonist used to manage moderate to severe pain, including cancer pain; postoperative, postextractional, and postpartum pain; and nonpain syndromes, such as restless leg and Tourette syndromes. Because of the potential for abuse or psychological dependence, oxycodone is not recommended for the long-term management of chronic arthritic pain.

E (rofecoxib) is incorrect. Rofecoxib is a selective cyclooxygenase-2 (COX-2) inhibitor that lacks a sulfonamide moiety in its structure. It was extensively used for the treatment of osteoarthritis and rheumatoid arthritis, especially in patients with NSAID-induced gastrointestinal distress or sulfonamide hypersensitivity. However in 2004, the manufacturer announced the removal of rofecoxib from the worldwide market based on data suggesting an increase in serious cardiovascular events, such as heart attacks and strokes, with continuous treatment with rofecoxib as compared with placebo. The selective inhibition of COX-2 will inhibit the production of PGI_2 but not of thromboxane A_2 (TXA$_2$), which is produced by COX-1. TXA$_2$ causes platelet aggregation, vasoconstriction, and vascular proliferation, whereas PGI$_2$ inhibits platelet aggregation, vascular smooth muscle contraction and proliferation, leukocyte endothelial cell interactions, and cholesteryl ester hydrolysis. Therefore, this shift in the TXA$_2$ to PGI$_2$ balance is likely to contribute to an increase in cardiovascular events.

46. **A** (allopurinol) is correct. The patient's clinical and laboratory findings are consistent with the diagnosis of gout. Allopurinol is used to prevent gout in patients who have experienced repeated attacks of the disorder. Allopurinol is also used to prevent hyperuricemia and uric acid nephropathy in cancer patients who are undergoing radiation therapy or chemotherapy. In these cancer patients, hyperuricemia is associated with rapid cell turnover and massive cell destruction. Allopurinol acts by inhibiting xanthine oxidase and thereby blocking the conversion of xanthine and hypoxanthine (oxypurines) to uric acid.

B (colchicine) is incorrect. Colchicine is the preferred agent for the treatment of acute gouty arthritis attacks, but allopurinol or probenecid is used to prevent future attacks. Colchicine possesses anti-inflammatory properties by binding to proteins in microtubules of neutrophils. This binding, in turn, inhibits the migration of neutrophils into the area of inflammation, thereby interfering with the inflammatory response to urate crystal deposition.

C (indomethacin) is incorrect. Because of its anti-inflammatory and pain-relieving properties, indomethacin is sometimes effective in terminating an acute attack of gout. However, the drug is not effective in preventing repeated attacks of gout.

D (probenecid) is incorrect. Probenecid is an oral uricosuric agent used to treat hyperuricemia associated with chronic gout, but it is contraindicated in patients with a renal creatinine clearance less than 50 mL/min. Probenecid is not effective for acute attacks of gout and actually can aggravate inflammation if administered during the initial stage of a gouty arthritic attack.

E (salicylates) is incorrect. Because salicylates interfere with the renal handling of uric acid, they should not be used in the management of gout.

47. **A** (set A) is correct. By acting on H$_2$ receptors, histamine evokes the copious secretion of gastric acid from parietal cells. It also increases the output of pepsin and intrinsic factor. Histamine characteristically dilates the small blood vessels, and this causes flushing, lowers the total peripheral resistance, and leads to a fall in systemic blood pressure. The fall in blood pressure evokes reflex tachycardia. Other changes induced by histamine include an increase in capillary permeability.

B (set B), **C** (set C), **D** (set D), and **E** (set E) are incorrect. Refer to the explanation for option A.

48. **E** (sumatriptan) is correct. The patient's complaints are consistent with the diagnosis of a migraine headache disorder, with migraine attacks preceded by an aura. Sumatriptan is approved for use in the treatment of migraine headaches with or without aura, but it is not indicated for the prevention of migraine attacks. Sumatriptan is a drug that is structurally similar to serotonin (5-hydroxytryptamine, or 5-HT) and acts by stimulating 5-HT_{1D} receptors. These receptors have been identified on basal arteries and in the vasculature of the dura mater. The drug's therapeutic effect is a result of selective vasoconstriction of inflamed and dilated cranial blood vessels in the carotid circulation.

A (buspirone) is incorrect. Buspirone exhibits the highest affinity for 5-HT_{1A} receptors. It is used to treat anxiety.

B (dihydroergotamine) is incorrect. Dihydroergotamine (DHE) is a semisynthetic ergot alkaloid that is administered parenterally or intranasally to terminate migraine headaches. Because less toxic agents are available, DHE is considered most appropriate for treating patients who have severe migraine disorder. DHE binds with high affinity to all known 5-HT_1 receptors and to a number of other biogenic amine receptors, including $5\text{-HT}_{2A/2C}$ receptors, α_1- and α_2-adrenergic receptors, and dopamine D_2 receptors. However, the drug's therapeutic effect in the treatment of migraine headaches is thought to be due primarily to its agonist activity at the 5-HT_{1D} receptor.

C (metoclopramide) is incorrect. Metoclopramide is a drug that enhances gastrointestinal motility and is an effective antiemetic. Its mechanism of action is complex. Unlike bethanechol, metoclopramide enhances motility without stimulating gastric secretions. Peripherally, metoclopramide augments cholinergic activity either by causing release of acetylcholine from postganglionic nerve endings or by sensitizing muscarinic receptors on smooth muscle. The net effect of the drug's activities is a remarkable coordination of gastric and duodenal motility. Metoclopramide is used to terminate severe migraine attacks. In patients who are responsive to DHE, metoclopramide is given prior to administration of DHE to offset DHE-induced nausea. In patients who are not responsive to DHE, metoclopramide is used as an alternative treatment.

D (ondansetron) is incorrect. Ondansetron selectively blocks serotonin 5-HT_3 receptors. It is used to control vomiting.

49. **C** (fexofenadine) is correct. The type and pattern of clinical manifestations are consistent with the diagnosis of nonseasonal rhinitis caused by an allergy to house dust. Fexofenadine, a histamine H_1-receptor antagonist, would be the drug of choice because it has a positive effect on all of the manifestations described. Fexofenadine is an active metabolite of terfenadine, a drug that was removed from the market because it caused severe cardiac side effects (torsades de pointes). Fexofenadine is nonsedating, and it is not associated with adverse cardiac effects.

A (cimetidine) is incorrect. Cimetidine is not used to treat uncomplicated allergic rhinitis. It is an oral histamine H_2-receptor antagonist similar to famotidine, nizatidine, and ranitidine used for management of peptic ulcer disease; note the common ending -tidine.

B (desensitization) is incorrect. Desensitization is much less effective in older individuals than in youths, and house dust allergy usually does not respond well to it.

D (fluticasone) is incorrect. Fluticasone is not used to treat uncomplicated allergic rhinitis. It is a medium-potency synthetic corticosteroid used (1) topically to relieve the inflammatory and pruritic manifestations of corticosteroid-responsive dermatoses and psoriasis; (2) intranasally for the management of symptoms of allergic and nonallergic rhinitis; and (3) by oral inhalation for the treatment of asthma.

E (naphazoline) is incorrect. Naphazoline is not used to treat uncomplicated allergic rhinitis. Because naphazoline is an α-adrenergic receptor agonist, it would cause vasoconstriction of the mucous membranes. Although this would reduce congestion in allergic rhinitis, long-term use of the drug would damage the mucous membranes.

50. **B** (desloratadine) is correct. The patient's clinical manifestations are consistent with the diagnosis of acute urticaria. Desloratadine, a second-generation H_1-receptor antagonist, is highly efficacious in the treatment of this condition. It is a nonsedating, long-acting histamine (H_1) receptor antihistamine. Because of its poor penetration into the CNS and a low affinity for brain H_1-receptors, CNS effects are much less with desloratadine than the traditional H_1-antagonsits, such as diphenhydramine. It is the active metabolite of loratadine and both loratadine and desloratadine are nonsedating; but desloratadine does not cause QT prolongation whereas loratadine does at higher doses. Desloratadine is used in adults and adolescents to relieve symptoms associated with seasonal allergic rhinitis, perennial allergic rhinitis, and chronic idiopathic urticaria.

A (chlorpheniramine) is incorrect. Chlorpheniramine is a competitive H_1-receptor antagonist of the propylamine group of antihistamines. It is effective for use in the treatment of histamine-mediated conditions, such as urticaria and allergic rhinitis. However, like other first-generation H_1-receptor antagonists, it has sedative effects. These effects, which result from antagonism at central histamine receptors, would interfere with driving an automobile.

C (famotidine) is incorrect. In patients with urticaria, H_2-receptor antagonists such as famotidine have little effect if given alone. Doxepin, a tricyclic antidepressant that acts as a combined H_1 and H_2 antagonist, is effective for use in the treatment of chronic idiopathic urticaria.

D (prednisone) is incorrect. Systemic corticosteroids, such as prednisone, have no role in the treatment of relatively innocuous conditions, such as acute urticaria, because their potential side effects outweigh their potential benefits.

E (triamcinolone cream) is incorrect. In cases of urticaria in which the itching is severe and prevents the patient from sleeping, a topical corticosteroid such as triamcinolone cream may be given as adjunct therapy to achieve more rapid relief, but the topical drug should be used for only a short period of time.

Index

Note: Page numbers followed by f indicate figures; those followed by t indicate tables; and those followed by b indicated boxed material.

Belladonna alkaloids, 33, 34b
Benzathine penicillin G, 195, 263
    for syphilis, 310
Benzisoxazoles, 71
Benzocaine, 60
Benzodiazepine(s), 50b, 51f, 52–53
    for preanesthetic medication, 59t
Benzodiazepine abuse, 231t
Benzodiazepine agonists, 53
Benzodiazepine antagonist, 53
Benzquinamide, 68
Benztropine, 33
    for Parkinson's disease, 80
β- and α$_1$-adrenergic receptor antagonists, 42b,
        43–44
Beta blockers, 41–44, 42b
    as antianginals, 98b, 98f, 99
    as antiarrhythmics, 86–87
    as antithyroid agents, 172
    for heart failure, 105
    with intrinsic sympathomimetic activity, 42b,
        44
    nonselective, 42b, 43
β$_1$ responses, 27
β$_2$ responses, 27
β-Adrenergic receptor(s), 16t, 23, 24
β-Adrenergic receptor agonists, 36, 39, 40
    as antihypertensives, 91–93, 91b
    for asthma, 138t
    for heart failure, 105
β$_1$-Adrenergic receptor agonists, 36, 40
β$_2$-Adrenergic receptor agonists, 39, 40
    as bronchodilators, 143–144, 143b, 144f
    uterine effect of, 186
β-Adrenergic receptor antagonists, 41–44, 42b
    as antianginals, 98b, 98f, 99
    as antiarrhythmics, 86–87
    as antithyroid agents, 172
    for heart failure, 103b, 105
    with intrinsic sympathomimetic activity, 42b, 44
    nonselective, 42b, 43
β$_1$-Adrenergic receptor antagonists, 42b, 43
β-lactam antibiotics, 194–197, 194b
β-lactamase inhibitor, 197
Betamethasone, 172b
    for asthma, 138t, 140b
Bethanechol, 30, 31b, 243, 268
Bextra. *See* Valdecoxib (Baxtra).
Bicalutamide, 190, 224
Biguanides, 179
Bile acid–binding resins, 99–101, 100f, 100t, 101b
Bioactivation, of chemotherapeutic drugs, 245,
        271–272
Bioavailability, 4–5, 6t, 268
Bioequivalence, 5
Biologic half-life, 12

Biotransformation, 2f, 5–9
    drug interactions and, 8
    genetic polymorphisms and, 8, 9t
    phase I, 7, 8f
    phase II, 7–8
    phase III, 8
    primary site of, 5
    products of, 7
    reactive metabolite intermediates in, 9
Bisacodyl, 156
Bismuth subsalicylate, 150, 151, 321
Bisphosphonates, 183–184
Bivalirudin, 118, 298
Bleach, poisoning from, 228t
Bleomycin, 219f, 220t, 221–222, 272
Blood pressure, autonomic effects on, 27–29
Blood redistribution, due to autonomic nerve activity, 29
Blood vessels, autonomic effect on, 27, 28t
Body compartments, drug distribution into, 5, 7t
Bone, drug concentration in, 7t
Bone disorders, 181–184, 182b, 182f, 182t
Bone marrow failure, anemia due to, 123t, 125
Bosentan, for heart failure, 105
Botulinum toxin, 23–24, 45–46
Bradycardia, reflex, 29
Brain tumor, highly malignant, carmustine for, 293, 319
Bromocriptine, 79, 169
Bronchiolar muscle, autonomic effect on, 28t
Bronchitis, chronic, 138
    bronchodilators for, 143–145, 143b, 144f
Bronchoconstriction, 243, 268–269
Bronchodilators, 143–145, 143b, 144f, 248, 279–280
Buccal administration, advantages and disadvantages of, 6t
Budesonide, for asthma, 140b
Bulk-forming laxatives, 154, 155t, 156b
Bumetanide, 109b, 255
Bupivacaine, 61
Buprenorphine, 133t, 136
Bupropion, 303
    for ADHD, 76
    as antidepressant, 74, 74t, 253
Buspirone, 54, 153t, 254, 327
Busulfan, 219, 220t, 271, 319
Butorphanol, 133t, 136
Butyrophenones, 69b, 70, 71t
BZ$_1$ benzodiazepine agonists, 53

C

Cadmium poisoning, 266
Caffeine, 231t
Calcineurin, 281, 297
Calcitonin, 181–183, 182f
Calcitriol, 183
Calcium (Ca^{2+}), 183
Calcium carbonate, 148f, 149
Calcium channel(s), 255

Quazepam, 52

Quetiapine, 71

Quinethazone, 109b

Quinidine
    adverse effects of, 258
    as antiarrhythmic, 83t, 85, 305
    and digoxin, 306
    for heart failure, 102

Quinine, 265

Quinupristin-dalfopristin, 201–202

R

"Rabbit syndrome," due to neuroleptics, 70

Rabeprazole, 148b

Radioactive iodine, 172

Raloxifene, 188
    for bone disorders, 184

Ranitidine, 148f, 149, 274

RAS (renin angiotensin system), drugs that affect, 91b, 95–96

Rasburicase, 163

Reabsorption, passive tubular, 9–10

Reactive metabolite intermediates, 9

Receptor(s), 16–19, 16t, 17f–19f

Receptor binding, degree of, 17

Receptor-linked enzymes, 16t

Recombinant human growth hormone (rhGH), 167–168

Rectal administration, advantages and disadvantages of, 6t

Redistribution, 5

Reduction, 7

Reflex bradycardia, 29

Reflex tachycardia, 29

Renal clearance, 10

Renal nephrons, functions of, 106

Renal toxicity
    of amphotericin B, 241, 263–264
    of antimicrobial drugs, 191
    of antineoplastic drugs, 271, 319

Renin angiotensin system (RAS), drugs that affect, 91b, 95–96

Repaglinide, 179, 323

Repetitive dosing kinetics, 12–13, 12t

Reproductive endocrinology, 185–190
    androgens and inhibitors in, 190
    contraceptives in, 189
    drugs that act on uterus in, 185–186, 186b
    estrogens and related drugs in, 187–189, 187b

Reserpine, 26

Resistance, microbial, 191

Respiratory depression, with general anesthetics, 238, 256

Respiratory effects, of muscarinic receptor agonists, 31t

Reteplase, 119–120

Retinoids, teratogenic effects of, 230t

Reuptake inhibitors, 38b

Reye's syndrome, 128

Rheumatic disorders, drugs for, 157–161, 158b, 159f

Rheumatoid arthritis, 157–161, 158b
    corticosteroids for, 157
    disease-modifying antirheumatic drugs for, 160–161, 295, 323–324
    NSAIDs for, 157, 247, 276
    pathogenesis and site of drug action for, 159f

rhGH (recombinant human growth hormone), 167–168

Rhinitis, allergic, 296, 327–328

Ribavirin, 210

Rickets, 183

Rifabutin, 207t, 208

Rifampin, 193t, 308
    adverse effects of, 312
    mechanism of action of, 210f
    thyroid effects of, 171t
    for tuberculosis, 206–208, 207t

Rimantadine, 209

Risedronate, 183

Risperidone
    adverse effects of, 252, 282, 301
    as antipsychotic, 71, 71t, 163t, 237, 253

Ritodrine, 37t, 38b
    uterine effect of, 186

Ritonavir, 211t, 212

Rituximab, 224

Rivastigmine, 32, 32b

Rofecoxib (Vioxx), 129
    cardiotoxicity of, 276
    for osteoarthritis, 325–326
    for rheumatoid arthritis, 157

Ropinirole, 79

Rosiglitazone, 179, 323

Routes of administration, advantages and disadvantages of, 5, 6t

RU 486, 175, 188

Rudins, 114t, 118

S

Salicylate(s)
    for inflammatory bowel disease, 154
    thyroid effects of, 171t
    and uric acid, 326

Salicylate poisoning, 228t, 313

Salicylism, 128

Saline cathartics, 154, 155t

Salmeterol, 40
    for asthma, 138t, 143–144

Saquinavir, 211t, 212

Sargramostim, 125

Sarin, 32, 32b, 33

Schilling test, 124

Schizophrenia, 282, 301
    antipsychotic drugs for, 68–72, 69b, 69t, 71t

Scopolamine, 33
    as antiemetic, 152b

Secalcifediol, 183